Melatonin: Clinical Perspectives and Pharmaceutical Applications

Melatonin: Clinical Perspectives and Pharmaceutical Applications

Edited by Hank Miller

STATES ACADEMIC PRESS
www.statesacademicpress.com

States Academic Press,
109 South 5th Street,
Brooklyn, NY 11249, USA

Visit us on the World Wide Web at:
www.statesacademicpress.com

ISBN: 978-1-63989-349-2

Cataloging-in-Publication Data

Melatonin : clinical perspectives and pharmaceutical applications / edited by Hank Miller.
p. cm.
Includes bibliographical references and index.
ISBN 978-1-63989-349-2
1. Melatonin. 2. Melatonin--Physiological effect. 3. Melatonin--Therapeutic use. 4. Hormones. I. Miller, Hank.
RM297.M44 M45 2022
615.36--dc23

Table of Contents

Preface

The world is advancing at a fast pace like never before. Therefore, the need is to keep up with the latest developments. This book was an idea that came to fruition when the specialists in the area realized the need to coordinate together and document essential themes in the subject. That's when I was requested to be the editor. Editing this book has been an honour as it brings together diverse authors researching on different streams of the field. The book collates essential materials contributed by veterans in the area which can be utilized by students and researchers alike.

Melatonin is a hormone that is associated with the control of sleep-wake cycle and is primarily secreted by the pineal gland at night. It is also taken orally as a dietary supplement to treat short-term insomnia such as from shift work or jet lag. Some melatonin receptor agonists are also available as medications that work as melatonin but may have some adverse effects for sleep conditions. Side-effects of melatonin use are headaches, somnolence, diarrhea, nausea, nervousness, irritability, abnormal dreams, psychomotor hypersensitivity, mouth ulcers, chest pain, mood swings, etc. These side-effects are minimal if taken at a low concentration for short durations. It is also involved in synchronizing circadian rhythms. This book provides significant information of this discipline to help develop a good understanding of the clinical perspectives of melatonin as well as its pharmaceutical applications. It unravels the recent studies in this field. This book will serve as a valuable source of reference for graduate and post graduate students.

Each chapter is a sole-standing publication that reflects each author´s interpretation. Thus, the book displays a multi-facetted picture of our current understanding of application, resources and aspects of the field. I would like to thank the contributors of this book and my family for their endless support.

Editor

1

Melatonin Modified Release Formulations Designed for Sleep Disorders

Marilena Vlachou and Angeliki Siamidi

Abstract

Melatonin (*N*-acetyl-5-methoxytryptamine, MLT), a hormone synthesized by the pineal gland and released at night, has a regulatory role on sleep in vertebrates, including humans. It has been shown to have a hypnotic action in animals and humans and it has been used as an agent for restoring circadian rhythms, disturbed by jet-lag, shift-work or aging. The physiological actions of melatonin in regulating seasonal and circadian rhythms are mediated through a family of specific, high affinity G protein-coupled membrane receptors. The beneficial effect of fast-release formulations on sleep initiation may come from the high amount of melatonin released immediately after administration, while the benefit of the sustained release systems comes from the release of melatonin in small dosages during the entire night period. This chapter covers the recent scientific work on melatonin modified release formulations.

Keywords: melatonin, sleep onset, sleep maintenance, modified release, formulations

1. Introduction

Melatonin (MLT), which was originally discovered in the bovine pineal gland in 1958, is a pleiotropic molecule with numerous cellular and physiological functions in vertebrates, including humans. MLT's production is regulated by a multisynaptic pathway from the biological clock in the suprachiasmatic nucleus (SCN), in the hypothalamus, to the pineal gland. The SCN is the primary site for both generation and integration of signals, which regulate melatonin's production by the pineal. Control at this central point ensures the high nocturnal concentration and extremely low diurnal melatonin synthesis.

Melatonin has been shown to have a hypnotic action in animals and humans, and there has been considerable recent interest in the therapeutic potential of melatonin and its analogues as hypnotics and as agents for restoring circadian rhythms, disturbed by jet-lag, shiftwork, and aging. The physiological actions of melatonin in regulating seasonal and circadian rhythms are thought to be mediated through a family of specific, high affinity, and G-protein-coupled cell membrane receptors. One of its main uses is insomnia treatment, particularly among the elderly, with up to 50% of people over the age of 65 reporting trouble sleeping. Night time insomnia is associated with increased daytime sleepiness, reduced motor and cognitive performance, and reduced productivity in the workplace and is an important cause of industrial and road traffic accidents. Current hypnotic drugs are recommended only for short-term treatment of insomnia, but concerns about "hangover" effects and problems upon withdrawal persist. Many people with occasional sleep problems resort to self-medication and over-the-counter sales of medicines for sleep problems are increasing rapidly [1].

The administration of exogenous melatonin is effected via different formulations, but at present, the most studied is the oral route. Also, there are different dosages of melatonin. Because of its pharmacokinetic characteristics, it is necessary to maintain melatonin's concentration for a long time to imitate its physiological release, especially for insomnia treatment. To this end, prolonged-release formulations of melatonin have been developed covering the entire night cycle and improving sleep disorders. As the toxicology of melatonin's formulations is concerned, very little is known. However, the acute toxicity of melatonin, as seen in both animal and human studies, is extremely low. Nevertheless, further research needs to be undertaken, including regulatory studies.

2. Formulations of melatonin

Melatonin is traditionally administered orally in immediate and modified release formulations, but has a poor and variable bioavailability. Apart from *per os* administration, melatonin is currently under research with respect to other routes of administration, such as sublingual, transbuccal/transmucosal, and intranasal for topical and systemic exposure, injectables (intravenous, i.v. bolus infusion, intramuscular, subcutaneous, and implant), topical preparations, and transdermal patches. This chapter aims at presenting an overview of all administration routes and different kinds of formulations of melatonin that are currently explored *in vitro* and *in vivo*, including experimental and clinical studies.

2.1. Melatonin *per os* immediate release formulations

Per os immediate release formulations imply that the full dose of the drug is absorbed into the bloodstream all at once. This pattern of fast released melatonin is most effective when against delayed sleep onset [2]. The immediate release dosage forms (fast released, orodispersible, sublingual tablets oral sprays, etc.) are usually administered to patients prior to sleep time in order to facilitate sleep onset. A research group has manufactured fast dissolving disintegrating tablets containing different dosages of melatonin for administration to pediatric patients that may have potential difficulties taking other oral dosage forms [3]. Dosages of 3 and 5 mg were intended for epileptic children, migraine prevention, neurodevelopmental disability, sleep disorders, and blindness, whereas dosages of 10 and 60 mg were used for Duchenne muscular dystrophy. Tablets have been produced with excipients for direct compression, having disintegration times of less than 25 s and with friability and hardness values that require no special storage or packaging conditions. The results indicated that these orodispersible tablets have been easily produced via direct compression, having low costs and optimal galenic assay results. To explore the therapeutic potential of melatonin, as an antioxidant agent, researchers have analyzed the red blood cell antioxidants and lipid peroxidation after 5 mg/daily immediate-release melatonin treatment of elderly with type 2 diabetes patients and healthy elderly subjects in comparison with 2 mg/daily sustained-release. The results suggest that both immediate and sustained release preparations may exert similar therapeutic effects related to melatonin's action as antioxidant [4].

2.2. Melatonin *per os* modified release formulations

Immediate release oral drug dosage forms are formulated in order to release the active substance immediately after oral administration. On the other hand, modified-release oral drug dosage forms are deliberately modified from those of an immediate release, to achieve a desired therapeutic objective or better patient compliance. The term modified release drug dosage forms is used to describe formulations that alter the time and/or the rate of release. With this in view, scientists have focused on modifying the release of melatonin especially to treat conditions that deal with circadian rhythmic disorders, like sleep syndrome, insomnia, jet lag, seasonal affective disease, shift work syndrome, etc. [5–7]. Modified-release melatonin treatment could be more useful to initiate and maintain sleep, compared with immediate-release therapy.

Many scientists have focused on different ways to manufacture modified release tablets. One of the most common ways is the use of various excipients that facilitate the prolong release when tablet manufacturing [8–13]. These excipients usually involve hydroxypropylmethylcellulose, polyvinylpyrrolidone, and sodium alginate in various molecular weights or forms. Another way to achieve modified release is the production of different tablet formulations, like multilayer or bilayer, coated or uncoated tablets [14–16]. Other researchers have studied the use of liposomal formulations [17] or nanoparticles [18]. Recently, electrospun nanofibrous systems, incorporating melatonin, have been used for its modified release [19]. Another way is to employ a variety of techniques, like for example, the experimental design [20] in order to facilitate the modified release tablet production and therefore, to improve quality of sleep in patients, with minimal side effects. Both in the development of these systems and the immediate release formulations, the fact that melatonin displays both a circadian and circannual rhythm and is secreted only during the night has been taken into account. This physiological rhythm needs to be conserved or modulated (advanced, reversed, diminished, or amplified) according to the appropriate therapeutic indications.

2.3. Melatonin sublingual/transbuccal formulations

The oral cavity is a perfect route of administration for both topical and systemic treatment. Considering melatonin, research has suggested that it is effective in treating pathologies like periodontitis, mucositis, cancers, and cytotoxicity from various drugs or biomaterials. Furthermore, melatonin has been observed to enhance osseointegration "functional ankylosis (bone adherence)" and bone regeneration, to promote the healing of tooth extraction sockets and may also impede the progression of oral cancer [21, 22]. On the other hand, sublingual and transbuccal/transmucosal administration of melatonin in the forms of sublingual tablets or oral sprays has shown comparable systemic results to other routes of administration.

Many scientists have considered the oral cavity as a route of administering melatonin and compared it to other routes. The effect of transdermal, in comparison to oral controlled release and oral transmucosal drug delivery systems, on plasma concentrations of melatonin and its principal metabolite, 6-sulfatoxymelatonin, was evaluated in 12 human volunteers, using a crossover, single dose design. Oral transmucosal delivery provided prompt systemic drug levels with less variability than oral or transdermal delivery and no indication of mucosal deposition. The results indicated that oral transmucosal delivery was able to mimic the physiological plasma profiles of both melatonin and its principal metabolite [23]. Another study involved 60 patients, who were randomly assigned to receive either sublingual melatonin (3 mg) or placebo, 60 min before cataract surgery. The dose of 3 mg of melatonin sublingually, 60 min before surgery, was chosen, because the onset of melatonin-induced sedation is reported to begin approximately 20–30 min after sublingual administration. The results concluded that sublingual melatonin premedication for patients undergoing cataract surgery, under topical anesthesia, reduced the anxiety scores and provided excellent operating conditions [24]. A prospective, randomized, double-blinded, placebo-controlled study was designed to compare the perioperative effects of different doses of melatonin and midazolam [25]. Doses of 0.05, 0.1, or 0.2 mg/kg sublingual midazolam or melatonin or placebo were given to 84 women, approximately 100 min before a typical anesthetic. Sedation, anxiety, and orientation were quantified before, 10, 30, 60, and 90 min after premedication and 15, 30, 60, and 90 min after admission to the recovery room. Patients who received premedication with either midazolam or melatonin had a significant decrease in anxiety levels and increase in preoperative levels of sedation, compared with control subjects. Premedication with 0.05 mg/kg melatonin was associated with preoperative anxiolysis and sedation without the impairment of cognitive and psychomotor skills or affecting the quality of recovery. To evaluate the analgesic dose response of the effects of melatonin on pressure and heat pain threshold, tolerance, and its possible sedative effects, the research group of Stefani et al. [26] recruited 61 healthy subjects aged 19–47 years old and placed them randomly into one of four groups: placebo, 0.05 mg/kg sublingual melatonin, 0.15 mg/kg sublingual melatonin, or 0.25 mg/kg sublingual melatonin. Serum plasma melatonin levels were found to be directly proportional to the melatonin doses given to each subject indicating that the sublingual melatonin has a well-defined dose-dependent antinociceptive activity. These results provided a correlation between the plasma melatonin drug concentration and acute changes in the pain threshold. To compare the perioperative effects of melatonin and midazolam, given in premedication, on sedation, orientation, anxiety scores, and psychomotor performance, melatonin 5 mg, midazolam 15 mg or placebo was administered 90 min prior to anesthesia, sublingually to 66 patients undergoing laparoscopic cholecystectomy [27]. Sedation, orientation, and anxiety were quantified before 10, 30, 60, and 90 min after premedication and 15, 30, 60 and 90 min after admission to the recovery room. The results indicated that melatonin premedication was associated with preoperative anxiolysis and sedation without postoperative impairment of psychomotor performance.

2.4. Melatonin intranasal formulations

Intranasal administration is a route of administration for drugs used primarily for the treatment of conditions affecting the nasal cavity, but can also be used for cases requiring systemic exposure, since drugs can be absorbed into the circulation through the nasal mucosa. This kind of systemic administration offers lots of advantages, such as rapid onset of action and avoidance of first-pass metabolism [28]. Many researchers have investigated melatonin's intranasal administration and tested their formulations *in vitro* and *in vivo* in rats, rabbits, and humans.

In another study, the role of inclusion complexes of melatonin with modified cyclodextrins (CDs) in order to improve melatonin's solubility and nasal absorption was investigated [29]. The formation of inclusion complex of melatonin with hydroxypropyl β-cyclodextrin (HPβCD) and randomly methylated β-cyclodextrin (RMβCD) was demonstrated in solution and solid state and both CD's at 1% w/v concentration were found to improve the nasal permeability (the *in vitro* permeability studies were carried out with EpiAirwayTM-100 cell cultures from MatTek Corporation) of melatonin from HPMC gel formulations.

Intranasal melatonin encapsulated in nanosized niosomes has been preclinically evaluated in male Wistar rats [30]. It was found that intranasal melatonin niosomes that were bioequivalent to intravenous injection of melatonin could provide therapeutic level doses, deliver melatonin to the brain to induce sleep, and delay systemic circulation. The cross-over study, including eight rats, examined the intranasal administration of melatonin from a nasal formulation consisted of melatonin (2.0 mg/ml), β-cyclodextrin (7.5 mg/ml) dissolved in saline that also contained benzalkonium chloride (0.01% w/v) and EDTA (0.1% w/v) as preservatives, in comparison to the administration from an intravenous bolus injection. Tmax was recorded at 2.5 min in both routes of administration and an almost zero plasma concentration after 120 min [31].

In another study, the research group [32] prepared melatonin gelatin microspheres (MLT-GMS) for intranasal administration and tested them in comparison to gelatin solution and i.v. injection. The *in vitro* release profile showed sustained effect, while the residence time of MLT-GMS in the rabbits' nasal cavity was longer than that of gelatin solution. After intranasal administration in rabbits, the bioavailability of MLT-GMS was 87.47%, while the bioavailability of melatonin solution was 69.72%, when compared to i.v. administration. The results showed that this formulation could meet the needs of intranasal administration, while increasing melatonin's bioavailability. Other scientists have studied the bioavailability of melatonin in rabbits after nasal administration of two formulations (1.5 mg melatonin in 40% PEG 300 in the presence and absence of 1% sodium glycocholate) in comparison to the i.v. route [33]. The results documented that the bioavailabilities in rabbits correspond to much higher values, which indicates a potential advantage of using nasal delivery for melatonin and the possibility of producing a clinically relevant nasal formulation. In another study, starch microspheres of melatonin for intranasal administration were prepared by an emulsification crosslinking technique using a uniform design to optimize preparation conditions [34]. The *in vitro* release experiments showed that melatonin was released from the microspheres in a sustained manner. Nasal clearance studies in six healthy, male rabbits showed that >80% of the radioactivity from the starch microspheres was present in the nasal mucosa 2 h after administration, compared to only 30% radioactivity from the solution. The absorption rate after intranasal administration of the microspheres was rapid, and the absolute bioavailability was high, compared to the intranasal solution and a significant correlation between *in vivo* and *in vitro* data was recorded.

In humans, a cross-over study in three volunteers, receiving either intranasally 0.4 mg melatonin or intravenously 0.2 mg on two separate study days, was undertaken. The study reported a Tmax value of 5 min for intranasal administration and 10 min for intravenous administration [35]. Other researchers [36] have formulated melatonin, as a thermoreversible Pluronic gel for nasal administration for treating sleep disorders. The comparative electroencephalogram (EEG) pattern, derived from five healthy volunteers who participated in this crossover study after administration of melatonin tablet and nasal gel, revealed that nasal absorption of melatonin was faster and the sleep produced resembled to one during nocturnal chronobiological melatonin secretion. The optimized formulation has provided bimodal drug release extending over 5 h at significantly low dose (1 mg intranasal dose) as compared to 3 mg oral dose. The use of the novel thermoreversible Pluronic gel showed the desired bioadhesion to the nasal mucosa, with no sensitizing effect in subjects and reproducible sleep characteristics thus making this formulation an agent with an excellent commercial potential.

2.5. Melatonin injectable formulations

Injectable formulations also play an important role as melatonin modified release systems. Many researchers have focused on intravenous (i.v. bolus infusion), intramuscular, subcutaneous, and implant administration of melatonin formulations in human volunteers, small laboratory animals, as well as in larger animals like ewes, goats, and deer.

A research work showed that during melatonin infusion (n = 4 bolus intravenous injection of 5 or 10 μg/person and after a 5-h infusion of 20 μg per person in six healthy subjects), the plasma hormone level reached a steady-state after 60 and 120 min, which was equal to the nocturnal level. This particular infusion regime could be valuable in replacing blunted hormonal secretion in disease states [37]. A human positron emission tomography (PET) study, performed in a healthy volunteer with ^{11}C-labeled melatonin, showed maximum activity in the brain 8.5 min following the injection, quite different from the curve observed for the plasma radioactivity (maximum at 3.5 min), confirming that melatonin crosses the blood-brain barrier and that 6-sulfatoxymelatonin is its main plasma metabolite [38]. The absolute bioavailability of melatonin was studied in 12 young healthy subjects (six males and six females) after administration at midday, on two separate occasions: 23 μg by intravenous infusion and 250 μg by oral solution of D7 melatonin (seven deuterium atoms replace seven hydrogen atoms in the melatonin molecule). Exogenous (D7) and endogenous (D0) melatonin were quantified simultaneously, but separately, by a highly specific assay, gas chromatography/negative ion chemical ionization mass spectrometry. After i.v. administration, the maximum plasma concentration (Cmax) and the area under the plasma concentration-time curve (AUC) values were found to be significantly different in male and female subjects, but there was no significant gender difference in total body clearance when normalized to body weight. After oral administration, pharmacokinetic parameters used to quantify bioavailability were near 3 times greater in female subjects than in males, with large inter-individual variations [39]. In the review article of Gómez-Moreno et al. [40], the use of melatonin in implant dentistry has been proved to increase the new bone formation and bone-to-implant values, around dental implants, leading to a more stable bone area around the implants. In view of these findings, researchers are currently exploring further possibilities as to how melatonin might benefit implant dentistry.

Two i.v. formulations of melatonin (5 mg/ml) have been tested in Wistar rats: one formulation with hydroxypropyl-β-cyclodextrin and propylene glycol to increase solubility and stability and the other with an antioxidant and chelating agent to minimize oxidation and hydrolysis. The pharmacokinetic profiles and the plasma antioxidant activity results suggested a potential for use in the clinical study for these two i.v. melatonin formulations [41]. Another research group [42] studied the possibility of using high-dose intravenous melatonin as an anesthetic adjuvant and compared its effects with thiopental and propofol using Sprague Dawley rats. By administering to the rats bolus or cumulative i.v. doses of melatonin, thiopental, or propofol, they assessed the righting reflex, hind paw withdrawal to a noxious stimulus, response to tail clamping and hemodynamic effects. The results showed that melatonin caused a dose-dependent increase in paw withdrawal. Melatonin was comparable to thiopental and propofol in terms of its rapid onset of hypnosis and it was concluded that intravenous melatonin can exert hypnotic effects similar to those observed with thiopental and propofol. Other researchers have injected mice daily with 50 μg of melatonin, 12 h after lights on, for 18 weeks. The results indicated that mice underwent gonadal regression after 4–7 weeks and reproductive recrudescence after 15 weeks [43].

The effect of differing doses and routes of administration of melatonin on plasma melatonin levels in sheep and goats has been examined by the researchers Kennaway and Seamark [44]. Melatonin injected subcutaneously in a saline or oil vehicle caused high transitory peaks in plasma melatonin, whereas oral administration, in either saline solution or adsorbed onto pelleted foodstuff, resulted in sustained elevated blood levels for periods exceeding 7 h. Oral dosages of about 2 mg proved adequate to raise the normal daytime plasma levels in both sheep and goats to levels within the normal night-time range. It was concluded that with ruminants the oral route of administration provides a facile and practical way of administering melatonin for physiological study. The review paper of Williams et al. [45] presents data from five research trials and 108 clinical trials conducted in three countries to validate the optimum use of melatonin to advance seasonal breeding patterns of a variety of breeds of sheep. In order to define the optimum time for treatment in breeding flocks, ewes of three different breeds were treated with controlled-release 18-mg melatonin implants (Regulin®), with treatments commencing at various times ranging from 9 to 3 weeks, prior to joining with fertile rams. Overall, the studies presented in this paper showed that melatonin pretreatment of spring and early summer joined ewe flocks resulted in both a modest decrease in the number of barren ewes and an increase in the number of multiple births concluding that this treatment strategy maximizes the potential advantages expected from the melatonin treatment.

2.6. Melatonin topical preparations

As mentioned previously, melatonin has shown antioxidant and immunological properties and therefore, it may be beneficial as a topical drug for the use against oxidative damage in the skin or even as a potential sun protection element, against UV-induced oxidative damage. Melatonin skin penetration properties have been studied in alcoholic solutions, creams, in various vesicular approaches (liposomes and ethosomes), in undecanoic, lauric, and oleic acids.

The skin penetration properties of melatonin from three galenic preparations (0.01% in a cream and 0.01 and 0.03% in a solution) were investigated by the evaluation of the serum melatonin levels over a 24-h time period in a clinical study (15 healthy volunteers) conducted by a research group [46]. The cumulative melatonin serum values for each preparation were 7.1, 8.6, and 15.7 pg/ml, respectively, showing that the alcoholic solution was superior to the cream formulation for melatonin delivery. The strongly lipophilic substance melatonin is able to penetrate through the skin, leading to dose- and galenic-dependent melatonin levels in the blood.

Novel ethanolic liposomes (ethosomes) bearing melatonin were evaluated for transdermal administration potential [47]. Melatonin loaded ethosomes were prepared and characterized for vesicular shape and surface morphology, vesicular size, entrapment efficiency, stability, *in vitro* skin permeation, and *in vivo* skin tolerability. The results suggested that ethosomes may offer a suitable approach for transdermal delivery of melatonin.

The effects of vehicles and enhancers on skin permeation and lag time were evaluated for a more effective transdermal delivery of melatonin [48]. Skin permeation study was conducted in Franz diffusion cells using excised hairless mouse skins and samples were analyzed by HPLC. As vehicles, ethanol (EtOH), polyethylene glycol 400 (PEG), or propylene glycol (PG) were used alone or mixed with a phosphate buffer. The results indicated that the use of binary vehicles could effectively modulate the skin permeability of melatonin (to the limited extent) and the lag time observed. As enhancers, fatty acids were used and when compared with the binary vehicles, the use of oleic acid drastically enhanced the skin permeation of melatonin as well as shortened its lag time.

Apart from being an established radioprotectant and anticancer agent [49], melatonin has also been found to counteract UV-induced solar damage, which includes the generation of reactive oxygen species, skin aging, mitochondrial, and DNA damage [50]. The presence of melatonin along with the UV filters could provide a synergistic effect for optimum sun protection as topical application of melatonin along with vitamin E and C in human volunteers has been found to counteract ultraviolet induced erythema and the generation and adverse effects of free radical species [51]. Another research work [52] has dealt with the preclinical safety evaluation of the sunscreen formulation comprising of four US FDA approved UV filters; namely avobenzone, octinoxate, oxybenzone, titanium dioxide along with melatonin and pumpkin seed oil. The results obtained from this study indicated that the sunscreen formulation is nontoxic and safe in animal models and alongside with additional preclinical evaluations may serve as a basis for considering the formulation, as a potential candidate for further trials to establish its efficacy, tolerability, and applicability.

2.7. Transdermal patches

The transdermal delivery of melatonin could be a good route for its administration, given the variability of absorption, short biological half-life, and extensive first-pass metabolism of melatonin when administered orally. The main obstacle is the barrier nature of the stratum corneum of the skin that requires the right choice of a suitable vehicle, where the drug can be dissolved, then released, and finally penetrate the skin.

A research group [53] prepared and evaluated monolithic drug-in-adhesive type transdermal patches of melatonin using Eudragit E 100 as the adhesive polymer, containing penetration enhancers such as fatty alcohols, fatty acids, and terpenes. The results indicated that the addition of enhancers in the patch increased the permeation of melatonin through hairless rat skin. Decanol and undecanoic acid showed the maximum permeation of melatonin among the fatty alcohols and fatty acids, respectively, while menthol showed the maximum permeation of melatonin among all the enhancers studied. The release profile of melatonin from the patches followed first order kinetics. A lag time of 4–6 h was observed before a steady-state flux of melatonin was reached.

The effect of transdermal in comparison to oral controlled-release and oral transmucosal drug delivery systems on plasma concentrations of melatonin and its principal metabolite (6-sulfatoxymelatonin (MT6s)) was evaluated in 12 human subjects using a crossover, single dose design [23]. The plasma concentrations of the parent drug and MT6s were measured by radioimmunoassay. Transdermal drug delivery resulted in a significant delay in systemic drug levels and a gradual decline in drug delivery after patch removal (patch dosage forms were removed after 10 h of application), possibly due to the deposition of melatonin in the skin.

Other researchers suggested that transdermal melatonin may have advantages over fast-release oral melatonin in improving sleep maintenance at adverse circadian cycles [54]. An experimental skin patch designed to deliver melatonin, such that plasma levels steadily increase for 6–8 h, and thus counteract the increasing circadian wake drive and improve daytime sleep was administered to 8 healthy subjects (2.1 mg melatonin or placebo, randomized, double-blind, crossover study) 1 h before an 8 h daytime sleep opportunity (09:00–17:00 h). The results indicated that transdermal melatonin delivery was effective in elevating plasma melatonin levels for an extended duration during the daytime.

Another group of researchers examined the pharmacokinetics of melatonin incorporated in solid lipid nanoparticles, administered by oral or transdermal route [18]. Solid lipid nanoparticles were used as a reservoir system, permitting a constant and prolonged release of melatonin. In comparison to the standard formulation of orally administered melatonin, the absorption and elimination after administration of the solid lipid nanoparticle-melatonin complexes through the transdermal route demonstrated to be slow and melatonin plasma levels above 50 pg/ml were maintained for at least 24 h. Therefore, these systems disclose a potential for the sustained delivery of melatonin.

3. Conclusions

In this chapter, a concise account of the different melatonin delivery routes is given. The choice of the most effective melatonin delivery system is circumstantial and depends on the dysfunction that needs to be treated. However, it seems that modified release formulations mimic closer the endogenous melatonin release pattern and thus a plethora of such systems are currently under thorough investigation.

Author details

Marilena Vlachou* and Angeliki Siamidi

*Address all correspondence to: vlachou@pharm.uoa.gr

School of Health Sciences, Department of Pharmacy, Division of Pharmaceutical Technology, National and Kapodistrian University of Athens, Athens, Greece

References

[1] Vlachou M, Tragou K, Siamidi A, Kikionis S, Chatzianagnostou AL, Mitsopoulos A, Ioannou E, Roussis V, Tsotinis A. Modified *in vitro* release of the chronobiotic hormone melatonin from matrix tablets based on the marine sulfated polysaccharide ulvan. Journal of Drug Delivery Science and Technology. 2018;**44**:41-48. DOI: 10.1016/j.jddst.2017.11.019

[2] Jan JE, Hamilton D, Seward N, Fast DK, Freeman RD, Laudon M. Clinical trials of controlled-release melatonin in children with sleep–wake cycle disorders. Journal of Pineal Research. 2000;**29**:34-39. DOI: 10.1034/j.1600-079X.2000.290105.x

[3] Muñoz H, Castan H, Clares B, Ruiz MA. Obtaining fast dissolving disintegrating tablets with different doses of melatonin. International Journal of Pharmaceutics. 2014;**5**(1-2): 84-89. DOI: 10.1016/j.ijpharm.2014.03.054

[4] Rybka J, Kędziora-Kornatowska K, Kupczyk D, Muszalik M, Kornatowski M, Kędziora J. Antioxidant effect of immediate- versus sustained-release melatonin in type 2 diabetes mellitus and healthy controls. Drug Delivery. 2014;**23**(3):804-807. DOI: 10.3109/10717544.2014.917343

[5] Lee BJ, Ryu SG, Cui JH. Formulation and release characteristics of hydroxypropyl ethylcellulose matrix tablet containing melatonin. Drug Development and Industrial Pharmacy. 1999;**25**(4):493-501. DOI: 10.1081/DDC-100102199

[6] Kumar A, Agarwal SP, Khanna R. Modified release bi-layered tablet of melatonin using b-cyclodextrin. Die Pharmazie. 2003;**58**(9):642-644

[7] Lyseng-Williamson KA. Melatonin prolonged release: In the treatment of insomnia in patients aged ≥55 years. Drugs and Aging. 2012;**29**(11):911-923. DOI: 10.1007/s40266-012-0018-z

[8] Filali S, Bergamelli C, Tall ML, Salmon D, Laleye D, Dhelens C, Diouf E, Pivot C, Pirot F. Formulation, stability testing, and analytical characterization of melatonin-based preparation for clinical trial. Journal of Pharmaceutical Analysis. 2017;**7**(4):237-243. DOI: 10.1016/j.jpha.2017.04.001

[9] Vlachou M, Eikosipentaki A, Xenogiorgis V. Pineal hormone melatonin: Solubilization studies in model aqueous gastrointestinal environments. Current Drug Delivery. 2006;**3**:255-265. DOI: 10.2174/156720106777731073

[10] Vlachou M, Tsiakoulia A, Eikosipentaki A. Controlled release of the pineal hormone melatonin from hydroxypropylmethylcellulose/sodium alginate matrices in aqueous media containing dioctyl sulfosuccinate. Current Drug Discovery Technologies. 2007;**4**:31-38. DOI: 10.2174/157016307781115449

[11] Vlachou M, Ioannidou V, Vertzoni M, Tsotinis A, Afroudakis P, Sugden D. Controlled release from solid pharmaceutical formulations of two nalkanoyl-4-methoxybicyclo [4.2.0]octa-1,3,5-trien-7-ethanamines with melatoninergic activity. Letters in Drug Design and Discovery. 2015;**12**:259-262. DOI: 10.2174/1570180811666141024005226

[12] Vlachou M, Papamichael M, Siamidi A, Fragouli I, Afroudakis PA, Kompogennitaki R, Dotsikas Y. Comparative in vitro controlled release studies on the chronobiotic hormone melatonin from cyclodextrins-containing matrices and cyclodextrin: Melatonin complexes. International Journal of Molecular Sciences. 2017;**18**:1641. DOI: 10.3390/ijms18081641

[13] Vlachou M, Stavrou G, Siamidi A, Flitouri S, Ioannidou V, Mavrokordopoulos S. N-acetylserotonin vs melatonin. in vitro controlled release from hydrophilic matrix tablets. Letters in Drug Design and Discovery. 2018;**15**. DOI: 10.2174/1570180815666180404125519

[14] Vlachou M, Siamidi A, Pareli I, Zampakola A, Konstantinidou S. An account of modified release of melatonin from mono- and bi-layer solid pharmaceutical formulations. Journal of Pharmaceutical Sciences. 2016;**1**(4):10-14. DOI: 10.24218/vjpps.2016.19

[15] Lee BJ, Min GH. Oral controlled release of melatonin using polymer-reinforced and coated alginate beads. International Journal of Pharmaceutics. 1996;**144**(1):37-46. DOI: 10.1016/S0378-5173(96)04723-0

[16] Lee BJ, Parrott KA, Ayres JW, Sack RL. Design and evaluation of an oral controlled release delivery system for melatonin in human subjects. The International Journal of Pharmaceutics. 1995;**124**(1):119-127. DOI: 10.1016/0378-5173(95)00088-Z

[17] Zampakola A, Siamidi A, Pippa N, Demetzos C, Vlachou M. Chronobiotic hormone melatonin: Comparative *in vitro* release studies from matrix tablets and liposomal formulations. Letters in Drug Design and Discovery. 2017;**14**(4):476-480. DOI: 10.2174/1570180813666161006162246

[18] Priano L, Esposti D, Esposti R, Castagna G, De Medici C, Fraschini F, Gasco MR, Mauro A. Solid lipid nanoparticles incorporating melatonin as new model for sustained oral and transdermal delivery systems. Journal of Nanoscience and Nanotechnology. 2007;**7**:3596-3601. DOI: 10.1166/jnn.2007.809

[19] Vlachou M, Kikionis S, Siamidi A, Tragou K, Kapoti S, Ioannou E, Roussis V, Tsotinis A. Fabrication and characterization of electrospun nanofibers for the modified release of the chronobiotic hormone melatonin. Unpublished results

[20] Vlachou M, Siamidi A, Konstantinidou S, Dotsikas Y. Optimization of controlled release matrix formulation of melatonin via experimental design. The Journal of Pharmaceutics and Drug Delivery Research. 2016;**5**(6):1-5. DOI: 10.4172/2325-9604.1000159

[21] Najeeb S, Khurshid Z, Zohaib S, Zafar MS. Therapeutic potential of melatonin in oral medicine and periodontology. The Kaohsiung Journal of Medical Sciences. 2016;**32**(8):391-396. DOI: 10.1016/j.kjms.2016.06.005

[22] Reiter RJ, Rosales-Corral SA, Liu XY, Acuna-Castroviejo D, Escames G, Tan DX. Melatonin in the oral cavity: Physiological and pathological implications. Journal of Periodontal Research. 2014;**50**(1):9-17. DOI: 10.1111/jre.12176

[23] Benes L, Claustrat B, Horriere F, Geoffriau M, Konsil J, Parrott KA, DeGrande G, McQuinn RL, Ayres JW. Transmucosal, oral controlled release, and transdermal drug administration in human subjects: A crossover study with melatonin. Journal of Pharmaceutical Sciences. 1997;**86**:1115-1119. DOI: 10.1021/js970011z

[24] Khezri MB, Merate H. The effects of melatonin on anxiety and pain scores of patients, intraocular pressure, and operating conditions during cataract surgery under topical anesthesia. Indian Journal of Ophthalmology. 2013;**61**:319-324. DOI: 10.4103/0301-4738.99637

[25] Naguib M, Samarkandi AH. The comparative dose-response effects of melatonin and midazolam for premedication of adult patients: A double-blinded, placebo-controlled study. Anesthesia and Analgesia. 2000;**91**(2):473-479. DOI: 10.1213/00000539-200008000-00046

[26] Stefani LC, Muller S, Torres ILS, Razzolini B, Rozisky JR, Fregni F, Markus R, Caumo W. A phase II, randomized, double-blind, placebo controlled, dose-response trial of the melatonin effect on the pain threshold of healthy subjects. PLoS One. 2013;**8**(10):e74107. DOI: 10.1371/journal.pone.0074107

[27] Acil M, Basgul E, Celiker V, Karagöz A, Demir B, Aypar U. Perioperative effects of melatonin and midazolam premedication on sedation, orientation, anxiety scores and psychomotor performance. European Journal of Anaesthesiology. 2004;**21**(7):553-557. DOI: 10.1017/S0265021504007094

[28] Grassin-Delyle S, Buenestado A, Naline E, Faisy C, Blouquit-Laye S, Couderc LJ, Le Guen M, Fischler M, Devillier P. Intranasal drug delivery: An efficient and non-invasive route for systemic administration: Focus on opioids. Pharmacology and Therapeutics. 2012;**134**:366-379. DOI: 10.1016/j.pharmthera.2012.03.003

[29] Babu RJ, Dayal P, Singh M. Effect of cyclodextrins on the complexation and nasal permeation of melatonin. Drug Delivery. 2008;**15**:381-388. DOI: 10.1080/10717540802006922

[30] Priprem A, Johns JR, Limsitthichaikoon S, Limphirat W, Mahakunakorn P, Johns NP. Intranasal melatonin nanoniosomes: Pharmacokinetic, pharmacodynamics and toxicity studies. Therapeutic Delivery. 2017;**8**:373-390. DOI: 10.4155/tde-2017-0005

[31] van den Berg MP, Merkus P, Romeijn SG, Verhoef JC, Merkus FWHM. Uptake of melatonin into the cerebrospinal fluid after nasal and intravenous delivery: Studies in rats and comparison with a human study. Pharmaceutical Research. 2004;**21**:799-802. DOI: 10.1023/B:PHAM.0000026431.55383.69

[32] Chen JM, Mao SR, Bi DZ. Studies on melatonin gelatin microspheres for intranasal administration. Yao Xue Xue Bao. 2000;**35**:786-789

[33] Bechgaard E, Lindhardt K, Martinsen L. Intranasal absorption of melatonin *in vivo* bioavailability study. International Journal of Pharmaceutics. 1999;**182**:1-5. DOI: 10.1016/S0378-5173(99)00019-8

[34] Mao S, Chen J, Wei Z, Liu H, Bi D. Intranasal administration of melatonin starch microspheres. International Journal of Pharmaceutics. 2004;**272**:37-43. DOI: 10.1016/j.ijpharm.2003.11.028

[35] Merkus P, Guchelaar HJ, Bosch DA, Merkus FWHM. Direct access of drugs to the human brain after intranasal drug administration? Neurology. 2003;**60**:1669-1671. DOI: 10.1212/01.WNL.0000067993.60735.77

[36] Pisal SS, Reddy P, Paradkar AR, Mahadik KR, Kadam SS. Nasal melatonin gels using Pluronic F-127for chronobiological treatment of sleep disorders. Journal of Biotechnology. 2004;**3**:369-377

[37] Mallo C, Zaidan R, Galy G, Vermeulen E, Brun J, Chazot G, Claustrat B. Pharmacokinetics of melatonin in man after intravenous infusion and bolus injection. European Journal of Clinical Pharmacology. 1990;**38**:297-301. DOI: 10.1007/BF00315035

[38] Le Bars D, Thivolle P, Vitte PA, Bojkowski C, Chazot G, Arendt J, Frackowiak RSJ, Claustrat B. PET and plasma pharmacokinetic studies after bolus intravenous administration of [^{11}C]melatonin in humans. International Journal of Radiation Applications and Instrumentation B. 1991;**18**(3):357-362. DOI: 10.1016/0883-2897(91)90132-5

[39] Fourtillan JB, Brisson AM, Gobin P, Gobin P, Ingrand I, Decourt JP, Girault J. Bioavailability of melatonin in humans after day-time administration of D7 melatonin. Biopharmaceutics and Drug Disposition. 2000;**21**:15-22. DOI: 10.1002/1099-081X(200001)21:1<15::AID-BDD215>3.0.CO;2-H

[40] Gómez-Moreno G, Aguilar-Salvatierra A, Boquete-Castro A, Guardia J, Piattelli A, Perrotti V, Delgado-Ruiz RA, Calvo-Guirado JL. Outcomes of topical applications of melatonin in implant dentistry: A systematic review. Implant Dentistry. 2015;**24**(1):25-30. DOI: 10.1097/ID.0000000000000186

[41] Johns J, Chenboonthai C, Pratheepawanit J, Saengkrasat A, Kuketpitakwong R, Porasupatana S. An intravenous injection of melatonin: Formulations, stability, pharmacokinetics and pharmacodynamics. Journal of Asian Association of Schools of Pharmacy. 2012;**1**: 32-43

[42] Naguib M, Hammond DL, Schmid III PG, Baker MT, Cutkomp J, Queral L, Smith T. Pharmacological effects of intravenous melatonin: Comparative studies with thiopental and propofol. BJA. 2003;**90**(4): 504-507. DOI: 10.1093/bja/aeg092

[43] Heath HW, Lynch GR. Effects of 18 weeks of daily melatonin injection on reproduction and temperature regulation in the mouse. Journal of Experimental Zoology. 1981;**216**(1):193-195. DOI: 10.1002/jez.1402160122

[44] Kennaway DJ, Seamark RF. Circulating levels of melatonin following its oral administration or subcutaneous injection in sheep and goats. Australian Journal of Biological Sciences. 1980;**33**:349-353. DOI: 10.1071/BI9800349

[45] Williams AH, McPhee SR, Reeve JL, Staples LD. Optimum use of subcutaneous melatonin implants to enhance the reproductive performance of seasonal and non-seasonal sheep joined in spring and early summer. Animal Reproduction Science. 1992;**30**:225-258. DOI: 10.1016/0378-4320(92)90012-3

[46] Fischer TV, Greif C, Fluhr JW, Wigger-Alberti W, Elsner P. Percutaneous penetration of topically applied melatonin in a cream and an alcoholic solution. Skin Pharmacology and Physiology. 2004;**14**:190-194. DOI: 10.1159/000078822

[47] Dubey V, Mishra D, Jain NK. Melatonin loaded ethanolic liposomes: Physicochemical characterization and enhanced transdermal delivery. European Journal of Pharmaceutics and Biopharmaceutics. 2007;**67**:398-405. DOI: 10.1016/j.ejpb.2007.03.007

[48] Oh HJ, Oh YK, Kim CK. Effects if vehicles and enhancers on transdermal delivery of melatonin. The International Journal of Pharmaceutics. 2001;**212**:63-71. DOI: 10.1016/S0378-5173(00)00598-6

[49] Shirazi A, Ghobadi G, Ghazi-Khansari M. A radiobiological review on melatonin: A novel radioprotector. Journal of Radiation Research. 2007;**48**(4):263-272. DOI: 10.1269/jrr.06070

[50] Kleszczynski K, Fischer TW. Melatonin and human skin aging. Dermatoendocrinol. 2012;**4**(3):245-252. DOI: 10.4161/derm.22344

[51] Dreher F, Gabard B, Schwindt DA, Maibach HI. Topical melatonin in combination with vitamins E and C protects skin from ultraviolet-induced erythema: A human study *in vivo*. The British Journal of Dermatology. 1998;**139**(2):332-339. DOI: 10.1046/j.1365-2133.1998.02447.x

[52] Bora NS, Pathak MP, Mandal S, Mazumder B, Policegoudra R, Raju PS, Chattopadhyay P. Safety assessment and toxicological profiling of a novel combinational sunprotective dermal formulation containing melatonin and pumpkin seed oil. Regulatory Toxicology and Pharmacology. 2017;**89**:1-12. DOI: 10.1016/j.yrtph.2017.07.004

[53] Kanikkannan N, Andega S, Burton S, Babu R, Singh M. Formulation and *in vitro* evaluation of transdermal patches of melatonin. Drug Development and Industrial Pharmacy. 2004;**30**(2):205-212. DOI: 10.1081/DDC-120028716

[54] Aeschbach D, Lockyer BJ, Dijk DJ, Lockley SW, Nuwayser ES, Nichols LD, Czeisler CA. Use of transdermal melatonin delivery to improve sleep maintenance during daytime. Clinical Pharmacology and Therapeutics. 2009;**86**:378-382. DOI: 10.1038/clpt.2009.109

2

Melatonin: A Silent Regulator of the Glucose Homeostasis

Cristina Manuela Drăgoi, Andreea Letiția Arsene,
Cristina Elena Dinu-Pîrvu, Ion Bogdan Dumitrescu,
Daniela Elena Popa,
George T.A. Burcea-Dragomiroiu,
Denisa Ioana Udeanu, Olivia Carmen Timnea,
Bruno Ștefan Velescu and Alina Crenguța Nicolae

Abstract

In the human organism, the circadian regulation of carbohydrates metabolism is essential for the glucose homeostasis and energy balance. Unbalances in glucose and insulin tissue and blood levels have been linked to a variety of metabolic disorders such as obesity, metabolic syndrome, cardiovascular diseases and type 2 diabetes. Melatonin, the pineal hormone, is the key mediator molecule for the integration between the cyclic environment and the circadian distribution of physiological and behavioral processes and for the optimization of energy balance and body weight regulation, events that are crucial for a healthy organism. This chapter reviews the interplay between melatonin modulatory physiological effects, glucose homeostasis and metabolic balance, from the endocrinology perspective. The tremendous effect of melatonin in the regulation of metabolic processes is observed from the chronobiology perspective, considering melatonin as a major synchronizer of the circadian internal order of the physiological processes involved in energy metabolism.

Keywords: melatonin, pineal gland, chronobiology, glucose homeostasis, metabolic syndrome

1. Introduction

Chronobiology depicts the temporal structure of biology. It integrates the rhythmic development and existence of the utmost majority of cells, comprising also cellular functions, as a fundamental property of the living matter, detectable at all levels of its organization, from the molecular level to rhythms in the integrity of the complex organisms. It regulates the species' biological clock, the circadian and seasonal biorhythms, synchronizing the existence of a cell within an organ, the functioning rationale of an organ within a system and the epigenetic temporal regulation of the whole living entity.

Synchronicity between external and internal circadian rhythms and harmony among molecular fluctuations within cells are essential for normal organ biology. Circadian clocks exist within multiple components of the metabolic, cardiovascular and immune systems, having the potential of affecting multiple cellular processes and, therefore, holding the promise of modulating various physiopathological aspects over the course of the 24 h cycle.

2. The pineal gland, a neuroendocrine transducer

Metabolic physiology undergoes diurnal variations, and serious pathologic events appear to be conditioned by the time of day. The suprachiasmatic nucleus imprints the control of circadian rhythms in peripheral tissues, by different neural and humoral signals, such as melatonin.

The molecular clock mechanism in mammals is currently understood as a transcriptional feedback loop involving several genes. The genes Clock and Bmal1 encode bHLH-PAS (basic helix-loop-helix) proteins that form the positive limb of the feedback circuit. The CLOCK:BMAL1 heterodimer initiates the transcription by binding to specific DNA elements, E-boxes (5′-CACGTG-3′) and E′-boxes (5′-CACGTT-3′) in the promoters of target genes. This set of activated genes includes members of the negative limb of the feedback loop including the PER (PER1 and PER2) and CRY (CRY1 and CRY2) genes. The resulting PER and CRY proteins dimerize and inhibit further CLOCK:BMAL1 transcriptional activity allowing the cycle to repeat from a level of low transcriptional activity. Thus, cellular metabolism may prove to play an important role in regulating the transcriptional state and therefore the phase of the clock. Degradation of the negative limb proteins PER and CRY is required to terminate the repression phase and restart a new cycle of transcription. The transcriptional feedback loop described above can be observed not only in the SCN, but also in nearly every mammalian cell. If viewed at the single-cell level, the molecular clockwork of transcription and translation can be observed as autonomous single-cell oscillators [1].

Melatonin (*N*-acetyl-5-methoxytryptamine) is synthesized by multiple tissues in the body, but the pineal gland is the major contributor to circulating melatonin concentration, as pinealectomy abolishes detectable melatonin in the blood.

In young- and middle-aged people, pineal melatonin is secreted based on a circadian pattern, with a high rhythm amplitude and a considerable nocturnal maximum.

Melatonin from extrapineal sites often oscillates with considerably lower amplitudes. According to current knowledge, some of the extrapineal sources are of particular importance, either in quantitative terms, such as the gastrointestinal tract or, with regard to functional aspects, some areas of the central nervous system (CNS) and several leukocytes. The physiological significance of other sites of melatonin biosynthesis is, at the moment, uncertain. Melatonin is secreted in small amounts from most of the extrapineal sites or only under specific conditions, for example, the postprandial release from the gastrointestinal tract, during which relatively high quantities can enter the circulation, being chronobiologically rather irrelevant. Thus, melatonin is not only a pineal hormone but also has additional functions as a local tissue factor and leukocyte-derived cell hormone with paracrine and autocrine actions [2].

The pineal gland or the epiphysis weighs about 150 mg, and it is located in the posterior part of the third cerebral ventricle. The pineal gland of mammals is a homogeneous tissue containing pinealocytes, glial cells, phagocytic cells and neurons. The pineal gland is innervated by nervous fibers of different origins. The gland was considered a vestigial organ until 1950s. Its position in the center of the brain and its presence in other species of vertebrates indicate its evolution in the evolutionary cerebral system of the humans, based on its absolute necessity on the overall organism development and important particular functions.

In the current scientific frame, it is generally acknowledged that the pineal organ is a neuroendocrine transducer. The pinealocytes, the main secretory pineal parenchymal cells, are fotoneuroendocrine cells, phylogenetically derived from primary sensory cells, having neural embryological origin. They primary respond to nervous-photic modulated stimulation and secondary to hormones in target organs. The endocrine secretory function is directly dependent on sympathetic innervation, the pinealocytes translating the nervous information in endocrine information.

In terms of phylogenetic evolution, the pinealocyte functions as a fotoneuroendocrine neuron. On some species of amphibians, reptiles and birds, the epiphysis is also called "parietal eye" or third eye because it has the form of a rudimentary eye fitted with a lens and a retina. Therefore, it is considered to be a vestigial of a sensory organ, functional in primitive vertebrates. Being directly affected by the light absorbed by the eye, the pineal gland regulates the sleep-wake states, the menstruation and the reproduction, the hibernation and the seasonal migration and other "instinctive" behaviors.

The role of the pineal gland, as an integral component of the brain, evolved on the phylogenetic scale from photoreceptor organ (fish, amphibians, reptiles), to neuroendocrine modulator of brain functions, in mammals and humans, thus having a role in the adaptation of reproductive conditions environment in some mammals (particularly rodents) and to a major role in the modulation of brain excitability in relation to the external environmental conditions in humans.

Nowadays, melatonin, the major pineal hormone, is considered the master hormone, regulating all other hormones within the human organism.

The main regulatory pathway is a complex one called the retinoic-hypothalamic-pineal axis that ends with the sympathetic transmission of the pineal parenchymal. The pineal gland receives neuronal transmissions of central and parasympathetic origin. These pineal nervous endings contain a great variety of neurotransmitters. The rhythm of melatonin synthesis depends on three interrelated factors: the endogenous circadian oscillator, located in the suprachiasmatic nucleus (SCN), the light/dark and day/night cycles that synchronize the endogenous oscillator and the light that dramatically inhibits the synthesis of melatonin [3].

In conclusion, the pineal gland is a connection point between various neural transmissions, its activity being under the high-fidelity control of the hypothalamic clock, the temporal message being delivered to the pineal gland via a polysynaptic path. However, new neuroanatomic and immunocytochemical proofs changed the concept according to which the pineal gland is innervated only by the sympathetic nervous system, presently, being unanimously accepted to be the target of several neurotransmitters of different origins.

3. Melatonin, the universal synchronizer

Melatonin biosynthesis at the level of pinealocytes occurs and is initiated by the absorption of tryptophan from the blood. Increased daytime tryptophan concentration at the pineal level precedes increased serum free and total tryptophan, suggesting that the essential amino acid is captured by the pineal against a concentration gradient. Once arrived in the pinealocyte, the major part of tryptophan is used for the synthesis of indole derivatives and the rest for protein synthesis (**Figure 1**).

The transformation of tryptophan into serotonin occurs in two stages: first, the hydroxylation into 5-hydroxytryptophan under the enzymatic action of tryptophan hydroxylase, this being a limiting step of the synthesis. The enzyme activity requires the presence of oxygen, tetrahydrobiopterin, $NADPH^+$ and a metal, iron or copper. Second, the decarboxylation of 5-hydroxytryptophan into serotonin by the action of L-aromatic amino acid decarboxylase, in the presence of pyridoxal phosphate (PLP).

The transformation of serotonin into melatonin also includes two stages: the acetylation of $-NH_2$ group by the *N*-acetyltransferase (NAT) enzyme to form *N*-acetyl-serotonin, and thereafter, the methylation of –OH group in position 5 by hydroxyl-indole-*O*-methyltransferase (HIOMT), an enzyme that catalyzes the transfer of methyl group from *S*-adenosyl methionine. This final step results in acetyl-5-methoxytryptamine or melatonin synthesis. The two enzymes, NAT and HIOMT, specific for this synthesis pathway, have different profiles of activity. The NAT enzyme is a limiting enzyme of reaction: it is subject to many mechanisms of transcriptional and/or posttranscriptional regulation depending on the species, which allows it to be active only during darkness. The NAT activity is strongly regulated by circadian alternation light/dark, contrary to HIOMT enzyme showing a constitutive activity along the nictemeral cycle. For example, in rats and humans, a short exposure to bright light during the dark period causes an inhibition of the NAT activity for the next 15 min [3].

The enzymes responsible for the melatonin production can be modulated in a circadian manner, in order to imprint its nictemeral synthesis cycle.

Extrapineal melatonin synthesis in mammals has been reported in the retina, Harderian glands, gastrointestinal tract and pancreas. In humans, melatonin has been reported outside the pineal gland in the follicles, the lining of the intestinal appendix, platelets and red blood cells. Melatonin is also produced by numerous nonendocrine cells, as is the case of the immune cells. In conclusion, while the pineal gland quantitatively accounts for most of the circulating melatonin, substantial local synthesis also occurs in retinal and peripheral tissues such as the gastrointestinal tract [4].

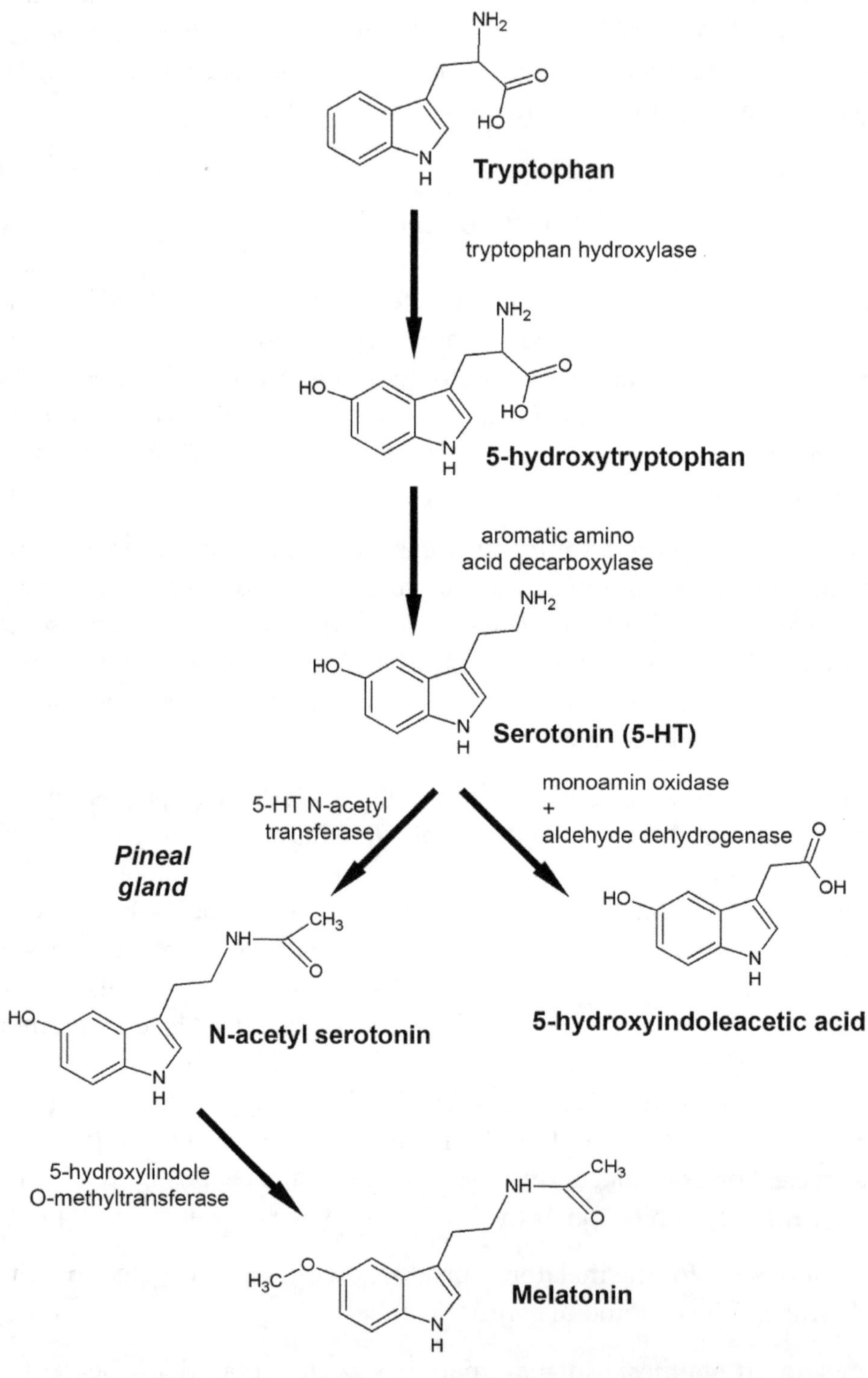

Figure 1. Melatonin biosynthesis pathway.

Melatonin appears to be secreted by the pineal gland in circulation by simple diffusion, because it is highly soluble in the cell membrane lipoproteins. Furthermore, melatonin may have effects on the pineal gland itself, as there are specific receptors for it, at this level. The cells of the suprachiasmatic nucleus also possess receptors for melatonin. In conclusion, melatonin has an inhibitory effect on the activity of the suprachiasmatic nucleus. So, melatonin is self-regulating its own synthesis. However, melatonin secreted into the bloodstream will send to all central and peripheral structures that possess receptors or melatonergic sites this information regarding the photoperiodicity, allowing the organism a physiological adaptation to alternations day/night or to the seasonal ones.

The circadian pacemaker within the suprachiasmatic nucleus triggers the pineal gland to produce high melatonin concentrations at night. There is a photic synchronized endogenous circadian biorhythm, allowing the maximum human melatonin production at night, between midnight and 3 a.m., and the serotonin during the day (**Figure 2a**). Initiating the melatonin synthesis in humans occurs between 9 and 11 p.m. and lasts for about 8–9 h in adults, these parameters being fairly constant from day to day. The daily and seasonal melatonin rhythms are involved in time of day and time of year signaling, and it is for this reason that they are considered to serve as a bioclock and biocalendar.

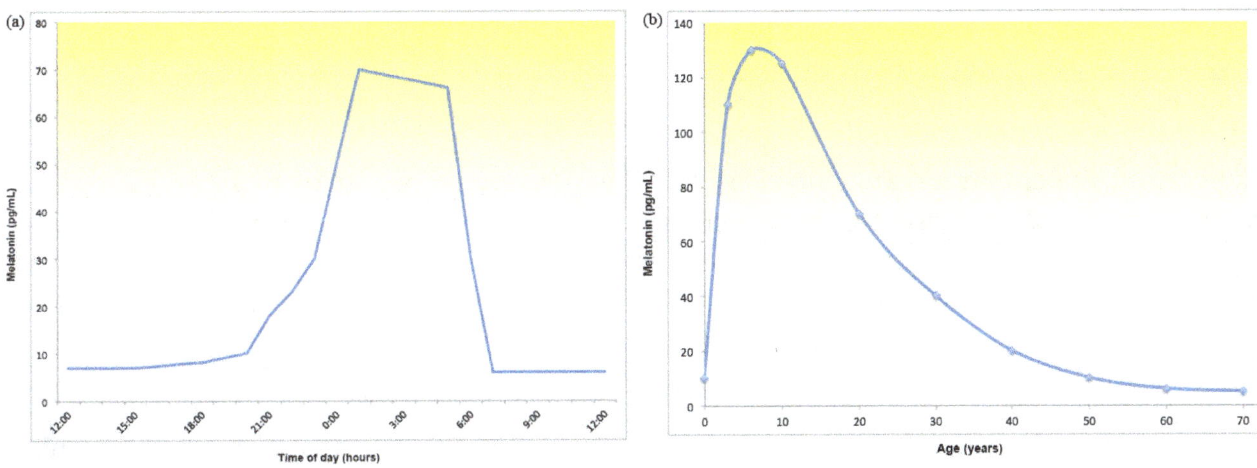

Figure 2. The daily (a) and lifetime (b) melatonin biosynthesis fluctuations.

In humans, it is required an intensity of light greater than in other mammals, over 1500 lux, for disrupting this synthesis biorhythm by external light. In all studied mammals, those with activity at day and at night, the nocturnal melatonin production is maximal and prevailing overnight.

In humans, blood levels of melatonin have a particular dynamics from birth (**Figure 2b**). The pineal synthesis begins in infants over 3 months old, to older age, and the time of puberty is very controversial whether it represents or not a particular step on the downward slope. It is of real interest the fact that melatonin synthesis decreases with the age of humans and has abnormal low levels in a series of age-related pathological disorders, as it is the case of cardiovascular and metabolic disease. Melatonin rhythmic profile has many implications in pathophysiological processes as inflammation, oxidative stress, hypertension and metabolic syndrome.

The half-life of blood melatonin is under 30 min, and the metabolic clearance is 630 mL/min in healthy men. Melatonin is a lipophilic substance metabolized in several compounds both in the liver (**Figure 3a**) and in the central nervous system (**Figure 3b**) [3, 5].

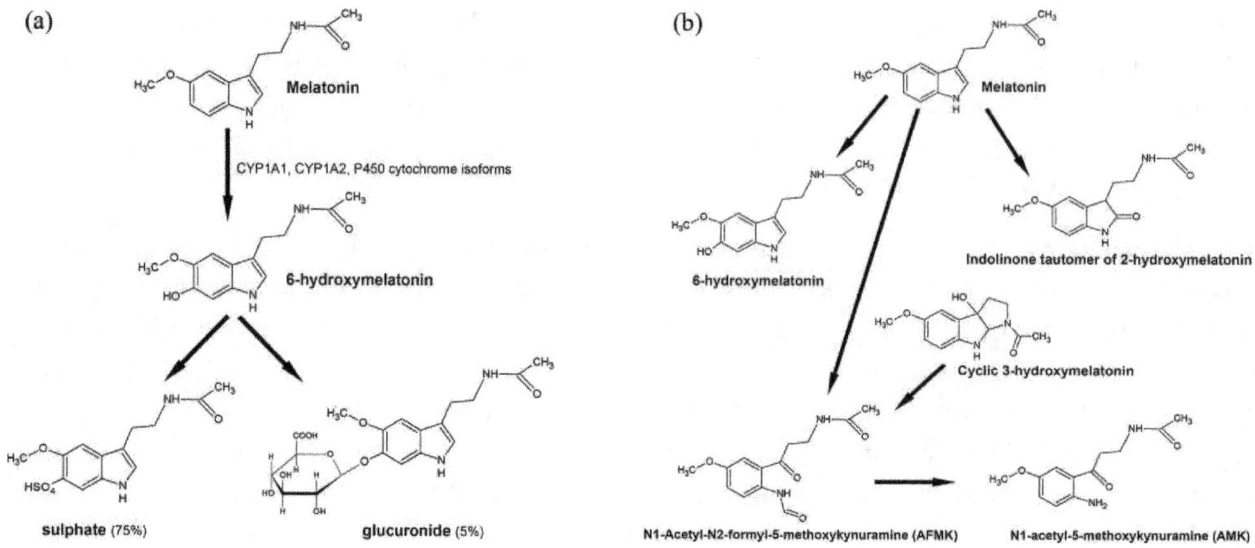

Figure 3. Melatonin hepatic (a) and cerebral (b) metabolism.

Circulating melatonin is catabolized in humans, under the action of hepatic microsomal hydroxylases in *N*-acetylserotonin, which is biologically inactive, and 6-hydroxymelatonin, which is urinary eliminated, as a sulfate (75%) or glucuronide (5%) conjugate. The rest of melatonin is eliminated under three forms: the native form (below 1%), as 5-metoxy indol-acetic acid (0.5%) or catabolized as *N*-acetyl-5-metoxy kynurenamine via *N*-formyl-5-metoxy kynurenamine in the central nervous system (15%).

In the brain, melatonin is metabolized in several compounds of which 5-metoxytriptamine is involved in the dreaming process and it will subsequently metabolize N, *N*-dimethyl-5-methoxytryptamine and other tryptamines.

Approximately 60–70% of the circulating melatonin in the bloodstream is bound to albumin, and about 30% is found in free state, this fraction being the one, that crosses the blood brain barrier [6, 7].

4. Melatonin's pleiotropic effects and the metabolic epigenetic regulation

Considered as nature's most versatile biological signaling and multitasking molecule, melatonin is a highly conserved molecule found in almost all types of organisms. Melatonin has several functions ranging from coordination of circadian activity, which is generally considered as a sleep-promoting effect, and melatonin administration induces hypothermic effects and heat loss via the distal skin regions, and stabilizes sleep-wake cycles [8].

Melatonin demonstrates properties of a powerful antioxidant, at sufficiently high concentrations as a direct radical scavenger, but, at lower, near-physiological levels, as a regulator of redox-relevant enzymes, suppressor of prooxidant excitatory and inflammatory processes and as a mitochondrial modulator [2]. Melatonin also acts on bone metabolism, activating its MT1 and MT2 specific receptors in an autocrine or paracrine fashion, near the target tissues. Melatonin may exert vasodilatatory (MT2) or vasoconstriction (MT1) effects, depending on the receptor type or the target cell, and it can also down-regulate the cortisol secretion [9].

Melatonin has a great influence on diabetes and associated metabolic unbalances by regulating insulin secretion, and also by scavenging reactive oxygen species, the pancreatic β-cells being highly susceptible to oxidative stress, and possessing only low-antioxidative potential. On the other hand, in several genetic studies, human MT2 receptor polymorphisms have been described as being causally linked to an elevated risk of developing type 2 diabetes [4].

5. Chronobiology, metabolic control and disease modulation by melatonin

It is universally accepted that social and industrial pressures, such as shift work, which opposes the physiological temporal circadian order, may be factors determining the occurrence or the development of chronic illnesses, such as metabolic disorders. In many disease states as diabetes mellitus and hypertension, neurohumoral circadian rhythms are chronically impaired and result in dyssynchrony of cellular order in different tissues and between the organism and the environment.

Diabetes mellitus is associated with a phase shift in the cardiac circadian clock. Shift workers have an increased incidence of cardiovascular disease, which might be related to alterations in cardiovascular and metabolic intracellular circadian clock function [5, 10].

The cardiovascular system actually exhibits significant daily variation regarding physiological, pathophysiological and molecular processes. Diurnal variations also affect gene and protein expression. Circadian clocks exist in cardiomyocytes, vascular smooth muscle cells and endothelial cells.

At molecular level, a complex interplay occurs between environmental influences and intrinsic mechanisms, which contributes to change in metabolic functions over the 24 h period.

Loss of synchronization occurs when there are changes in feeding or sleep patterns and during exposure to light at abnormal times, at night, considering this phenomenon as "light-at-night pollution." Such dyssynchronization is seen in patients with hypertension, diabetes mellitus, obesity and shift workers, in whom there is an elevated risk of cardiovascular disease [5, 11].

Melatonin is the key mediator molecule in the in vivo scenario, mediating the integration between the cyclic environment and the circadian distribution of physiological and behavioral processes.

The relation between pineal gland, melatonin and energy metabolism was initially studied in both humans and rodents. Over 70 years ago, one of the first references to the functional connection between the pineal gland and carbohydrates metabolism was made by the Romanian researcher Constantin I. Parhon, followed by his coworkers, endocrinologists Milcu and Nanu. They conducted animal experiments on "pinealin," a pineal peptide, described as having metabolic effects similar to insulin, displaying hypoglycemic, anabolic, anticholesterolemic and glomerulotrophic characteristics. In the following years, a controversial discussion was carried out in many publications on the importance of pineal extracts on glucose metabolism. Even after the isolation and identification of the molecular structure of melatonin, by Aron Lerner and colleagues, this discussion continued [12].

6. The functional synergism between melatonin and insulin

The scientific literature states that first experimental injections with pineal extracts led to hypoglycemia, increased glucose tolerance, and hepatic and muscular glycogenesis. The metabolic disruption caused by the absence of melatonin in the pinealectomized animals was characterized as a diabetogenic syndrome depicted by glucose intolerance and insulin resistance, both expressed peripherally: hepatic, adipose, and skeletal muscle, and centrally, at the level of the hypothalamus. This pathological picture can be reverted by melatonin replacement therapy or restricted feeding.

In addition to this dramatic finding, insulin resistance, glucose intolerance, and several other metabolic disorders can be seen in some physiological or pathological states associated with reductions in blood melatonin levels, as aging, diabetes, shift work, and environmental illumination during the night and the so-called phenomenon of light pollution. An adequate melatonin replacement therapy alleviates most of these alterations.

Emphasizing the functional synergism between melatonin and insulin, it is considered that the pinealectomy-induced insulin resistance and glucose intolerance are related to the mechanistic consequences of the depletion of melatonin, perceived at the molecular level as a deficiency in the insulin-signaling pathway and reduction in GLUT4 gene expression and protein content. It was shown that melatonin, acting through MT1 membrane receptors, induces rapid tyrosine phosphorylation and activation of the tyrosine kinase beta-subunit of the insulin receptor, succeeding to overcome several intracellular transduction steps of the insulin-signaling pathway [6, 7].

7. Melatonin effects on adipocytes

The melatonin-insulin synergism was described in an in vitro experiment which supposed the incubation of isolated visceral white adipocytes with melatonin, the peripheral function of insulin being potentiated by the action of melatonin, and, in addition, this was the first evidence of a direct action of melatonin on adipocytes [6].

All in all, this was a proof that the adipose tissue is a peripheral target of melatonin for the regulation of the overall metabolism. Similarly, it was demonstrated that melatonin activation of MT2 receptors in human adipocytes modulates glucose uptake by these cells. Considering the adipose tissue physiology, it was possible to document synergistic effect of melatonin on several other insulin actions in addition to glucose uptake: insulin-induced leptin synthesis and release in isolated adipocytes is potentiated by the MT1-mediated melatonin action, and melatonin regulates other aspects of adipocyte biology that influence energy metabolism, lipidemia and body weight, as lipolysis, lipogenesis, adipocyte differentiation and fatty acids uptake [6].

Melatonin also exerts different effects on the carbohydrates metabolism, considering various targets: it stimulates glucose uptake in muscle cells by phosphorylation of insulin receptor substrate-1 through MT2 signaling, MT2 receptors are expressed in hepatocytes, and melatonin therapy elevates glucose release from the liver [9].

Another major site of melatonin's action in reference to the regulation of energy metabolism is the pancreatic islets where it influences insulin and glucagon synthesis and release.

Molecular and immunocytochemical studies confirmed the presence of melatonin receptors MT1 and MT2 in the islets of Langerhans and also in human pancreatic tissue [13]. MT1 and/or MT2-mediated melatonin action decreases glucose-stimulated insulin secretion in isolated rat pancreatic islets and rat insulinoma beta-cells.

Melatonin influences exocytosis of insulin by β-cells as concluded from experiments via nonhydrolyzable guanosine-5′-trisphosphate (GTP) analog and luzindole, a melatonin antagonist, both of which inhibit the melatonin action on secretion of insulin from neonatal rat islets.

The intracellular signal transduction pathways of the pancreatic β-cell influenced by melatonin via MT1 and MT2 membrane receptors include cAMP, cGMP and IP3 signaling pathways. The activation of these receptors inhibits glucose- and forskolin-induced insulin secretion, showing that melatonin acts by inhibiting the adenylate cyclase/cAMP system and reducing the content of PKA.

The pineal indolamine induces IGF-1 receptor phosphorylation, which participates in the integrity of islet cells. Moreover, it has been demonstrated, as well, that melatonin stimulated glucagon synthesis and secretion.

Above all considerations, these actions of melatonin are required to build the circadian profile of insulin secretion, synchronizing the pancreatic metabolic rhythms with the circadian rhythm of the activity/rest profile. And it should be also noted that insulin is able to regulate pineal melatonin synthesis by potentiating norepinephrine-stimulated melatonin production.

Interestingly, the association between melatonin and type 2 diabetes could be based on the observation that insulin secretion is inversely proportional to plasma melatonin concentration. These two hormones, melatonin and insulin, exhibit a circadian rhythm, but there is negative correlation between their synthesis dynamics.

Decreased abnormally regulated melatonin levels have been related to diabetes, which suggests that the melatonin signal is critical for glucose homeostasis. In patients with type 2 diabetes, gluconeogenesis and endogenous glucose production exhibit circadian rhythms that impose fasting high blood glucose and do not exist in healthy humans.

Melatonin inhibits glucose-mediated release of insulin from pancreatic cells emphasizing its activity in the function of insulin. Suppression of melatonin secretion by nocturnal light exposure could be a trigger for type 2 diabetes development (**Figure 4**) [9].

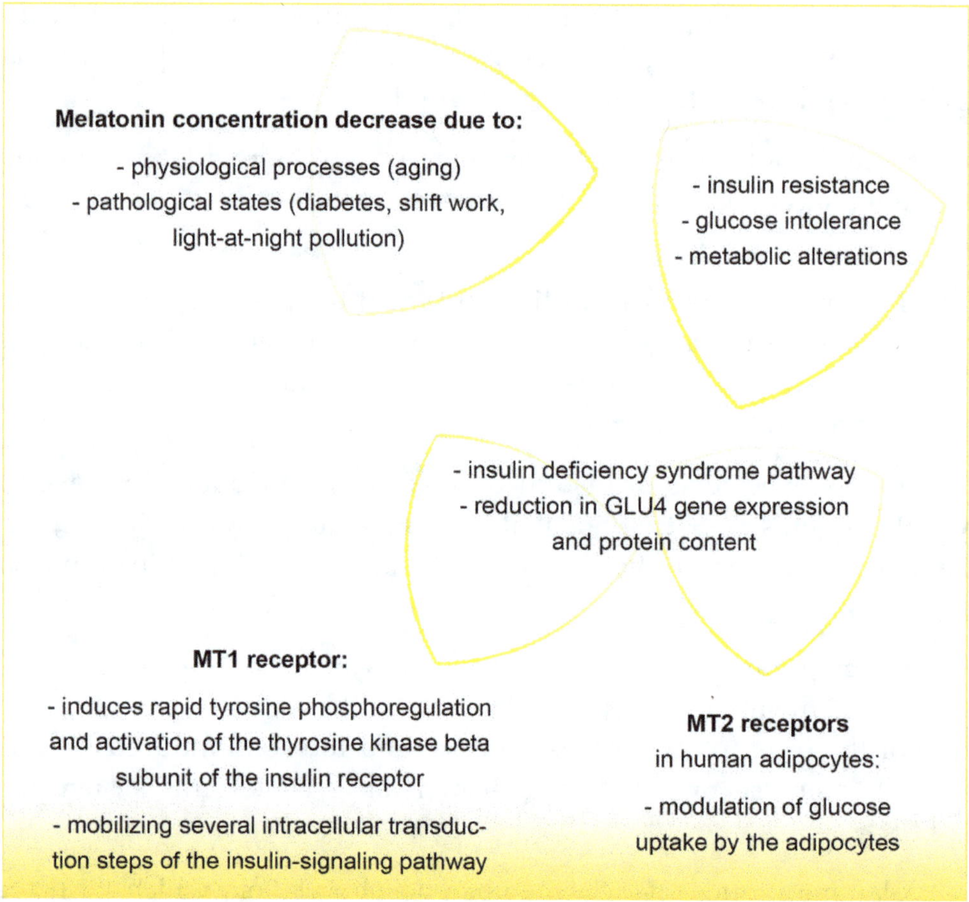

Figure 4. Melatonin depletion induced pathological consequences.

As an addition to the importance of melatonin on the regulatory processes in energy metabolism, it was recently demonstrated that the intrauterine metabolic programming is completely disturbed by the deficiency of melatonin in the pregnant mother. The adult child of a melatonin unpaired mother presents glucose intolerance, insulin resistance and a serious delay in the glucose-induced insulin secretion by isolated pancreatic islets [6, 13, 14].

This in once more a clear evidence that melatonin has a crucial role in the metabolic epigenetic regulation of a healthy organism that undergoes vicious trials and environmental demands that are, to a certain extent, meant to test the physiological robustness.

Robustness is one of the fundamental organizational principles of biological systems, this being the major characteristic involved in their adaptation, survival and reproduction. Metabolic diseases are considered a breakdown in the robustness in biological systems, the continuous maintenance of physiological functions being of extreme importance, despite external and internal disturbances [4].

Melatonin is a powerful chronobiotic, regulating the daily metabolic processes so that the activity/feeding phase of the day is assimilated with high insulin sensitivity, and the rest/fasting is synchronized to the insulin-resistant metabolic phase of the day. Melatonin is the key mediator molecule for the nictemeral integration of physiological and behavioral processes and for the modulation of energy balance and body weight regulation, all crucial for a healthy life [6].

The hypothalamus controls a great variety of physiological processes, including sleep/wake cycles, sexual behavior and reproduction, and metabolic control such as thermoregulation, glucose metabolism, lipid metabolism, energy intake/expenditure, and food and water intake, all these functions following circadian rhythms.

The hypothalamus identifies nutrients such as glucose and lipids, and via a specialized area of the blood brain barrier in the arcuate nucleus it also detects circulating metabolic hormones such as leptin, insulin, thyroid hormone, adiponectin and ghrelin. Researchers showed that SCN lesions abolished the daily rhythms in plasma concentrations of glucose and insulin and revealed the existence of a pronounced day/night difference in the response to 2-deoxy glucose, a glucose-utilization inhibitor, proving that the SCN is involved in the daily rhythm of glucose metabolism. SCN-lesioned rats do not have a rhythm in food intake either, so it should not be excluded an indirect effect of the lack of a feeding rhythm on glucose metabolism [11].

The chronobiotic nature of energy balance and energy metabolism is depicted by the two separated phases that exist during a 24 h period. The first one is characterized by energy harvesting and eating that results in energy intake, utilization, and storage, a period associated with high central and peripheral sensitivity to insulin and high glucose tolerance, elevated insulin secretion, high glucose uptake by the insulin-sensitive tissues, glycogen synthesis and hepatic and muscular glycolysis, blockade of hepatic gluconeogenesis, and increased adipose tissue lipogenesis and adiponectin production.

In opposition, the second one, the rest/sleep phase of the day, is characterized by fasting periods that require the use of stored energy for maintaining the cellular homeostasis, exhibiting insulin resistance, accentuated hepatic gluconeogenesis and glycogenolysis, adipose tissue lipolysis, and leptin secretion [6].

Other hormones exerting modulatory effects on cellular metabolism, as glucocorticoids, growth hormone and catecholamines, present circadian rhythmic fluctuations in their secretion and activity. Melatonin, as an orchestrating factor in the circadian organization of the metabolic processes, prepares and modifies the central and peripheral metabolic tissues in order to respond to these hormones.

The antiobesogenic effect of melatonin is, in part, a result of its regulatory role on the balance of energy, acting mainly on the regulation of the energy mobilization from the stores and in energy expenditure. It was demonstrated that in healthy young animals, melatonin supplementation therapy reduces long-term body weight gain and the size of the visceral fat deposits, effects independent on the reduction in food intake. The same antiobesity protective effect of melatonin was seen in experiments of diet-induced obesity [6, 15, 16].

The adequate supplementation of melatonin lowers body weight and regulates body weight gain as well as the intra-abdominal visceral fat accumulation, as a result of the reestablishment of the circadian distribution of energy metabolism, the insulin signaling pathway reinstatement, the consequent disappearance of insulin resistance and glucose intolerance and, most importantly, the accentuation of the energy expenditure over the energy intake.

8. Conclusions

Melatonin is the key modulatory molecule responsible for the integration between the cyclic environment and the circadian distribution of physiological and behavioral processes, assuring a healthy metabolism and the optimization of energy balance and body weight regulation.

The circadian system may be a tractable target for decreasing the prevalence of metabolic disturbances. Melatonin acts by potentiating central and peripheral insulin action either due to regulation of GLUT4 expression or triggering the insulin-signaling pathway. Melatonin is responsible for maintaining an adequate energy balance mainly by regulating energy flow and the energy expenditure through the activation of brown adipose tissue. It also assures the metabolic processes respect the nictemeral physiology of the two major phases existent during 24 h, the activity/wakefulness/feeding state versus the rest/sleep/fasting phase.

The decline in melatonin synthesis, during physiological processes as aging, or pathology associated events as shift-work or illuminated environments during the night, induces insulin resistance, glucose intolerance, sleep disturbances and metabolic circadian disorganization, depicting a state of chronodisruption and metabolic imbalances, aggravating the general health state.

The present evidence that melatonin induces insulin secretion and can improve β-cell function certify melatonin supplementation as an accurate therapeutic approach for glucose homeostasis reestablishment. The available scientific proofs support the suggestion that melatonin replacement therapy, if adequately carried out, in terms of dose, formulation and time of the day of administration, might contribute to maintaining optimal blood glucose levels in diabetic patients and restore the chronobiotic order for achieving a more robust healthy state of the organism.

Acknowledgements

This study was partially funded by the University of Medicine and Pharmacy "Carol Davila," through the research project "Young Researchers" number 33886/11.11.2014.

Author details

Cristina Manuela Drăgoi[1], Andreea Letiţia Arsene[2], Cristina Elena Dinu-Pîrvu[3], Ion Bogdan Dumitrescu[4], Daniela Elena Popa[5], George T.A. Burcea-Dragomiroiu[5], Denisa Ioana Udeanu[6], Olivia Carmen Timnea[7], Bruno Ştefan Velescu[8] and Alina Crenguţa Nicolae[1*]

*Address all correspondence to: alinanicolae29@gmail.com

1 Department of Biochemistry, Faculty of Pharmacy, University of Medicine and Pharmacy "Carol Davila," Bucharest, Romania

2 Department of General and Pharmaceutical Microbiology, Faculty of Pharmacy, University of Medicine and Pharmacy "Carol Davila," Bucharest, Romania

3 Department of Physical and Colloidal Chemistry, Faculty of Pharmacy, University of Medicine and Pharmacy "Carol Davila," Bucharest, Romania

4 Department of Pharmaceutical Physics and Informatics, Faculty of Pharmacy, University of Medicine and Pharmacy "Carol Davila," Bucharest, Romania

5 Department of Drug Control, Faculty of Pharmacy, University of Medicine and Pharmacy "Carol Davila," Bucharest, Romania

6 Department of Clinical Laboratory and Food Safety, Faculty of Pharmacy, University of Medicine and Pharmacy "Carol Davila," Bucharest, Romania

7 Department of Medical Sciences, Faculty of Physical Education and Sports, Ecologic University of Bucharest, Romania

8 Department of Pharmacology and Clinical Pharmacy, Faculty of Pharmacy, University of Medicine and Pharmacy "Carol Davila", Bucharest, Romania

References

[1] Johnston J.D., Skene D.J. Regulation of mammalian neuroendocrine physiology and rhy thms by melatonin. Journal of Endocrinology. 2015;JOE-15-0119. doi:10.1530/JOE-15-0119

[2] Hardeland R. Neurobiology, pathophysiology, and treatment of melatonin deficiency and dysfunction. The Scientific World Journal. 2012;640389. doi:10.1100/2012/640389

[3] Drăgoi C.M. Tryptophan, serotonin, melatonin-the spectacular triad: physiological, pathological and therapeutic implications of some bio-compounds with indolic structure. LAP Lambert Academic Publishing, Germany; 2013.

[4] Espino J., Pariente A.J., Rodríguez A.B. Role of melatonin on diabetes-related metabolic disorders. World Journal of Diabetes. 2011 June 15;2(6):82–91. doi:10.4239/wjd.v2.i6.82

[5] Dominguez-Rodriguez A., Abreu-Gonzalez P., Sanchez-Sanchez J.J., Kaski J.C., Reiter R.J. Melatonin and circadian biology in human cardiovascular disease. Journal of Pineal Research. 2010;49:14–22. doi:10.1111/j.1600-079X.2010.00773.x

[6] Cipolla-Neto J., Amaral F.G., Afeche S.C., Tan D.X., Reiter R.J. Melatonin, energy metabolism, and obesity: a review. Journal of Pineal Research. 2014;56:371–381. doi:10.1111/jpi.12137

[7] Drăgoi C.M. Biochemical mechanisms of action of some bio-compounds with indolic structure [thesis]. Bucharest; 2012.

[8] Nduhirabandi F., du Toit E., Lochner A. Melatonin and the metabolic syndrome: a tool for effective therapy in obesity-associated abnormalities? Acta Physiologica. Forthcoming. doi:10.1111/j.1748-1716.2012.02410.x

[9] Cardinali D.P., Hardeland R. Inflammaging, metabolic syndrome and melatonin: a call for treatment studies. Neuroendocrinology. Forthcoming. doi:10.1159/000446543

[10] Kalsbeek A., la Fleur S., Fliers E. Circadian control of glucose metabolism. Molecular Metabolism. 2014;3(4):372–383.

[11] Peschke E., Bähr I., Mühlbauer E. Melatonin and pancreatic islets: interrelationships between melatonin, insulin and glucagon. International Journal of Molecular Sciences. 2013;14(4):6981–7015. doi:10.3390/ijms14046981

[12] Owino S., Contreras-Alcantara S., Baba K., Tosini G. Melatonin signaling controls the daily rhythm in blood glucose levels independent of peripheral clocks. PLos One. 2016;11(1). doi:10.1371/journal.pone.0148214

[13] Sharma S., Singh H., Ahmad N., Mishra P., Tiwari A. The role of melatonin in diabetes: therapeutic implications. Archives of Endocrinology and Metabolism. 2015;59(5). doi:10.1590/2359-3997000000098

[14] Nicolae A.C., Drăgoi C.M., Ceaușu I., Poalelungi C., Iliescu D., Arsene A.L. Clinical implications of the indolergic system and oxidative stress in physiological gestational homeostasis. Farmacia. 2015;63(1):46–51.

[15] Drăgoi C.M., Nicolae A.C., Grigore C., Dinu-Pîrvu C., Arsene A.L. Characteristics of glucose homeostasis and lipidic profile in a hamster metabolic syndrome model, after the co-administration of melatonin and irbesartan in a multiparticulate pharmaceutical formation. In: March; Bucharest. Book of abstracts: ASRMN; 2016. p. 25.

[16] Suzana E.V., Diana L.D., Adrian E.R., Vlad Z., Diana M.C., Andreea L.A., Cristina M.D., Alina C.N., Leon Z., Torsten S., Ana-Maria Z. Behavioral and molecular effects of prenatal continuous light exposure in the adult rat. Brain Research. 2016;1650:51–59.

3

Measurement of Plasma Tryptophan Metabolites: Clinical and Experimental Application for Depression and Stress States Assessment

Akikazu Takada, Fumiko Shimizu and
Junichi Masuda

Abstract

There are three pathways in tryptophan (TRP) metabolism. Serotonin (5-hydroxytryptamine; 5-HT) pathway is important in mood, anxiety, memory, and cognition and is impaired in depression. Kynurenine (KYN) pathways are involved in immunity, inflammation, muscles movement, and mental health. We investigated changes in TRP metabolites in plasmas of stressed rats and in depressive patients. TRP metabolite levels in 5-HT and KYN pathways in various brain areas and plasma were increased soon after electric foot shock given to rats but returned to normal 24 h later. Plasma levels of 5-HT were very low or undetectable in patients of monopolar depression. 5-hydroxyindole acetic acid (5-HIAA)/TRP ratios or KYN/TRP ratios were not different between healthy controls and depressive patients, indicating 5-HT quickly being degraded into 5-HIAA in patients of depression but KYN levels were not changed in depression. These results indicate that TRP metabolism changes upon stress application and in patients of depression.

Keywords: tryptophan, serotonin, 5-hydroxyindole acetic acid, kynurenine, 3-hydroxykynurenine, kynurenic acid

1. Introduction

Tryptophan (TRP) is one of the essential amino acids, which must be taken as food. It is not only needed for protein synthesis but serves as a substrate for bioactive component with important physiological roles.

There are three pathways in TRP metabolism: serotonin (5-HT), kynurenine (KYN), and indole-3-acetic acid pathways.

Since 5-HT is known as an important neurotransmitter and derived from TRP, many people know about TRP to some extent. 5-HT is really involved in the adaptive responses in the central nervous system and considered to be related to mood, anxiety, or cognition [1].

5-HT is further converted in the pineal body and the retina to N-acetyl serotonin (NAS) and melatonin which controls circadian rhythm [2].

In mammals, most of the free TRP is converted to KYN and generates metabolites involved in inflammatory, immune, responses, and neurotransmission [3].

We have recently succeeded in simultaneous measurements of almost all TRP metabolites including melatonin by using an ultrahigh speed liquid chrom`atography and mass spectrometry (LC-MS) [4], which is the first time in the world.

In this chapter, we report about the precise methodology of the simultaneous measurements and some results obtained from stressed rats and depressive patients.

1.1. Measurements of TRP metabolites using LC-MS

1.1.1. Background

Since 5-HT and its derivatives have the strong fluorescence, high-sensitive analyses of some TRP metabolites can be performed by liquid chromatography with fluorescence detection. However, it is very limited to analyze the total metabolites including kynurenine by photometric detection although kynurenic acid (KYNA) can be detected as zinc chelate compound under zinc acetate solution.

In the past years, liquid chromatograph mass spectrometry (LC-MS) has been widely spread in many areas including clinical and biological analyses. Since LC-MS with electrospray ionization (ESI) is suitable for determination of metabolites of TRP, LC-MS is expected as a powerful tool for this type of analysis.

In addition, the tandem mass spectrometer also has widely used in recent years with its high sensitivity and selectivity.

There are several researches for the simultaneous analyses of TRP metabolites using LC-MS or LC-MS/MS methods for clinical samples such as human serum and plasma [5, 6]. In general, isotope-labeled internal standards are used in LC-MS/MS analysis to improve the accuracy, although isotope-labeled regents are expensive and limited availability [7, 8]. Even though less accurate, acceptable results can be obtained without internal standards for the screening purposes. In this chapter, the simultaneous determination of TRP metabolites in human plasma by LC-MS/MS technique combined with simple pretreatment procedure is described.

1.1.2. Regents and instrumentation

The simultaneous analytical method was developed for major metabolites of TRP including melatonin.

The targets are 17 of major metabolites, tryptophan (TRP), L-5-hydroxytryptophan (5-HTP), serotonin (5-HT), kynurenine (KYN), 5-hydroxy-tryptophol, tryptophol, 5-hydroxyindoleacetic acid (5-HIAA), indole-3-acetic acid, anthranilic acid (AA), kynurenic acid (KYNA), quinaldic acid, 3-indolebutyric acid, 3-hydroxykynurenine (3-HKYN), 3-hydroxyanthranilic acid (3-HAA), xanthurenic acid (XA), melatonin, and quinolinic acid (QA). Each compound is commercially available from major chemical regent manufacturers, such as Fujifilm-Wako chemical (Osaka, Japan) and Sigma-Aldrich (St. Louis, MO, USA).

Analysis was performed by a liquid chromatograph tandem mass spectrometer, the LCMS-8060 mass spectrometer equipped with Nexera X2 liquid chromatograph system (Shimadzu Corporation, Kyoto, Japan).

The targets are separated by reversed phase mode using ODS analytical column, L-Columns ODS (2.1 mm x 150 mm, CERI, Tokyo, Japan) with a gradient elution. Mobile phases were 0.1% formic acid solution and acetonitrile with 5% concentration of acetonitrile to 3 min, then 5–95% in 6 min followed by 5% in 3 min (12 min analytical cycle) at total flow rate of 0.4 mL/min. The

			Qualification (m/z)		Qualification (m/z)	
Compound	**Molecular weight**	**Monoisotopic mass**	**Precursorion**	**Production**	**Precursorion**	**Production**
DL-Trypotophan	204.225	204.090	205.10	188.10	205.10	146.10
L-5-Hydroxytrypotophan	220.225	220.085	221.10	204.05	221.10	162.00
Serotonin	176.215	176.095	177.10	160.10	177.10	115.05
L-Kynurenine	208.214	208.085	209.10	192.00	209.10	94.05
5-Hydroxytrypotophol	177.200	177.079	178.10	160.10	178.10	115.05
Trypotophol	161.200	161.084	162.10	144.05	162.10	117.10
5-Hydroxyindole -3-acetic acid	190.176	190.051	192.10	146.05	192.10	110.00
Indole-3-acetic acid	175.184	175.063	176.10	130.05	176.10	77.05
Anthranilic acid	136.129	136.040	138.10	120.05	138.10	65.05
Kynurenic acid	189.167	189.043	190.10	144.05	190.10	89.10
Quinaldic acid	172.161	172.040	174.10	128.05	174.10	156.05
Indole-3-acetic acid	202.230	202.087	204.10	186.10	204.10	130.10
3-Hydroxykynurenine	224.213	224.080	225.15	208.20	225.15	162.15
Hydroxyanthranilic acid	152.128	152.035	154.15	136.20	154.15	80.15
Xanthurenic acid	205.167	205.038	206.15	160.20	206.15	132.20
Melatonin	232.279	232.121	232.20	174.10	232.20	130.05
Quinolinic acid	167.120	167.022	168.00	78.10	168.00	150.00

Table 1. MRM transition.

temperature of the column was 40°C. For LC-MS, electrospray ionization (ESI) was used with multi-reaction monitoring (MRM) mode.

Flow rate of the neutralizer and the drying gas were 2 L/min and 10 mL/min, respectively. The temperature of desolvation line (heated capitally tube) was 250°C. ESI interface was used at 400°C with 10 L/min of heating gas flow. Each MRM transition was optimized using each standard solution. Optimized results are shown in **Table 1**.

All mother solution of 1 mg/mL had been stocked under −80°C and standard samples for calibration curve were prepared before use as mixture solution by consideration of each range of measurement concentration.

1.1.3. Analysis of human plasma

Aliquot of 50 μL human plasma was used for each sample analysis. The procedure including deproteinization is shown in **Figure 1**. The typical chromatograms of 17 major metabolites are shown in **Figure 2** as standard solution and in **Figure 3** as human plasma sample. These chromatograms demonstrate the usefulness of the developed method for simultaneous analysis of TRP metabolites.

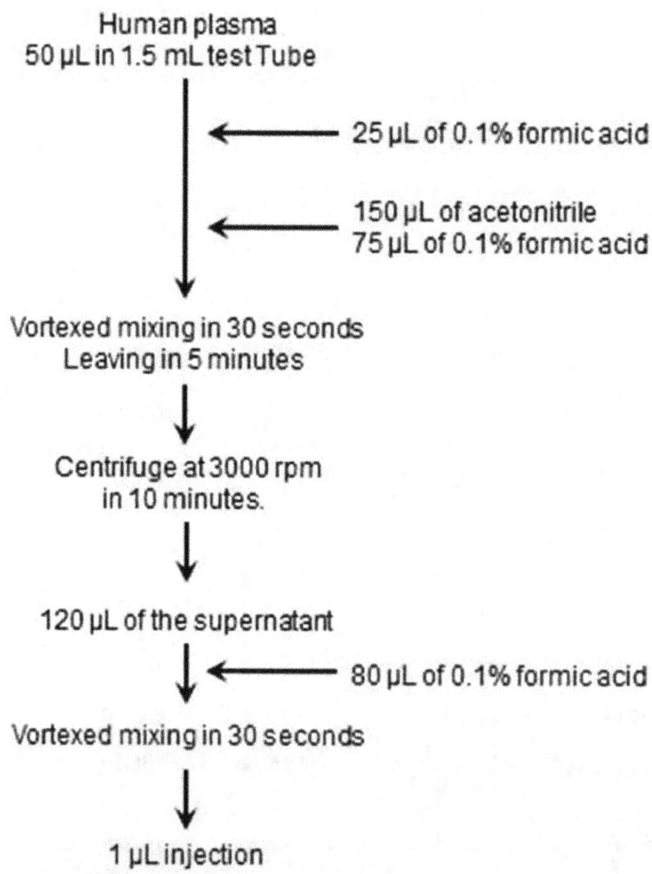

Figure 1. The procedure of deproteinization.

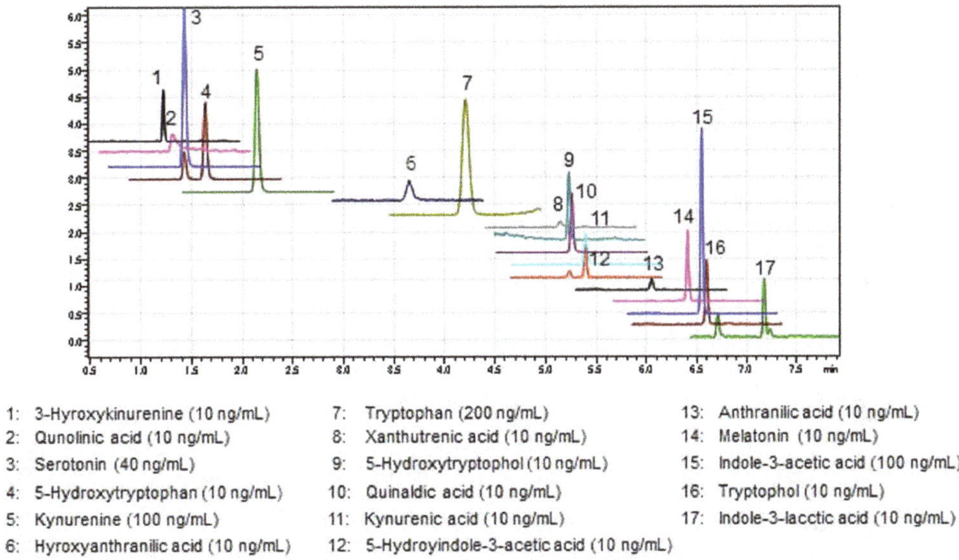

Figure 2. Chromatograms of 17 major metabolites of tryptophan.

1.2. Stress and TRP metabolism

Stress influences many functions related to mental and body health. We have shown that the application of electric shock increased plasma and brain TRP, 5-HT, and 5-HIAA levels [9, 10] and changed nicotine-induced release of 5-HT or dopamine in rats [11–14]. We also examined changes in serotonergic and kynurenic pathways in rats exposed to foot shock [15].

Stress induces a number of changes in the central system of neurotransmitters, particularly noradrenaline and 5-HT [16, 17].

A pathologic overabundance of endogenous excitotoxin, quinolinic acid, or hypofunction of KYNA has been hypothetically linked to the occurrence of seizures and nerve cell death [18, 19].

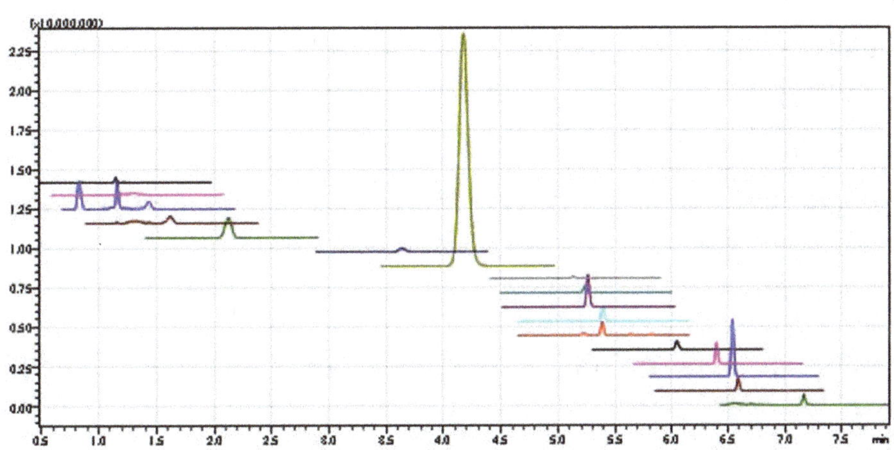

Figure 3. Chromatogram of human plasma sample.

1.2.1. Stress and TRP metabolites in the brain

Animals: Male Wistar rats (9 weeks old) were fed with standard laboratory foods and tap water *ad libitum*. Two weeks later, rats were randomly divided into two groups. One group received foot shock, which was given as a series of 10-s shock (o.19 mA) followed by 50 s intervals during a 60-min period. CT 110 cycle timer and NS-SG01 shock generator scrambler (Neuroscience Inc., Tokyo, Japan) were used. Samples of 10 rats were taken immediately after the foot shock and samples of another 10 rats were taken 24 h after the shock. Ten rats were used as controls.

Blood: Rats were anesthetized with pentobarbital, and blood was taken by heart puncture and put into a tube containing 3/13% sodium citrate. Plasma was obtained by centrifugation at 3000 rpm for 20 min.

Brain sampling: The brains were removed and chilled on ice. Eight regions (cerebellum, medulla, hypothalamus, striatum, midbrain, hippocampus, cortex, and frontal cortex) were dissected and samples were immediately frozen. Frozen brain samples were homogenized in 0.15 N perchloric acid containing 0.025% EDTA (pH 3.0). The samples were centrifuged at 14,000 rpm for 20 min at 4°C. After centrifugation, the supernatant was filtered (0.45 μm Millipore filter) and stored at −80°C until assayed.

Figure 4 shows TRP pathway and its metabolites.

Figure 5 shows that 5-HT levels increased significantly at hypothalamus and midbrain soon after the shock but returned normal 24 h later.

5-HT levels were not increased in cerebellum, medulla, striatum, hippocampus, cortex, and frontal cortex.

Figure 6 shows 5-HIAA levels of various brain areas after foot shock.

5-HIAA levels significantly increased in all the brain areas except striatum but returned normal 24 h later.

Figure 7 shows KYN levels in various brain areas after foot shock.

KYN levels significantly increased in all the brain areas after foot shock but returned to normal 24 h later.

Figure 8 shows plasma levels of TRP, 5-HT and 5-HIAA after foot shock.

Plasma levels of TRP, 5-HT, and 5-HIAA significantly increased after foot shock but returned to normal 24 h later.

Figure 9 shows plasma levels of KYN,3-HKYN, and KYNA after foot shock.

Plasma levels of KYN, 3-HKYN, and KYNA increased significantly after foot shock but returned to normal 24 h later.

1.3. TRP metabolites in plasma of patients of depression

We asked male and female acquaintances older than 50 years old and male and female college students to participate in the experiments. We checked their health carefully and

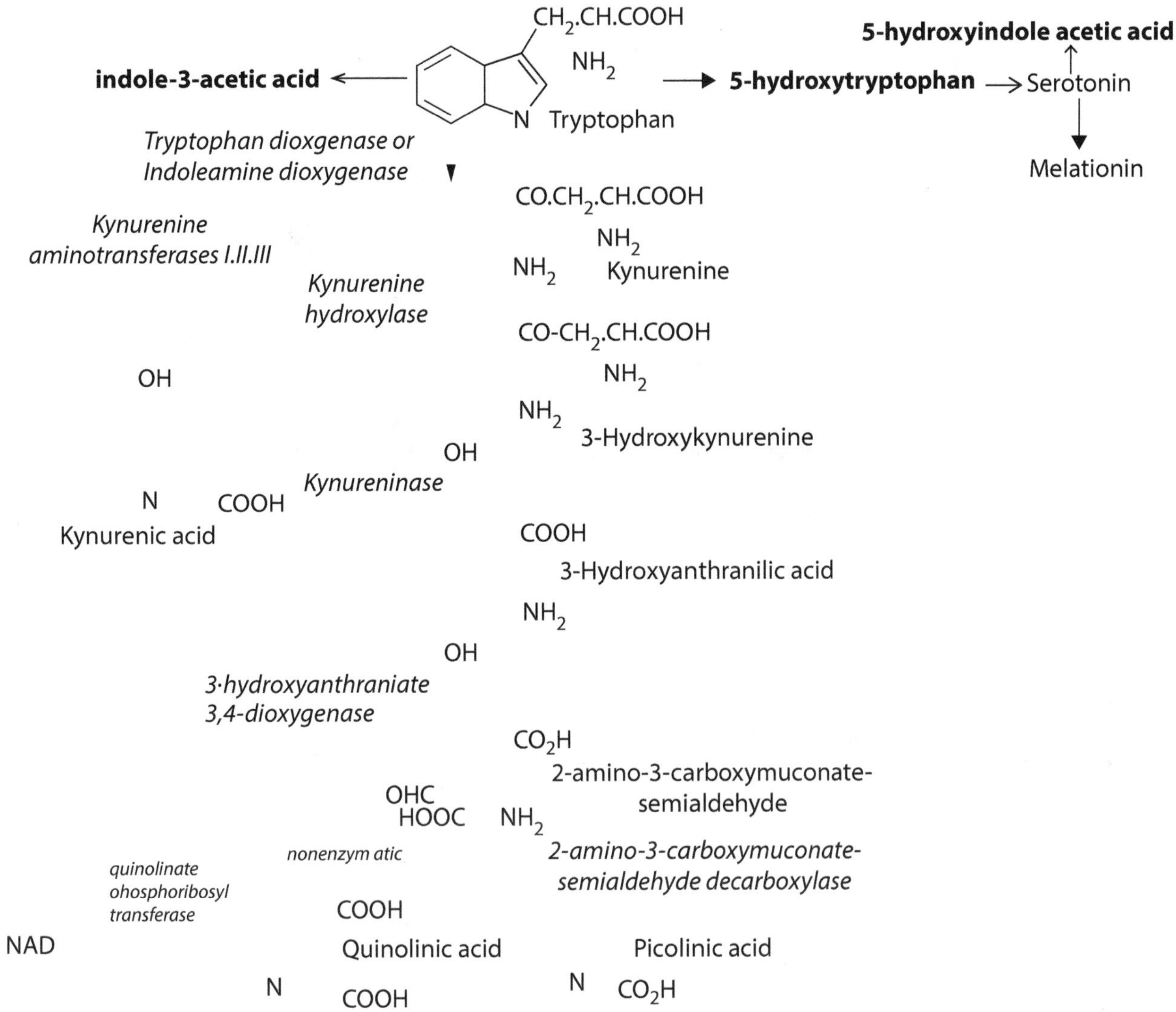

Figure 4. TRP pathways.

recruited them if there were no health problems such as diabetes, hypertension, or no serious diseases experienced in the past. They did not smoke in the past. We also excluded people who took drugs for dyslipidemia, hyperglycemia, or hypertension. We collected blood samples early morning. Participants were asked not to eat anything after 21.00 PM the previous evening. Plasma specimens were collected for assays of blood parameters. We obtained an informed consent prior to conducting the protocol which had been approved by the Ethical Committee of Showa Women's University and Yokohama North Hospital of Showa University.

Patients were diagnosed to be monopolar depression at the psychiatry clinic of Yokohama North Hospital of Showa University. The Zung Self-Rating Depression Scale [20] was used, which is a short self-administered survey to quantify the depressed status of a patient. There are 20 items on the scale that rate the affective, psychological, and somatic symptoms associated with depression. We took blood from five male patients (26, 30, 45, 47, and 56 years old) and four female patients (23, 25, 41, and 60 years old).

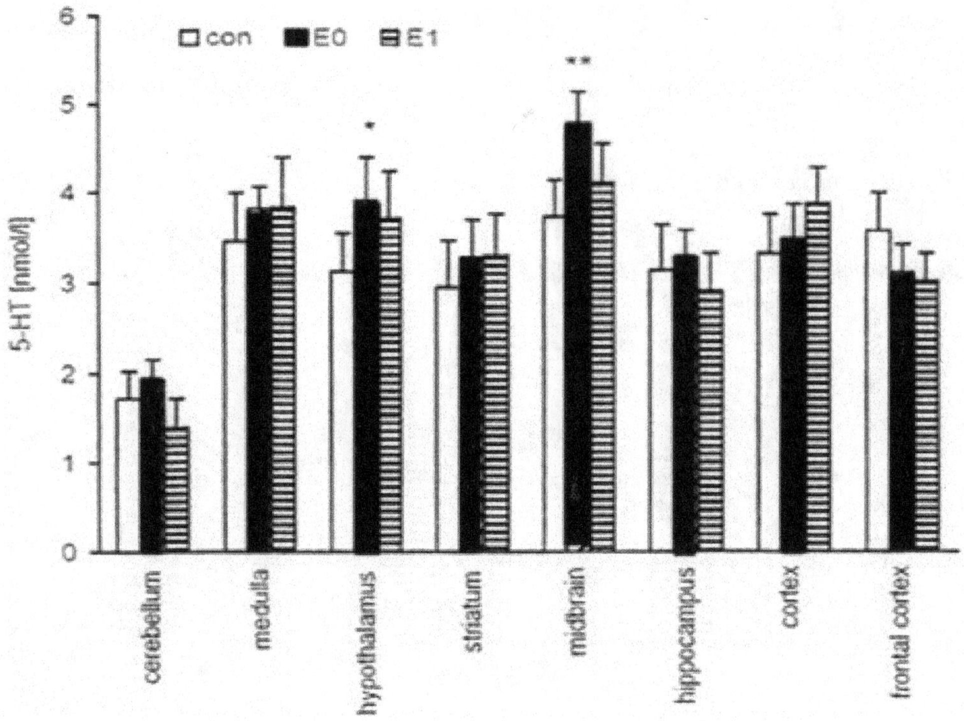

Figure 5. Serotonin (5-HT) levels in various brain areas after electric foot shock. con, control; E0, soon after the shock; E1, 24 h after the shock. $^{*}p < 0.05$ and $^{**}p < 0.01$.

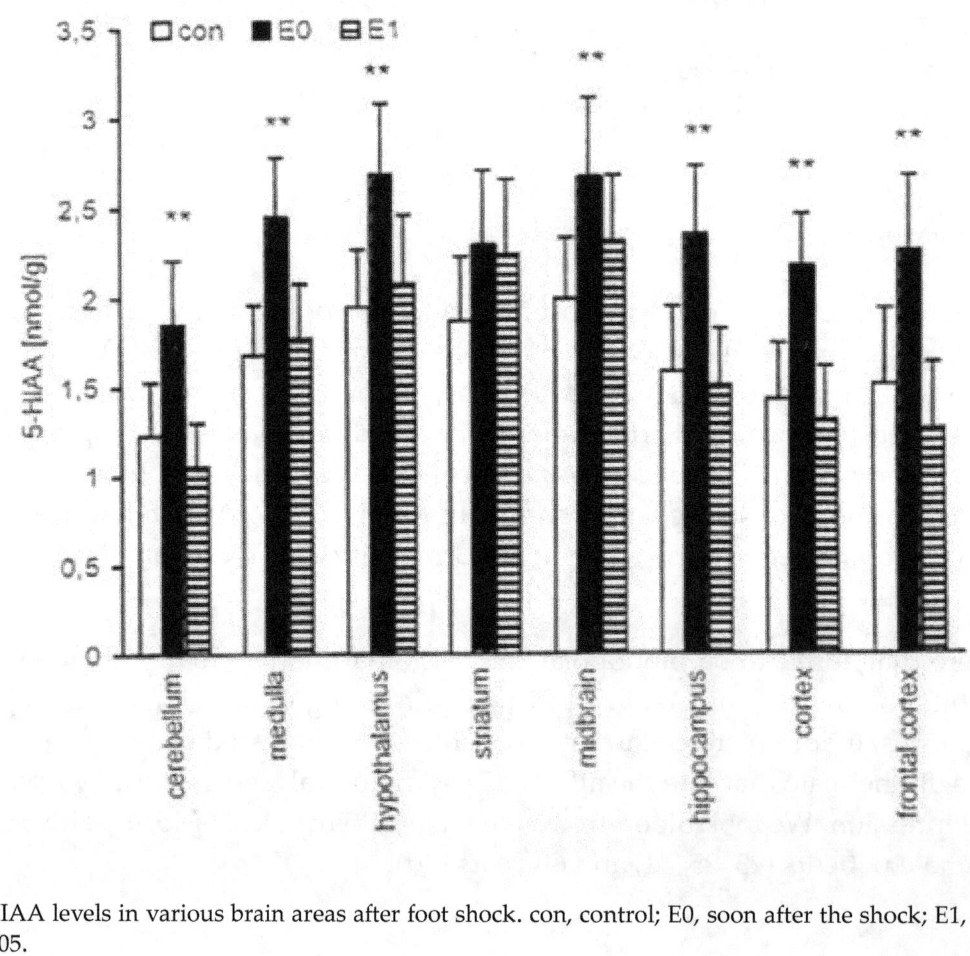

Figure 6. 5-HIAA levels in various brain areas after foot shock. con, control; E0, soon after the shock; E1, 24 h after the shock. $^{*}p < 0.05$.

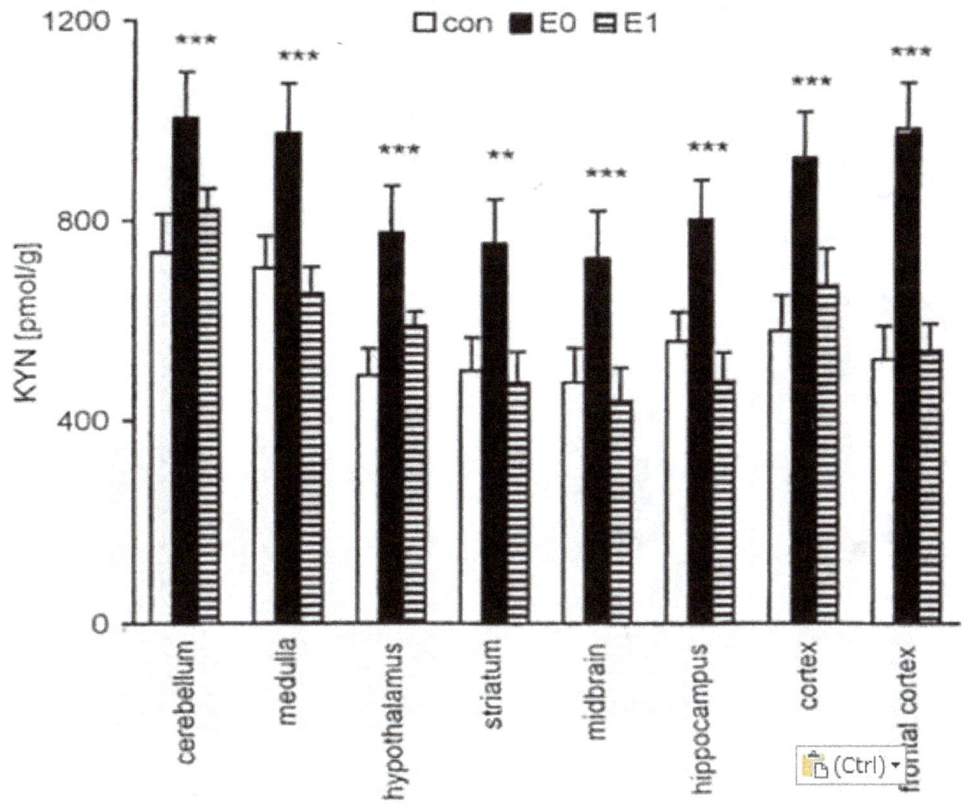

Figure 7. Kynurenine levels in various brain areas after foot shock. con, control; E0, soon after the shock; E1, 24 h after the shock. **p < 0.01 and ***p < 0.001.

5-HT was detected only in plasma of two patients. Both of them were young females. A 60-year-old woman took Jay Zoloft 25 mg and ethyl loflazepate 1 mg, and another 41-year-old woman took Cymbalta 20 mg and Luran 3 mg. 5-HT was not detected in plasmas of these women.

The number of healthy old men and young women were 20, and the number of depressive patients were 9.

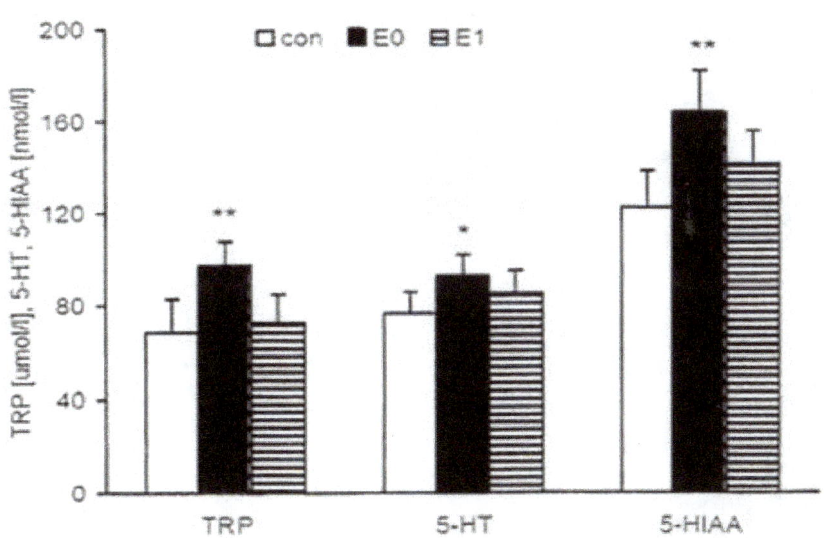

Figure 8. Plasma levels of TRP, 5-HT, and 5-HIAA after electric foot shock. con, control; E0, soon after the shock; E1, 24 h after the shock. *p < 0.05 and **p < 0.01.

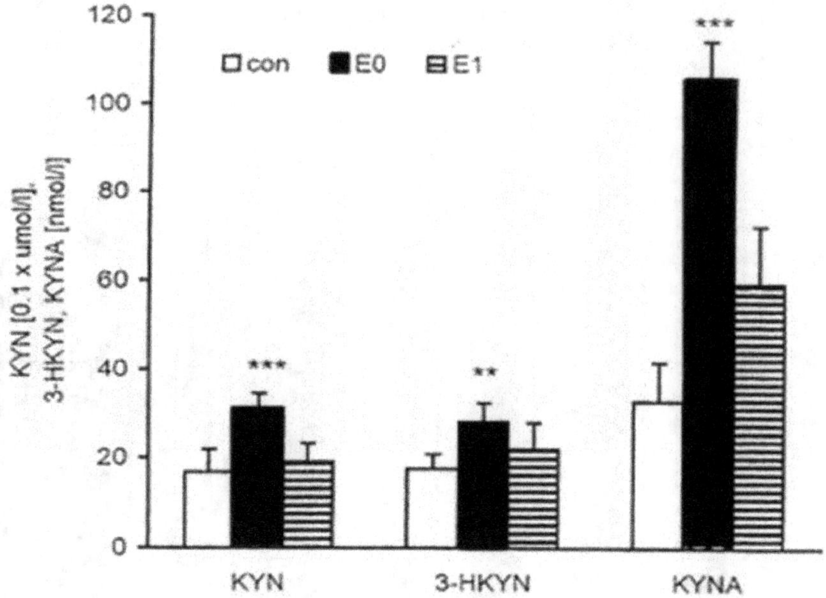

Figure 9. Plasma levels of KYN (kynurenine), 3-HKYN (3-hydroxykynurenine), and KYNA (kynurenic acid). con, control; E0, soon after the shock; E1, 24 h after the shock. $^{**}p < 0.01$ and $^{***}p < 0.001$.

	Young men (n = 20)	Young women (n = 20)	Old men (n = 20)
Age	20.7 ± 1.5	21.2 ± 0.7	60.8 ± 9.9
Height (m)	1.72 ± 0.06	1.58 ± 0.05	1.69 ± 0.07
Weight (kg)	65.1 ± 8.9	51.4 ± 5.8	71.1 ± 13.1
BMI	22.1 ± 3.1	20.4 ± 1.6	24.9 ± 3.7

Table 2. Basic backgrounds of healthy participants.

Patients	Sex	Serotonin detection	Visit (age)	Medication
H1	Male	–	45	None
H2	Male	–	47	None
H3	Female	–	60	Jay Zoloft 25 mg, ethyl loflazepate1 mg
H4	Female	+	23	None
H5	Female	+	25	None
H6	Male	–	30	None
H7	Female	–	41	Cymbalta 20 mg, Luran 3 mg
H8	Male	–	56	None
H9	Male	–	26	None

Table 3. Various parameters of patients.

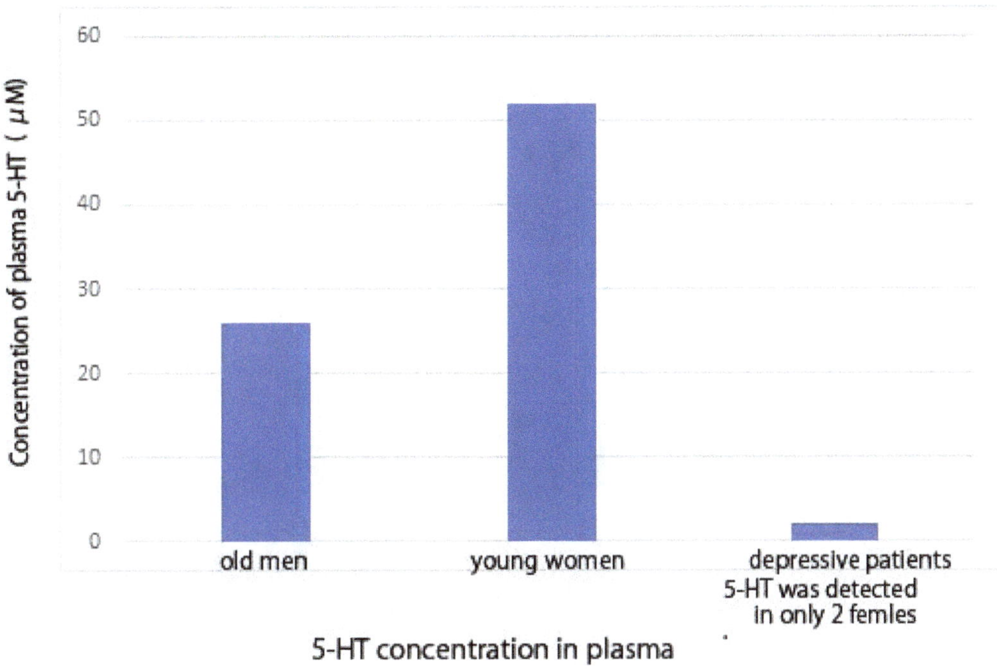

Figure 10. 5-HT levels in plasmas of depressive patients and controls.

Tables 2 and **3** show the background data of these patients.

Figure 10 shows plasma levels of 5-HT of healthy young women, old men and depressive patients.

Plasma levels of 5-HT in depressive patients were very low compared to those of old men and young women. 5-HT was detected in plasmas of only two young females.

Figure 11 shows 5-HT/TRP and 5-HIAA/TRP ratios.

Although 5-HT/TRP ratio of depressive patients was low compared to that of old men and young women, 5-HIAA/TRP ratio was almost the same as that of old men and young women.

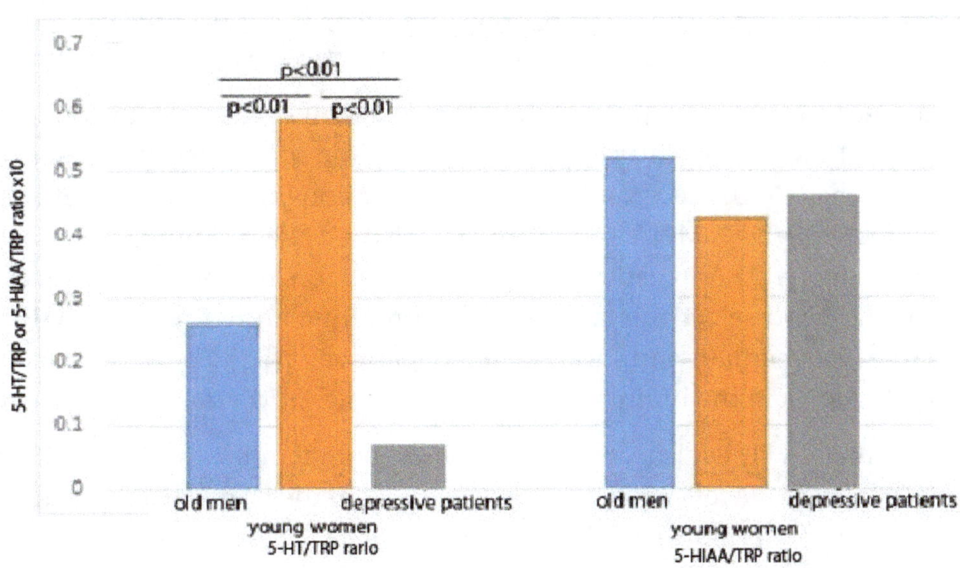

Figure 11. 5-HT or 5-HIAA/TRP ratio.

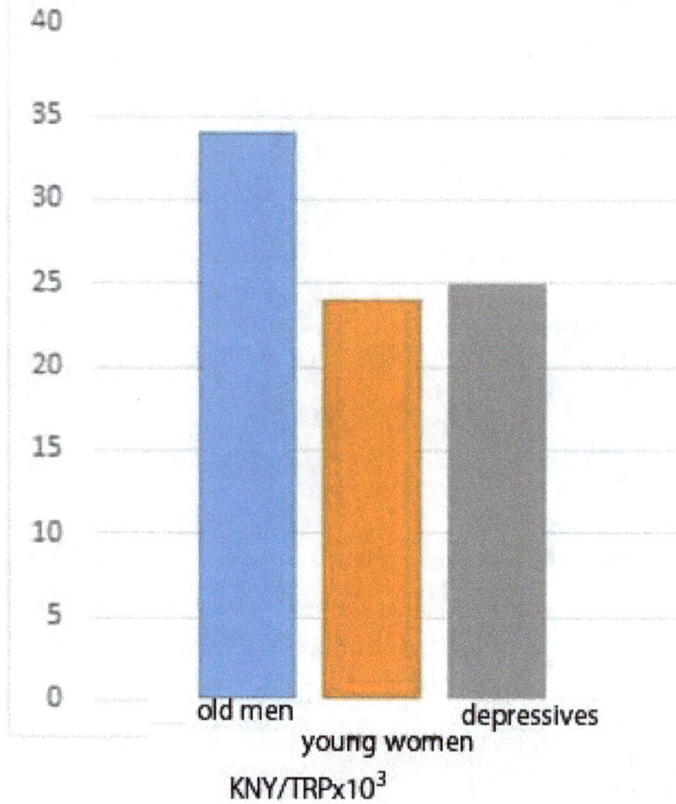

Figure 12. KYN/TRP ratio.

Figure 12 shows that there were no differences in KYN/TRP ratios between that of old men, young women, and depressive patients.

2. Discussion

As stated above, most of the metabolites of KYN pathway are found in the brain [1, 21–23]. Some metabolites of KYN pathway are neurotoxic and some are neuroprotective.

KYNA is an endogenous neuroprotective agent that is usually present in the brain at nanomolar concentration [24]. KYNA is an antagonist to quinolinic acid (QA) and acts on the glycine modulatory site of the NMDA receptor at low concentration [22] and at higher concentration at the glutamate site of the NMDA receptors and also on the a-amino3-hydroxy-5-methyl-4-isoxazolepropionate (AMPA) receptors [25]. It also antagonizes the alpha 7 nicotinic acetylcholine receptors [26] and selectively activates a G-protein-coupled receptor, GPR35–48 [27]. Many neuroactive intermediates are shown in KYN pathways [28]. So, we decided to measure some of TRP metabolites in the brain and plasma in the stressed rats.

Our results show that 5-HT levels increased only in hypothalamus and midbrain, but its degradation product, 5-HIAA levels, increased in every part of the brain. These results may imply that 5-HT is quickly converted to 5-HIAA soon after shock, so that 5-HT levels apparently did not increase after shock. This finding is important in the explanation of plasma 5-HT and 5-HIAA levels in patients of depression.

Some of TRP metabolites were shown to be neuroexcitatory and convulsive, thus toxic [29]. One of such neuroexcitatory factors in KYN pathway is 3-HKYN [24]. Its synthesis is catalyzed by kynurenine 3-hydroxylase. Although data of brain analyses were not shown here, 3-HKYN levels increased in all the brain areas and plasma (**Figure 6**).

3-HKYN is said to be the most toxic substance in TRP metabolism [30]. So stress induces disturbances in the central nervous system by increasing levels of 3-HKYN (**Figures 4–9**).

KYN is usually hydroxylated to 3-HKYN and then further converted to 3-hydroxyanthranilic acid (3-HAA). 3-HAA is rapidly converted to QN by the non-enzymatic reaction and further to NAD^+.

The other pathway of KYN, the production of KYNA and xanthurenic acid (XA), is minor under normal conditions. KYNA is an endogenous antagonist of excitatory amino acid receptors and may serve as a modulator of excitatory nerve transmission. This study may suggest that stress induces the indirect modulation of excitatory amino acids in the central nervous system by increasing KYNA.

KYNA has an antagonist activity of the three ionotropic excitatory amino acid receptors [22, 31]. At low concentrations, KYNA blocks the glycine co-agonist site of N-methyl-D-aspartate receptor and may serve to prevent the overactivation of glutamic acid receptor. When brain kynurenic acid levels were increased experimentally, neuroprotection and seizure reduction have been reported [32].

The roles of various metabolites of KYN pathway are reviewed [28], so we do not discuss these roles in detail.

As to relationships between serotonin levels and depression, we analyzed plasma levels of TRP metabolites in patients of depression.

Although the concentration of 5-HT has been considered to be low in depressive patients [33], 5-HT concentration in the brains of suicide victims was not low [34]. Therefore, it is not known if 5-HT concentration is decreased in the brains of depressive patients (**Table 2**).

We decided to measure TRP metabolites in patients of monopolar depression. **Table 3** shows five male patients participated in the experiments. The age is 44–61 years old (41.2 ± 11.3). Plasma serotonin levels were detected only in two young female patients. We could not measure 5-HT in plasma in seven persons, which is shown in **Figure 10**.

Although plasma serotonin levels and 5-HT/TRP ratio were low in depressive patients, the levels of 5-HIAA/TRP were not lower in depressive patients. This result indicates that 5-HT is degraded to 5-HIAA in depressive patients almost to the same extent to healthy old and young women (**Figures 11** and **12**).

We measured the levels of KYN in healthy old men and young women and depressive patients. TRP seems to be degraded to KYN pathways to the same extent in these three groups.

These results suggest that in depressive patients 5-HT was quickly degraded to 5-HIAA, and this seems to be a reason of low 5-HT levels in depressive patients.

As to a relationship between serotonin pathway and KYN pathway, Lapin IP suggested that in depression tryptophan 2,3-dioxygenase in the liver shunted metabolism of serotonin away from 5-HT production to KYN production, resulting in serotonin deficiency [35]. KYN,

QN, and 3-HKYN were shown to be anxiogenic and KYNA were anxiolytic [36]. From these results, he tried to explain the effects of antidepressive drugs.

Our results do not support this hypothesis. Metabolites of KYN pathways were not high in depressive patients.

There have not been enough studies as to 5-HT levels in the brain of patients of bipolar depression. Serotonin levels in cerebrospinal fluids of patients of bipolar depression were shown to be high [37] or normal [38]. So it seems to be very important to discriminate monopolar and bipolar depression to study roles of serotonin in the pathogenesis of disease.

Our results show that plasma 5-HT levels were low and metabolites of KYN pathway were not changed in patients of monopolar depression.

3. Statistics

Standard ANOVA methodology was used and $p < 0.05$ was considered as significant difference. Results are expressed as mean ± SD. Bars of figures represent standard deviations.

4. Ethics

This work has been approved by the Ethical committees of Showa Women's University, Showa University School of Medicine, and NPO "International projects on food and health" and has been carried out in accordance with The Code of Ethics of the World Medical Association (Declaration of Helsinki) for experiments.

Acknowledgements

Experiments were designed and performed by all of the authors. AT wrote the manuscript. Statistical analyses were done by FS. All authors read the manuscript and approve the final manuscript. All the authors had responsibilities for a final content. A part of the work was reported in Japanese (http://www5c.biglobe.ne.jp/~takada-a/protein%20and%20brain.pdf).

Author details

Akikazu Takada[1]*, Fumiko Shimizu[2] and Junichi Masuda[3]

*Address all correspondence to: takadaa@mwd.biglobe.ne.jp

1 International Projects on Food and Health (NPO), Tokyo, Japan

2 Faculty of Life and Environmental Sciences, Showa Women's University, Tokyo, Japan

3 Global Application Development Center, Shimadzu Corporation, Kanagawa-ken, Japan

References

[1] Canli T, Lesch KP. Long story short: The serotonin transporter in emotion regulation and social cognition. Nature Neuroscience. 2007;**10**:1103-1109. DOI: 10.1038/nn1964pmid: 17726476

[2] Yates CA, Herbert J. Differential circadian rhythms in pineal and hypothalamic 5-HT induced by artificial photoperiods or melatonin. Nature. 1976;**262**:219-220. DOI: 10.1038/262219a0pmid:934338

[3] Stone TW, Stoy N. Darlington LG an expanding range of targets for kynurenine metabolites of tryptophan. Trends in Pharmacological Sciences. 2013;**34**:136-143. DOI: 10.1016/j.tips.2012.09.006pmid:23123095

[4] Matsuoka K, Kato K, Takao T, Ogawa M, Ishii Y, Shimizu F, Masuda J, Takada A. Concentrations of various tryptophan metabolites increase in patients of diabetes mellitus compared to healthy aged male adults. Diabetology International. 2016;**8**:69-72. DOI: 10.1007/s13340-016-0282-y

[5] Hervè E, Beyne E, Jamault H, Delacoux E. Determination of tryptophan and its kynurenine pathway metabolites in human serum by high-performance liquid chromatography with simultaneous ultraviolet and fluorimetric detection. Journal of Chromatography B. 1996;**675**:157-161

[6] Marklová E, Makovičková H, Krákorova I. Screening for defects in tryptophan metabolism. Journal of Chromatography. A. 2000;**870**:289-293

[7] Zhu W, Stevens AP, Dettmer K, Gottfried E, Hoves S, Kreutz M, Holler E, Canelas AB, Kema I, Oefner PJ. Quantitative profiling of tryptophan metabolites in serum, urine, and cell culture supernatants by liquid chromatography-tandem mass spectrometry. Analytical and Bioanalytical Chemistry. 2011;**401**:3249-3261

[8] Zhang A, Rijal K, Kah S, Ravid K, Chitalia V. A mass spectrometric method for quantification of tryptophan-derived uremic solutes in human serum. The Journal of Biological Methods. 2017;**4**:e75

[9] Malyszko J, Urano T, Takada Y, Takada A. Amino acids, serotonin, and 5-hydroxyindole acetic acid following foot shock to rats. Brain Research. 1995;**36**:137-140

[10] Malyszko J, Urano T, Yan D, Serizawa Y, Koima Y, Takada Y, Takada A. Foot shock induced changes blood and brain serotonin and related substances in rats. The Japanese Journal of Physiology. 1994;**44**:35-47

[11] Takahashi H, Takada Y, Nagai N, Urano T, Takada A. Effects of nicotine and foot shock stress on dopamine release in the striatum and nucleus accumbens. Brain Research Bulletin. 1998;**145**:157-162

[12] Takahashi H, Takada Y, Nagai N, Urano T, Takada A. Nicotine increase stress-induced serotonin release by stimulating nicotinic acetylcholine receptors in rat striatum. Synapse. 1998;**28**:212-219

[13] Pawlak R, Takada y, Takahashi H, Urano T, Ihara H, Nagai N, Takada A. Differential effects of nicotine against stress induced changes in dopaminergic system in rat striatum and hippocampus. European Journal of Pharmacology. 2000;**387**:171-177

[14] Takahahi H, Takada Y, Nagai N, Urano T, Takada A. Previous exposure to foot shock stress attenuates nicotine-induced serotonin release in rat striatum during the subsequent stress. Brain Research Bulletin. 2000;**52**:285-290

[15] Pawlak D, Takada Y, Urano T, Takada A. Serotonergic and kynurenic pathways in rats exposed to foot shock. 2000;**53**:197-205

[16] Adel A, Trullas R, Gelpi E. Time course of changes in serotonin and noradrenaline in rat brain after predictable and unpredictable shock. Brain Research. 1988;**459**:54-59

[17] Dunn AJ. Changes in plasma and brain tryptophan and brain serotonin and 5-hydroxy indole acetic acid after foot shock stress. Life Science. 1988;**42**:1847-1853

[18] Harris C, Miranda AF, Tanguay JL, Beninge RJ, Jhamands K. Modulation of atrial quioline neurotoxicity by elevation of endogenous brain kynurenic acid. British Journal of Pharmacology. 1998;**124**:391-399

[19] Hodkins MP, Schwarcz R. Metabolic control of kynurenic acid formation in the rat brain. Developmental Neuroscience. 1998;**20**:408-416

[20] Zung WW. A self-rating depression scale. Archives of General Psychiatry. 1965;**12**:63-70

[21] Freese A, Swartz KJ, During MJ, Martin JB. Kynurenine metabolites of tryptophan:Implication for neurologic diseases. Neurology. 1990;**40**:691-695

[22] Stone TW. Neuropharmacology of quinolinic acid and kynurenic acid. Pharmacological Reviews. 1993;**45**:309-379

[23] Saito K, Heyes MP. Kynurenine pathway enzymes in brain. In Fillipini GA, editor. Recent Advances in Tryptophan Research. New York: Prenum Press. 1996;485-492

[24] Moroni F, Russi P, Lombardi G, Beni M, Carla V. Presence of kynurenic acid in the mammalian brain. Journal of Neurochemistry. 1988;**51**:177-180.45

[25] TW S, Addae JI. The pharmacological manipulation of glutamate receptors and neuroprotection. European Journal of Pharmacology. 2002;**447**:285-296

[26] Hilmas C, Pereira EF, Alkondon M, Rassoulpour A, Schwarcz R, Albuquerque EX. The brain metabolite kynurenic acid inhibits alpha7 nicotinic receptor activity and increases non-alpha7 nicotinic receptor expression: Physiopathological implications. Journal of Neurosurgical Sciences. 2001;**21**:7463-7473

[27] Wang H, Liao H, Ochani M, et al. Cholinergic agonists inhibit HMGB1 release and improve survival in experimental sepsis. Nature Medicine. 2004;**10**:1216-1221

[28] Chen Y, Guillemin GJ. Kynurenine pathway metabolites in humans: disease and healthy States. International Journal of Tryptophan Research. 2009;**2**:1-19

[29] Okuno E, Nishikawa T, Nakamura M. Kynurenine aminotransferases in the rat. Localization and characterization. Advances in Experimental Medicine and Biology. 1996;**398**:455-464

[30] Okuda S, Nishiyama N, Saito H, Katsuki H. Hydrogen peroxide-mediated neuronal cell death induced by an endogenous neurotoxin, 3-hydroxykynurenine. Proceedings of the National Academy of Sciences. 1996;**93**:12533-12558

[31] Schwarcz R, Du F. Quinolinic acid and kynurenic acid in mammalian brain. Advances in Experimental Medicine and Biology. 1991;**294**:185-199

[32] Connick JH, Heywood JC, Sills GJ, Thompson GG, Brodie MJ, Stone TW. Nicotinylalanine increases central kynurenic acid content and anticonvulsant activity. General Pharmacology. 1992;**23**:235-239

[33] Mann JJ, Arango V, Marzuk PM, Theccanat S, Reis DJ. Evidence for the 5-HT hypothesis of suicide. A review of postmortem studies. The British Journal of Psychiatry. 1989;**155**(Suppl 8):7-14

[34] Oquendo MA, Sullivan GM, Sudol K, Baca-Garcia E, Stanley BH, et al. Toward a biosignature for suicide. The American Journal of Psychiatry. 2014;**171**:1259-1277

[35] Lapin IP. Kynurenines as probable participants of depression. Pharmakopsychiatr-Neuropsychopharmakol. 1973;**6**:273-279

[36] Lapin IP. Antagonism of kynurenic acid to anxiogens in mice. Life Sciences. 1998;**63**: 231-236

[37] Pålsson E, Sellgren C, Rydén E, Kizza R, Pelanis A, Zetterberg H, Blennow K, Landén M. Cerebrospinal fluid monoamine metabolite profiles in bipolar disorder, ADHD, and controls. Journal of Neural Transmission (Vienna). Sep 2017;**124**(9):1135-1143. Epub 2017 Jun 27. PMID: 28656371. DOI: 10.1007/s00702-017-1746-3

[38] Berrettini WH, Nurnberger JI Jr, Scheinin M, Seppala T, Linnoila M, Narrow W, Simmons-Alling S, Gershon ES. Cerebrospinal fluid and plasma monoamines and their metabolites in euthymic bipolar patients. Biological Psychiatry. 1985;**20**:257-269

4

Role of Melatonin in Reproductive Seasonality in Buffaloes

Tamer Awad Ramadan

Abstract

Buffaloes are characterized by seasonal reproductive activity. Anestrus buffalo heifers and lactating buffaloes were used to study the effect of melatonin treatment on the resumption of ovarian activity during out-of-breeding season. Buffaloes of treated group were injected or implanted with melatonin (18 mg melatonin/50 kg body weight). Using CIDR-eCG protocol preceded with melatonin successfully achieved estrus behavior and induced conception rate during out-of-breeding season. Furthermore, the reproductive performance of buffaloes during out-of-breeding season was clearly improved by melatonin implantation in conjunction with CIDR-eCG protocol due to the luteotrophic effect of melatonin expressed as increasing diameter of CL (corpus luteum) and progesterone concentration. This improvement resulted in greater values of conception rate, in melatonin implanted compared to not implanted buffaloes. Melatonin implantation in anestrus buffalo heifers increased the diameter of largest follicles and melatonin concentration but progesterone and luteinizing hormone (LH) concentrations were decreased. In addition, melatonin implantation in anestrus lactating buffaloes increased the SOD (superoxide dismutase) enzyme activity. Sustained release of exogenous melatonin significantly protects against oxidative stress while increasing beneficial total antioxidant capacity (TAC) concentration in summer-stressed anestrus buffaloes. Melatonin implantation in conjunction with CIDR-eCG protocol successfully improved some blood metabolites, in anestrus buffalo heifers during out-of-breeding season under tropical conditions.

Keywords: melatonin, CIDR, buffalo, reproductive seasonality, ovarian activity, oxidative stress

1. Introduction

Even though buffaloes are able to breed throughout the year in tropical regions, but with distance from the equator they show a seasonal breeding pattern [1, 2], that is determined by melatonin secretion in response to short-day length [3]. In general, reproductive activity of buffaloes is mainly determined by day length, climate (ambient temperature and relative humidity) and nutrition [2]. During summer, poor nutrition coupled with high ambient temperature was implicated with anestrus condition in buffaloes [4]. Heat stress in the hot summer months is an important driver of anestrus in buffalo, whose effects are mediated by increased blood concentrations of prolactin [1], leading to decreased progesterone secretion, and, consequently, extended calving to conception intervals due to repeated breeding and, generally, reduced reproductive performance [5].

In buffalo (*Bubalus bubalis*), reduced sexual activity has been reported as coincident with an increase in ambient temperature and day length [6], in either heifers or mature buffaloes. The proportion of buffaloes exhibiting estrus during the period of short-day length was significantly greater than that in the long-day period (74% versus 26%, respectively) [6]. Also, the conception rates are usually lower between February and August [7], and the number of services per conception are higher in animals calving in summer compared to animals calving at all the other seasons [7]. Decreasing day length may be a stronger determinant of the onset puberty and postpartum ovarian activity, whereas ambient temperature and relative humidity may have relatively lesser impact [8]. Nevertheless, the species physiological characteristics adversely affect buffalo dairy industry and result in a typical seasonal calvings that impair milk supply throughout the year [9].

To overcome seasonality and discipline milk production, it is necessary to implement suitable management schemes, particularly for out-of-season breeding [10]. Hormonal therapies to induce estrus and ovulation in anestrus buffaloes became important breeding strategies to achieve these goals. Hormonal treatments, adapted from other seasonal ruminant species, have been designed to control follicular and luteal functions, to synchronize estrus and ovulation and, more importantly, to eliminate estrus detection by scheduled of timed artificial insemination (TAI).

In deep anestrus buffaloes, out-of-season breeding requests the use of melatonin. Melatonin is a hormone produced and stored in the pineal gland during the day and secreted during the dark, starting after sunset and ending at sunrise. Melatonin controls the reproductive rhythm in diverse ruminant species, like goats and sheep (short-day species), and also in horses (long-day species), especially at higher latitudes [11]. Melatonin-mediated pathways regulate GnRH pulsatibility and, therefore, the activity of the reproductive neuroendocrine axis. It also modulates prolactin secretion by acting on the hypophysis. In addition to melatonin, the concomitant application of estrus/ovulation protocols suggests that controlled internal drug release systems (CIDR) gave better results for anestrus buffaloes [12]. The priming of hypothalamo-hypophysial-gonadal (HHG) axis with adequate amounts of P4 is beneficial for the recovery of reproductive function after calving and, hence, a better display of estrus behavior at the induced estrus [13]. Furthermore, the sufficient priming of endometrium with

P4 might be necessary to enhance the conception rate [14]. Melatonin implantation in conjunction with CIDR-eCG protocol successfully induced estrus behavior and enhanced conception rate in anestrus heifers and anestrus lactating buffaloes during out-of-breeding season under tropical conditions [12, 15].

The objectives of this study were to revise the efficacy of melatonin-based treatments for alleviation of the summer-induced decline in ovarian activity in anestrus heifers and lactating buffaloes and also to evaluate its effects on blood hormonal levels and metabolites concentrations, as well as those of antioxidant enzyme activities, as indicators of sustainability of buffaloes to the expenditure of melatonin treatment for preventing summer-induced decline in ovarian activity in true anestrus buffaloes.

2. Characterization of the buffalo reproductive cycle

The reproductive patterns of an animal are a result of the interaction of the endogenous regulatory mechanisms, mainly endocrine, with environmental signals. This complex interaction may deeply affect the reproductive function, e.g., females suspend cyclic ovarian activity in some periods of the year, or respond to the presence of a dominant individual on the group, or they can ovulate and come into estrus during the non-reproductive season. Bashir (2006) [16] has reported that buffaloes calving in summer (June–August) had a shorter calving interval than those calving in other seasons. The longest calving interval observed in buffaloes was calving in winter (December–January). This means that the buffaloes that had calved just before the onset of their breeding season (October–November) had more chances of getting bred than those calving after passing their breeding season. The buffalo heifers attaining their proper weight just before their breeding season are more likely to get bred than those passing this period and thus, may have lower age at puberty and consequently at calving than those attaining proper weight after this season. Based on this hypothesis, while raising the replacement buffalo heifers, efforts should be made to keep an eye on both critical weight of buffaloes for attaining the age at puberty and also the season in which this weight is attained. In this regard, adjustments in feeding regime may be required to get the critical weight of buffalo heifers just before their breeding season. Because once this breeding season is over, then feeding for accelerated growth may not reduce the age at their puberty and then one has to wait for their next breeding season to see the puberty in the heifers.

The normal interestrous interval in buffaloes may vary from 16 to 28 days, the estrus lasting for 10–20 h during breeding season [17]. The interval between the onset of estrus and LH surge is 1–12 hours and ovulation occurs 18–40 h after the LH surge [18]. The reduced intensity of heat symptoms recorded in buffaloes as compared to cows is possibly associated with lower estradiol levels due to smaller size pre-ovulatory follicles [17], in a mechanism that is further exaggerated by low P4 during luteal phase, a reduced pulsatile LH secretion, growth of ovulatory follicle and low estradiol production during summer months [19].

The stress and adverse environmental factors exert a direct effect on the neuroendocrine set-up, resulting in hyperprolactinemia, reduced pulsatile gonadotrophin secretion, poor follicular maturation and poor estradiol production, thereby culminating in poor heat expression and anestrus [20]. The postpartum anestrus has been differentiated into temporary (less than 150 days) and deep anestrus (more than 150 days), according to the time elapsed between calving and conception [3], or into superficial and deep anestrus based upon the presence or absence of follicular turnover [21].

3. Mechanisms regulating seasonal reproduction in buffaloes

The place of origin and gestation length undoubtedly influence the way in which reproductive seasonality occurs. The natural necessity to coincide calving and weaning with the most suitable time of year represents one of the causes of this 'adaptation' process [22]. This time of year should satisfy the nutritional requirements of the offspring through a period in which etiologic agents (infectious and parasitic) are less aggressive and/or present. Those born under the most favorable conditions have brought about the natural selection of individuals endowed with a more ideal reproductive seasonality that promotes the survival of the species [23].

In domestic animals, spring calving (March–May), which guarantees good availability of forage to offspring in temperate zones occurs whenever reproduction takes place in autumn in species with 5-month gestation (sheep and goats) or in the previous spring in the case of 11- and 12-month gestation (horses and donkeys). The same calving period, therefore, is conditioned by the neuroendocrine system. The reactivation of the reproductive cycle with regard to the length of gestation [short day breeder (negative photoperiod) or long breeder (positive photoperiod)] is therefore controlled.

Researchers in Italy [24] showed that buffaloes displaying stronger seasonality showed high plasma melatonin concentrations 2 hours after sunset, even when they were moved to another farm where other females showed low plasma melatonin concentrations and less sensitivity toward light stimulation [25]. The plasma melatonin concentrations had a repeatability of 0.733 [26]. If the heredity of plasma melatonin turns out to be high, as expected on the base of the high repeatability, the determination of plasma melatonin could be incorporated into genetic selection programmes for buffalo [22]. Lincoln [27] showed that sheep presenting continuous cyclic activity throughout the year retain this characteristic even if living at latitudes where other genotypes were sensitive to the light:dark ratio.

The differences between night and day concentrations of plasma melatonin in March were lower in heifers (5.0 times) than in adult buffaloes (28.3 times) [28]. It has been shown that buffaloes that calve in spring were more adaptable to out-of-breeding-mating strategy [26] and the heifers were less sensitive to the photoperiod [22, 28]. Heifer fertility is not compromised by season [22]. During the summer and when daylight hours are more than the dark, there is an increase in blood prolactin, but contrary to the assertions by Madan [7], buffalo regularly conceive. It is believed that hyperprolactinemia is secondary to hypothyroidism [29] during the warm months. Hypothyroidism exerts a positive feedback on thyroid stimulating hormone and hence on thyrotropin-releasing hormone, which in turn promotes an increase in prolactin [22, 23].

4. Methods to manipulate the out-of-season breeding in buffaloes

In small ruminants, induction of 'out-of-season' estrous cycles may be practiced, enabling spring breeding and, therefore, fall lambing/kidding, resulting in winter production of milk and lambs/kids for the winter markets. Several methods to control the reproduction of small ruminants involve the manipulation of the environmental light (extension of hours of light in a day) [30]. Some others are based on the administration of exogenous hormones that modify the physiologic chain of events involved in the sexual cycle (pharmacologic methods) and ultimately modify the luteal phase of the cycle (progesterone/progestagen and prostaglandins) or the annual pattern of reproduction (melatonin). Synchronization of estrous allows the control and short ending of lambing and kidding, with synchronization of weaning and uniform batching of animals to slaughter; it also allows more efficient use of labor and animal facilities. An appropriate management of reproduction allows ewes and does to breed in the spring to increase the supply of product to the market place on a year-round basis. Pharmaceutical control of reproduction is possible, usually through administration of hormones related to the natural estrous cycle, such as progesterone and/or melatonin [31]. Similar treatments can be used to tame the reproductive cycle in buffaloes.

In buffalo, during the out-of-breeding season (spring and summer), the greater light:dark ratio (long days) suppresses the estrus behavior and the occurrence of ovulation. Anestrus buffaloes have insufficient pulsatile secretion of LH to support the final stages of follicular development, and subsequently, estrus behavior and ovulation do not occur, limiting reproductive efficiency, especially in artificial insemination (AI) programs [32]. Therefore, hormonal therapies to induce estrus and ovulation in anestrus buffaloes became important breeding strategies. These hormonal treatments have been designed to control follicular and luteal functions, to synchronize estrus and ovulation and, more importantly, to eliminate estrus detection by preplanned scheduled of timed artificial insemination (TAI).

In most studies, the success rate was lower when treatment was performed in periods of low breeding activity or during seasonal anestrus, and various modified protocols have been tried to improve pregnancy rates. Among the hormonal therapies developed for cattle, GnRH plus PGF2α-based TAI protocols resulted in a reduced ovulatory response when applied in anestrus buffalo [33]. Also, during the out-of-breeding season, when a high incidence of anestrus is expected, lower pregnancy rates are encountered in buffalo cows synchronized with the Ovsynch protocol for TAI [33]. Recent studies in buffalo have demonstrated that similar pregnancy rates at TAI in both breeding and out-of-breeding seasons can be obtained with the use of progesterone (P4), estradiol (E2) and (eCG)-based protocols [34].

Melatonin implants for subcutaneous application have been commercially available in several countries. These implants have been widely used to advance the breeding season of anestrus ewes and goats. Melatonin implants induce high plasma concentrations of melatonin for 24 h every day, without suppressing the endogenous secretion of the pineal hormone during the night. Thereby, implants cause a short day-like response by lengthening the duration of the melatonin signal [35]. The implants contain 18 mg of melatonin and are designed to maintain high plasma melatonin concentrations for at least 60 days, although most of them continue to release the hormone for longer than 100 days [36].

The mechanisms by which melatonin improves reproductive performance are not fully understood, as the pineal hormone can act at different body sites. Effects at hypothalamus-hypophysis level have been previously mentioned, and an effect at ovary level seems to be consistent, either by reducing atresia during late folliculogenesis to increase ovulation rate [16] or by acting as luteotropic agent [37] to improve fertility. The time of treatment is important to guarantee a good efficacy. Melatonin implants inserted around the summer solstice have been widely used as a means of advancing the out-of-breeding season in buffaloes in areas with high latitude.

In buffalo reproduction, few investigations have been made to clarify a relationship between plasma melatonin concentrations and seasonal reproductive pattern. The Mediterranean buffaloes showing seasonal reproductive trend had highest night-time plasma melatonin concentrations in winter and lowest in summer [24]. In another study carried out on heifers and buffaloes, the melatonin levels showed remarkable differences between seasons. In peak summer because of the shortest night, the lowest plasma melatonin with less persistence of melatonin peak were found, whereas the highest concentrations were noted in early winter corresponding to the start of hypothalamic-hypophysial-ovarian axis (HPO) activity [28]. Moreover, low plasma melatonin was associated with a low seasonal ovulatory activity in buffaloes [24]. This decrease in ovulatory activity during long days happens despite the presence of follicles with ovulatory size (12–14 mm) on the ovaries of nulliparous and pluriparous Mediterranean buffaloes [3, 21].

Melatonin appears to act at hypothalamic sites to increase the release of GnRH pulses by modulating the negative feedback potency of estradiol [38], which acts at hypothalamic and hypophysial loci to reduce luteinizing hormone secretion [39]. The photoperiod modulates KiSS-1 expression via melatonin, strongly suggesting that kisspeptin relays photoperiodic information to the HPO axis. Kisspeptin stimulates LH secretion in a GnRH-dependent manner by increasing GnRH secretion into the hypophysial portal blood [40]. Kisspeptin neurons express estrogen and progesterone receptors [41], which are directly regulated by these steroids in a manner consistent with both positive and negative feedback regulation of pulsatile GnRH secretion [41].

The protocol for melatonin application is simple and less demanding than the traditional treatment of induction-synchronization of estrus using progestogens. Administration of melatonin during anestrus seems to improve the fertility. It has been reported that melatonin implants in buffaloes can improve conception rate [12, 15]. Melatonin treatment in buffalo is necessary to induce cyclicity during anestrus in out-of-breeding season in which evidenced an improvement in conception rate [42, 43]. Ramadan et al. [12, 15] found that melatonin implantation alone did not affect the post-treatment reproductive performance in either anestrus buffalo or lactating buffaloes during out-of-breeding season. On the other hand, combined melatonin and CIDR treatments induced cyclicity and enhanced the reproductive performance of anestrus buffalo heifers and anestrus lactating buffaloes during out-of-breeding season [12, 15] (**Figure 1**).

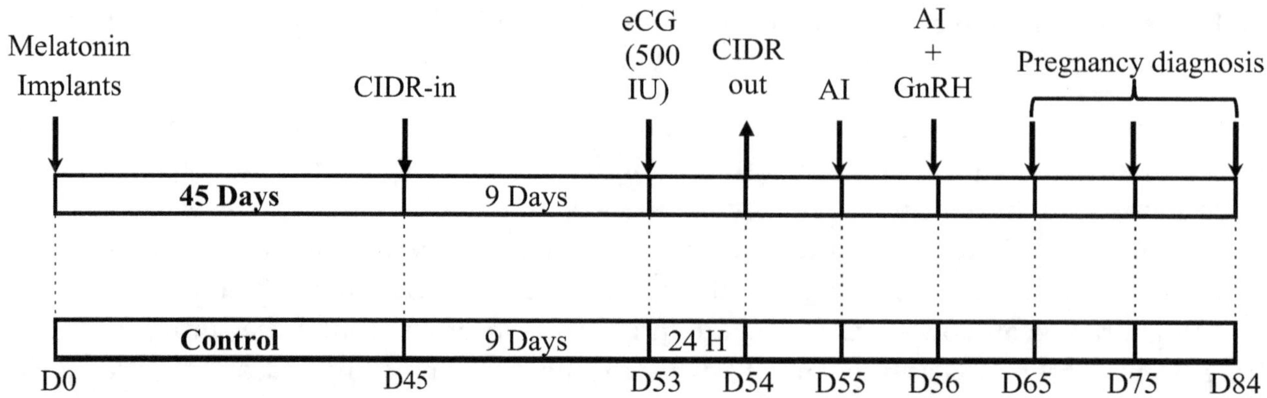

Figure 1. Experimental design to evaluate the effect of melatonin implantation and CIDR-GnRH-based synchronization protocol in heifers and lactating buffaloes. CIDR, controlled internal drug release device (1.38 g progesterone); GnRH, gonadotropin-releasing hormone (10 μg Receptal, i.m); eCG, equine chorionic gonadotropin (500 IU Folligon, i.m) and AI, artificial insemination. Ramadan et al. [12, 15].

5. The effect of exogenous melatonin on hormonal levels and blood metabolites in buffaloes

In anestrus lactating buffaloes injected with melatonin, the serum P4 concentrations increased (0.71 ng/ml) after melatonin injection compared with control group (0.28 ng/ml) at days 12 and 16 post-treatment (post-AI), during the summer season, suggesting a luteotrophic effect of melatonin [42]. Also, exogenous melatonin might improve uterine expression of P4 receptors or their binding capacity, which would result in higher reproductive efficiency [42]. Melatonin implants plus CIDR in buffalo heifers and lactating buffalo were able to maintain the corpus luteum at day 21 of estrous cycle [12, 15]. In addition, the plasma P4 was highest at the second ovulation post-treatment than the first ovulation in implanted anestrus heifers in summer [43] (**Table 1**).

The decrease in P4 concentrations in anestrus lactating buffaloes compared with buffalo heifers was attributed to a prolactin effect. Misztal et al. [44] reported that in lactating ewes the melatonin concentration decreases, whereas prolactin, responsible for the initiation and maintenance of lactation, increases. Prolactin may block the hypothalamic mechanism responsible for episodic release of LH or inhibit the positive feedback of estrogen on LH secretion, and it can even affect ovarian steroidogenesis by altering the number of LH receptors [45].

Lactating buffaloes treated with melatonin alone present higher E_2 concentrations recorded (16 pg/ml) after melatonin treatment in comparison to the control group (9.02 pg/ml) [42]. The pattern of serum E_2 profile in the induced estrous cycle was highest on the day of estrus and decreased in the second week of the cycle [46]. The elevated levels of E_2 4 days before estrus may mediate the LH surge, as demonstrated in cattle [47]. The reducing effect of melatonin on estradiol concentration has also been reported in sheep [38]. Moreover, melatonin decreases the estradiol receptor expression in deep endometrial stroma of ewes, where E2-estradiol receptor complex acts as a luteolytic agent [48]. In ewes, estradiol concentration has also been correlated with the mean response of prostaglandins to oxytocin, via the estrogenic stimulation of uterine oxytocin receptors [49].

Route of administration[1]	Associated treatment	Animal type	P_4 (ng/ml)	E_2 (pg/mL)	LH (mlU/mL)	Melatonin (pg/mL)	Ref(s)
Injection	-	Lactating (n=20)	0.71	16	-	412.3	[42]
Implantation	-	Heifers (n=12)	0.66	-	-	-	[43]
Implantation	CIDR eCG GnRH	Heifers (n=8)	0.72	-	3.44	9.10	[12]
Implantation	CIDR eCG GnRH	Lactating (n=6)	0.97	-	-	6.80	[15]

[1](18 mg/50 kg BW).

CIDR, controlled internal drug release device (1.38 g progesterone); eCG, equine chorionic gonadotropin (500 IU Folligon, i.m at day before CIDR removal) and GnRH, gonadotropin-releasing hormone (10 μg Receptal, i.m at day after CIDR withdrawal).

Table 1. Hormonal levels in anestrus Murrah buffalo before synchronization with melatonin during the non-breeding season.

Melatonin treatment interferes with the effects of melatonin directly in buffalo's hypophysis. In anestrus heifers, with the advancement of melatonin treatment, on days 28 and 42, it resulted in a decrease in serum LH (3.44 mlU/mL) [12]. Melatonin had no effect on the frequency of LH pulses [12]. In sheep, the rise in circulating melatonin is responsible for the increase in GnRH and gonadotropins, thus leading to follicular growth and ovulation [50]. However, this finding is inconsistent with the reduction of LH serum concentration observed in the melatonin-treated buffalo heifers. The failure of high concentrations of serum melatonin to increase LH concentration might be explained by the reduction of buffalo estradiol concentration in summer [51]. Estradiol seems to be positively linked with the action of melatonin on the female reproductive activity, where melatonin exerts a modulatory effect on LH secretion, stimulating its release in the presence of estradiol feedback (cyclic animals) and inhibiting it during steroid deprivation (animals in anestrus) [52]. Also, the presence of low concentrations of plasma GnRH and gonadotropins during the summer period in buffaloes [53] might disturb the development of LH receptors and the synthesis of adequate estradiol in the dominant follicle [51] required to induce the ovulatory surge of gonadotropins [54].

The administration of slow-release melatonin (implants) was responsible for an increase in serum melatonin concentration, ranging from 14.34 to 412.31 pg/ml in treated lactating buffaloes [42]. Administration of exogenous slow-release melatonin induced the restoration of the ovarian activity in summer anestrus buffaloes, which can be explained by a 'cascading effect' of at least a 10-fold increase on the plasma concentrations of GnRH and gonadotrophins, which provides the necessary boost for follicular growth and ovulation [50]. It has been shown that treatments with melatonin implants tend to originate an increase in serum melatonin concentration (9.10 pg/ml) in anestrus buffalo heifers [12] and in anestrus lactating buffalo (6.80 pg/ml) (**Table 1**), which could be associated with the antiprolactinic action of melatonin, as it was suggested in another species [55].

Singh et al. [56] showed that, in anestrus lactating buffalo, melatonin treatments decrease plasma albumin (2.7 g/dl), compared to pre-treatment concentrations. In contrast, Ramadan et al. [57] found higher albumin values (3.41 g/dl) in treated anestrus buffalo heifers implanted with melatonin. Ramadan et al. [57] also reported that the combined treatment of melatonin and CIDR resulted in an increase in plasma concentrations of albumin, glucose, high-density lipoprotein (HDL), alanine aminotransferase (ALT) and reduction in plasma alkaline phosphate (ALP) compared with control animals (**Table 2**). Because of the interaction of melatonin with various endocrine systems [58], it was proposed that melatonin treatment may initiate ovarian cyclicity in true anestrus buffalo heifers through its influence on body metabolism [59]. Albumin, being the most abundant plasma protein, could play a major role as an antioxidant in plasma, mediating thiol oxidation and carbonyl formation [60].

Plasma concentrations of glucose (65.16 mg/dl) were increased by melatonin and CIDR treatment [57]. Glucose is the primary energy source for the ovary and it is possibly metabolized in the ovary through anaerobic pathways. It also stimulates the ovarian follicular growth [61]. Furthermore, plasma glucose is a positive metabolic signal for the central control of GnRH release [62].

Increased lipolysis during lactation is hormonally regulated and not an expression of energy deficiency. Plasma concentrations of HDL (62.29 mg/dl) were increased by melatonin treatment combined with CIDR [57]. The concentration of transaminase enzyme ALT (98.72 IU/L) was increased with treatment of melatonin and CIDR in anestrus buffalo heifers during out-of-season breeding [57]. Singh et al. [56] found that exogenous melatonin did not record any alterations in plasma concentration of AST and ALT enzyme activities in anestrus lactating buffaloes. Thus, minor alterations in AST during treatment period in spite of elevated plasma activities of ALT suggested that hepatic functions were not impaired in the buffalo [63]. Follicular growth is a dynamic process in which follicular development is continuous but accelerates during the later stages of the estrous cycle [64]. Plasma concentrations of ALP (97.99 IU/L) were increased by melatonin treatment combined with CIDR in anestrus buffalo heifers [57]. The ALP content in serum may changes during the estrous cycle [64]. ALP is a lysosomal enzyme that catalyzes various reactions in the body, including synthesis of proteins and DNA turnover within the nucleus [65].

Route of administration[1]	Associated treatment	Animal type	Albumin (g/dl)	Glucose (mg/dl)	HDL (mg/dl)	ALT (IU/L)	ALP (IU/L)	Ref(s)
Implantation	-	Lactating (n=5)	2.7	62.1	35.1	56.4	-	[56]
Implantation	CIDR eCG GnRH	Heifers (n=8)	3.41	65.16	62.29	98.72	97.99	[57]

[1](18 mg/50 kg BW).

CIDR, controlled internal drug release device (1.38 g progesterone); eCG, equine chorionic gonadotropin (500 IU Folligon, i.m at day before CIDR removal); GnRH, gonadotropin-releasing hormone (10 μg Receptal, i.m at day after CIDR withdrawal); HDL, high-density lipoprotein; ALT, alanine aminotransferase and ALP, alkaline phosphate.

Table 2. Serum metabolites and some enzyme activities in anestrus Murrah buffalo synchronized with melatonin during out-of-breeding season.

6. The effect of exogenous melatonin on the antioxidant enzyme activity in buffaloes

Metabolic pressures of adaptation to high milk yield and environmental conditions, especially high ambient temperature, exert a retrograde effect on buffalo reproduction. High temperature-humidity index (THI) predisposes buffaloes to develop oxidative stress [66] with anti-gonadotropic and anti-steroidogenic actions [67]. This in turn is involved in modulation of estrous cycle and uterine environment causing defective embryo development and reproductive failure in buffaloes [68] and also contributes to the elongation of the postpartum anestrus [69]. Jan et al. [70] found that overall greater concentrations of biomarkers of oxidative stress coupled with the reduced concentrations of total antioxidant capacity (TAC) in follicular fluid of acyclic buffaloes are indicative of the involvement of oxidative stress in the suspension of the ovarian activity. Further evidence showed that the oxidative stress and the depletion of the antioxidant activity play a significant role in diminished ovarian function, as evidenced by the significant increment in circulatory malondialdehyde (MDA) and simultaneous decline of TAC in buffalo heifers [71].

Melatonin affects membrane fluidity in different cells under conditions of high oxidative stress, indicating that its mechanism of action relates to possible due to an antioxidant activity associated to the directly scavenging of free radicals and the inhibition of lipid peroxidation [72] and thereby the decrease in MDA concentration. A wide range of antioxidant enzymes are also induced [73], counteracting the generation of free radicals due to inhibition of the activity of some pro-oxidant enzymes such as nitric oxide (NO) synthase and lipoxygenase [72]. Moreover, melatonin stimulates the activity of several enzymes related to the antioxidative defense system [74].

Several authors reported that exogenous melatonin increased blood melatonin level, which has a positive correlation with antioxidant capacity [75]. Kumar et al. [76] refer that the total antioxidant capacity (TAC) in the serum of melatonin-treated female buffalos during summer anestrus tends to be higher (2.22 mmol/L) on days 12 and 24 after the onset of melatonin treatment, compared with the control group (1.42 mmol/L), supporting the previous studies of Ahmed et al. [77]. In the same study [76], it was also shown that the concentrations of serum MDA and NO tend to decrease (3.97 mmol/L and 42.41 mmol/L, respectively) (**Table 3**).

The beneficial effect of a sustained release of melatonin on the increase in TAC and the reduction in MDA and NO concentrations [76] suggests a beneficial effect of melatonin in mitigating the oxidative stress effects on fertility, alike that reported in women [78]. The beneficial effect of exogenous melatonin in the resumption of estrus may be related with the facilitation of cellular functions in the growing follicles, because NO, an important intra-ovarian factor, regulates the process of follicular development through its multifaceted role in angiogenesis, vasodilation, regulation of normal follicular growth and function, steroidogenesis and ovulation [79].

Ramadan et al. [15] observed that melatonin treatment resulted in an increase in blood plasma of SOD (superoxide dismutase, 4.72 U/mg protein) activity in anestrus lactating buffaloes under tropical conditions (**Table 3**). Therefore, the increased activity of erythrocytic SOD in

Route of administration[1]	Associated treatment	Animal type	MDA (μmol/L)	SOD (U/mg protein)	GPx (IU/gHb/m)	Nitric oxide (μmol/L)	TAC (mmol/L)	Ref(s)
Injection	-	Lactating (n=20)	3.97	-	-	42.41	2.22	[76]
Implantation	-	Lactating (n=41)	-	10.14	5.67	-	-	[83]
Implantation	CIDR eCG GnRH	Heifers (n=8)	3.40	4.12	-	-	-	[12]
Implantation	CIDR eCG GnRH	Lactating (n=6)	1.95	4.72	-	-	-	[15]

[1](18 mg/50 kg BW).

CIDR, controlled internal drug release device (1.38 g progesterone); eCG, equine chorionic gonadotropin (500 IU Folligon, i.m at day before CIDR removal); GnRH, gonadotropin-releasing hormone (10 μg Receptal, i.m at day after CIDR withdrawal); MDA, malondialdehyde; SOD, superoxide dismutase; GPx, glutathione peroxidase and TAC, total antioxidant capacity.

Table 3. Antioxidant enzymes, nitric oxide and total antioxidant capacity in anestrus Murrah buffalo synchronized with melatonin during out-of-breeding season.

treated anestrus bovine heifers could be attributed to the physiological upregulation of this enzyme to mitigate superoxide radical challenge [80]. It has been established that, in bovine, the SOD and catalase activities in the CL (corpus luteum) parallel the P4 plasma patterns: the enzymatic activity of catalase and SOD present a sixfold to eightfold increase from day 6 to day 16 of the estrous cycle thereafter decreasing through the luteal regression [80]. SOD plays important roles in the maintenance of luteal function, possibly by rescuing the corpus luteum when pregnancy occurs [81]. It has been reported that SOD acts protectively against superoxide radicals to stimulate P4 production by the corpus luteum [82].

The results of Singh et al. [83] are consistent with the results reported by Kumar et al., in summer anestrus buffaloes [76], which also documented the potential of exogenous melatonin to augment the antioxidative capacity of summer anestrus buffalo [76]. Reactive nitrogen species are another category of potentially destructive substances that react with melatonin. It was suggested that melatonin acts by binding with calmodulin and suppresses the gene transcription of NO synthase enzyme [84]. The enzyme is involved in a rate limiting step in the synthesis of nitric oxide; a known oxidant suggested being a major free radical causing follicular damage, thereby resulting in anovulatory condition in summer anestrus buffalo [84].

7. The effects of exogenous melatonin on the reproductive performance in buffaloes

7.1. Effect of melatonin alone

Estrus response and fertility in melatonin-treated female is largely dependent on the animal status, the association of a progesterone treatment and of animals' management at onset of treatment. According to Kumar et al. [42], a single subcutaneous injection of melatonin

(18 mg/50 kg BW in sterilized corn oil) in summer anestrus water buffalo showed a definite influence on the interval to induced estrus (18 days), obtaining a 90% estrus induction rate. In addition, treatments with melatonin implant (18 mg/50 kg BW) in delayed pubertal buffalo heifers during summer successfully induced estrus within 6–36 days [43]. Also Ghuman et al. [43] reported a successful estrus induction in 100% anestrus buffalo heifers implanted with melatonin in summer season (**Table 4**). However, in other studies on buffalo, melatonin implants alone failed to induce estrus signs for the first 45 days after implantation in either anestrus heifers or lactating buffaloes during summer season [12, 15].

Ghuman et al. [43] showed that melatonin treatment increased the diameter of the largest follicle (14.55 mm) compared to control group (12.2 mm), which might be due to the inability to ovulate even after attaining normal pre-ovulatory diameter (>9 mm) [43]. This suggests that the follicle diameter itself may not be determinant of ovulation. The failure of ovulation of largest follicles could be a drive of a lack of sufficient LH stimulus. The amplitude and frequency of GnRH pulses and, therefore, those of gonadotropins, required to induce the growth of follicles are different from those required for ovulation [85]. The wide extension of the period until estrus induction might be derived from the ovarian structures presented at the ovary at starting of treatment in summer anestrus buffalo heifers. Early responders might have, on the day of melatonin treatment, dominant follicles or follicles emerging in the ovaries, whereas in the later responders the follicles developing in the ovaries still not reached divergence. This hypothesis implies an individual variation in the requirements for exogenous melatonin to attain the threshold level necessary to activate hypothalamus-hypophysial-ovarian axis, as defended by Ghuman et al. [43].

Buffalo heifers in anestrus implanted with melatonin revealed larger CL diameter (15.16 mm) at second ovulation than at first [43]. Ghuman et al. [43] hypothesized that in the absence of a strong negative-feedback effect of estradiol on the hypothalamus, the sustained release of

Route of administration[1]	Associated treatment	Animal type	EIR (day)	Estrus %	LF (mm)	CL (mm)	CR (%)	Ref(s)
Injection	-	Lactating (n=20)	18	90	-	-	-	[76]
Injection	-	Lactating (n=20)	18	90	-	-	32.4	[42]
Implantation	-	Heifers (n=12)	6-36	100	14.55	15.16	-	[43]
Implantation	-	Lactating (n=41)	-	65.8	-	-	-	[83]
Implantation	CIDR eCG GnRH	Heifers (n=8)	-	100	10.04	16.40	37.5	[12]
Implantation	CIDR eCG GnRH	Lactating (n=6)	-	100	13.90	18.33	100	[15]

[1](18 mg/50 kg BW).

CIDR, controlled internal drug release device (1.38 g progesterone); eCG, equine chorionic gonadotropin (500 IU Folligon, i.m at day before CIDR removal); GnRH, gonadotropin-releasing hormone (10 μg Receptal, i.m at day after CIDR withdrawal); EIR, estrus induction response; LF, largest follicle; CL, corpus luteum and CR, conception rate.

Table 4. Estrus response, ovarian activity and conception rate in anestrus Murrah buffalo synchronized with melatonin during out-of-breeding season.

exogenous melatonin in summer anestrus buffalo heifers could stimulate the hypothalamus-hypophysial-ovarian axis triggering the early induction of estrus. Lactating Murrah buffaloes treated with single subcutaneous injection of melatonin during summer evidenced an improvement in conception rate (32.4%) compared to untreated animals (0 %) [42].

7.2. Effect of melatonin plus CIDR

When melatonin treatments are associated to CIDR and eCG, the estrus rate after the progesterone removal recorded 100% in either the buffalo heifers or cows during out-of-breeding season. Also, the diameter of the follicle at the day of AI is higher after melatonin treatment plus CIDR in anestrus heifers and anestrus lactating buffaloes [12, 15]. Moreover, compared to the use of CIDR alone, the association of melatonin treatment and CIDR presented a superior ability to maintain CL for 21 days post-AI (12.5% vs. 37.5 %, respectively) in anestrus heifers or between 21 and 30 days post-AI (33,3% vs. 100 %, respectively) in anestrus lactating buffaloes [12, 15]. The increase in CL size paralleled the increased serum progesterone concentration in either treated buffalo heifers or cows [12, 15] (**Table 4**). Furthermore, melatonin may act directly on the corpus luteum to increase progesterone production [37], instead of decreasing the uterine secretion of prostaglandin F2α [86] or modifying prostaglandin biosynthesis in the hypothalamus [87].

Combined melatonin and CIDR treatments enhanced the reproductive performance of buffalo heifers during out-of-breeding season in comparison with CIDR treatments only [12, 15], which could be explained by the deepness of anestrus. The percentage of conception at day 30 post-AI was threefold higher in the melatonin with CIDR-treated anestrus heifers compared to untreated group (37.5% *vs.* 12.5%) [12], as well as in anestrus lactating buffaloes (100% vs. 33.3%, respectively in the melatonin treated and non-treated groups) [15].

8. Conclusion

So far, it has been believed that milk yield in buffaloes is determined by genetic and environmental factors. In recent years, a special focus has been placed on melatonin treatment on reproductive seasonality. In farm animals, day light changes play a very important role as they establish their yields. The length of day light, and in particular the melatonin profile, is of special importance in buffaloes as they determine reproductive process, in which lactation is the last stage of reproductive physiology. Experiments carried out in buffaloes demonstrated that buffaloes are characterized by seasonal reproductive activity. They become sexually active in response to a decreasing day length in late summer to early autumn. During the out-of-breeding season, buffaloes often exhibit anestrus, which extends the calving to conception interval and, consequently, reduces reproductive performance resulting in seasonal calving and a dramatic disturbance to milk supply throughout the year. To avoid seasonality-related constraints, it is necessary to implement management schemes to overcome reproductive seasonality and regulate production of milk throughout the year. Thus, hormonal therapies to induce estrus and ovulation in anestrus buffaloes are important strategies to overcome seasonality. These hormonal treatments have been designed to control follicular and luteal functions synchronizing estrus and ovulation and, more importantly, to eliminate estrus detection by preplanned scheduled of timed artificial insemination. Melatonin implantation in conjunction with CIDR-eCG protocol successfully induced estrus behavior and enhanced conception rate in anestrus heifers and anestrus lactating buffaloes during out-of-breeding season under tropical conditions.

Author details

Tamer Awad Ramadan

Address all correspondence to: tamereweda1174@yahoo.com

Animal Production Research Institute, Agricultural Research Center, Giza, Egypt

References

[1] Perera BMAO. Reproductive cycles of buffalo. Animal of Reproduction Science. 2011; **124**:194-199. DOI: 10.1016/j.anireprosci.2010.08.022

[2] Singh J, Nanda AS, Adams GP. The reproductive pattern and efficiency of female buffaloes. Animal of Reproduction Science. 2000;**60-61**:593-604. DOI: 10.1016/s0378-4320(00)00109-3

[3] Zicarelli L. Reproductive seasonality in buffalo. In: Proceedings of Third Course on Biotechnology of Reproduction in Buffaloes, Caserta, Italy; 6-10 October, (Issue II). 1997;. p. 29-52

[4] Shah SNH. Comparative studies of seasonal influence on breeding behaviour and conception rate of dairy buffalo and zebu cattle. In: Proceedings 11th International Congress on Animal Reproduction and Artificial Insemination. Book of congress, Dublin, Ireland. 1988;**3**:538-542.

[5] Zicarelli L. Can we consider buffalo a non-precocious and hypofertile species? Italian Journal of Animal Science. 2007;**6**:143-154. DOI: 10.4081/ijas.2007.s2.143

[6] Tailor SP, Jain LS, Gupta HK, Bhatia JS. Oestrus and conception rates in buffaloes under village conditions. Indian Journal Animal Science. 1990;**60**:1020-1021

[7] Madan ML. Status of reproduction in female buffalo. In: Proc. Second World Buffalo congress, Buffalo Production and Health: a compendium of latest research information based on Indian studies. New Delhi, India: ICAR Publication; 1988;**3**(12-16): pp. 89-100

[8] Singh R. Studies on the onset of postpartum ovarian activity in relation to climatic and nutritional status in buffaloes. MVSc thesis. India: Punjab Agriculture, University of Ludhiana; 1993

[9] Neglia G, Gasparrini B, Caracciolo di Brienza V, Di Palo R, Zicarelli L. First pregnancies carried to term after transfer of vitrified buffalo embryos entirely produced in vitro. Veterinary Research Communication. 2004;**1**:233-236. DOI: 10.1023/b:verc.0000045414.65331.6a

[10] Zicarelli L. Enhancing reproductive performance in domestic dairy water buffalo (Bubalus bubalis). In: Lucy MC, Pate JL, Smith MF, Spencer TE, editors. Eighth International Symposium on Reproduction in Domestic Ruminants. Anchorage, Alaska: Nottingham University Press; 2010. p. 443-455. DOI: 10.7313/upo9781907284991.034

[11] Chemineau P, Malpaux B, Delgadillo JA. Control of sheep and goat reproduction: use of light and melatonin. Animal of Reproduction Science. 1992;**30**:157-184. DOI: 10.1016/0378-4320(92)90010-B

[12] Ramadan TA, Sharma RK, Phulia SK, Balhara AK, Ghuman SS, Singh I. Effectiveness of melatonin and controlled internal drug release device treatment on reproductive performance of buffalo heifers during out-of-breeding season under tropical conditions. Theriogenology. 2014;**82**:1296-1302. DOI: 10.1016/j.theriogenology.2014.08.014

[13] De Rensis F, Ronci G, Guarneri P, Nguyen BX, Presicce GA, Huszenicza G, Scaramuzzi RJ. Conception rate after fixed time insemination following ovsynch protocol with and without progesterone supplementation in cyclic and non-cyclic Mediterranean Italian buffaloes (*Bubalus bubalis*). Theriogenology. 2005;**63**:1824-1831. DOI: 10.1016/j.theriogenology.2004.07.024

[14] Stevenson JS, Pursley JR, Garverick HA, Fricke PM, Kesler DJ, Ottobre JS, Wiltbank MC. Treatment of cycling and non-cycling lactating dairy cows with progesterone during ovsynch. Journal of Dairy Science. 2006;**89**:2567-2578. DOI: 10.3168/jds.s0022-0302(06)72333-5

[15] Ramadan TA, Sharma RK, Phulia SK, Balhara AK, Ghuman SS, Singh I. Manipulation of reproductive performance of lactating buffaloes using melatonin and controlled internal drug release device treatment during out-of-breeding season under tropical conditions. Theriogenology. 2016;**86**:1048-1053. DOI: 10.1016/j.theriogenology.2016.03.034

[16] Bashir MK. Genetic and phenotypic aspects of some performance traits of Nili-Ravi buffaloes in Pakistan. PhD Thesis. Univ. Agri., Faisalabad, Pakistan; 2006

[17] Baruselli PS, Mucciolo RG, Vistin JA, Viana WG, Arruda RP, Maduriera EH, Oliveira CA, Molero- Filho JR. Ovarian follicular dynamics during estrus cycle in buffalo. Theriogenology. 1997;**47**:1531-1547. DOI: 10.1016/s0093-691x(97)00159-3

[18] Prakash BS, Sarkar M, Paul Vijay Mishra DP, Mishra A, Meyer HHD. Postpartum endocrinology and prospects for fertility improvement in the lactating riverine buffalo (*Bubalus bubalis*) abd yak (*Poephagus grunniens* L.). Livestock Science. 2005;**98**:13-23. DOI: 10.1016/j.livprodsci.2005.10.014

[19] Awasthi MK, Khare A, Kavani FS, Siddiquee GM, Panchal MT, Shah RR. Is one-wave follicular growth during the estrous cycle a usual phenomenon in water buffaloes (*Bubalus bubalis*). Animal of Reproduction Science. 2006;**92**:241-253. DOI: 10.1016/j.anireprosci.2005.05.024

[20] Phogat JB, Smith RF, Dobson H. The influence of stress on neuroendocrine control of the hypothalamic-pituitary-ovarian axis—A review. Veterinary Bulletin. 1997;**67**:551-567

[21] Presicce GA, Senatore EM, De Santis G, Bella A. Follicle turnover and pregnancy rates following oestrus synchronization protocols in Mediterranean Italian buffaloes (*Bubalus bubalis*). Reproduction in Domestic Animals. 2005;**40**:443-447. DOI: 10.1111/j.1439-0531.2005.00606.x

[22] Zicarelli L, Campanile G, Esposito L, Di Palo R, Boni R, Spadetta M, Montemurro N, Pacelli C, Borghese A, Barile VL, Terzano GM, Annicchiarico G, Allegrini S, De Benedetti A, Malfatti A, Lucaroni A, Todini L Anaestro e induzione dell'estro in bufale acicliche, (Anoestrus and oestrus induction in acyclic buffaloes), Agriculture Ricerca. 1994;**153**:25-40

[23] Zicarelli L, Esposito L, Campanile G, Di Palo R, Armstrong DT. Effect of using vasectomized bulls in A.I. practice on the reproductive efficiency of Italian buffalo cows. Animal Reproduction Science. 1997;**47**:171-180. DOI: 10.1016/s0378-4320(97)00008-0

[24] Parmeggiani A, Di Palo R. Melatonina e stagionalità riproduttiva della bufala. Atti Conv. su "Miglioramento dell'efficienza produttiva e riproduttiva della specie bufalina" Agricolture e Ricerca. 1994;**153**:41-48

[25] Di Palo R, Parmeggiani A, Spadetta M, Campanile G, Esposito L, Seren E, Zicarelli L. Influence of changing farm on the repeatability of melatonin plasma level in Italian Mediterranean buffalo. In: Proceedings of the Fifth World Buffalo Congress, Caserta, Italy. 1997; p. 758-761

[26] Di Palo R, Parmeggiani A, Campanile G, Zicarelli L. Repeatability of melatonin plasma levels in buffaloes bred in Italy. Atti della Societa Italiana delle Scienze Veterinarie. 1993;**47**:331-335

[27] Lincoln GA. Photoperiod-pineal-hypothalamic relay in sheep. Animal Reproduction Science. 1992;**28**:203-217. DOI: 10.1016/0378-4320(92)90107-o

[28] Borghese A, Barile VL, Terzano GM, Pilla AM, Parmeggiani A. Melatonin trend during season in heifers and buffalo cow. Bubalus bubalis 1995;**1**:61-64

[29] Campanile G, Avallone L, d'Angelo A, Di Palo R, Di Meo C. Influence of the season and of the number of days after calving on the pattern of thyroid hormones in buffalo cows. In: Proceedings of the Fourth World Buffalo Congress, São Paulo, Brazil, June. 1994; p. 564-566

[30] Vesely JA. Induction of lambing every eight months in two breeds of sheep by light control with or without hormonal treatment. Animal Production. 1975;**21**:165-174. DOI: 10.1017/s0003356100030580

[31] Abecia J A, Forcada F, González-Bulnes A. Pharmaceutical Control of Reproduction in Sheep and Goats. Veterinary Clinics of North America: Food Animal Practice. 2011;**27**:67-79. DOI: 10.1016/j.cvfa.2010.10.001

[32] Carvalho NAT, Julia GS, Pietro SB. Strategies to overcome seasonal anestrus in water buffalo. Theriogenology. 2016;**86**:200-206. DOI: 10.1016/j.theriogenology.2016.04.032

[33] Souza DC, Carvalho NAT, Soares JG, Monteiro BM, Madureira EH, Baruselli PS. Effect of the presence of corpus luteum in lactating buffaloes on the response to the ovsynch

protocol during the breeding season (preliminary results). 29th Annual Meeting of the Brazilian Embryo Technology Society (SBTE). Gramado, RS, Brazil: Animal Reproduction. 2015; p. 629

[34] Carvalho NAT, Soares JG, Porto Filho RM, Gimenes LU, Souza DC, Nichi M, et al. Equine chorionic gonadotropin improves the efficacy of a timed artificial insemination protocol in buffalo during the nonbreeding season. Theriogenology. 2013;**79**:423-428. DOI: 10.1016/j.theriogenology.2012.10.013

[35] Malpaux B, Viguié C, Skinner DC, et al. Control of the circannual rhythm of reproduction by melatonin in the ewe. Brain Research Bulletin. 1997;**44**:431-438. DOI: 10.1016/s0361-9230(97)00223-2

[36] Forcada F, Abecia JA, Zúñiga O, et al. Variation in the ability of melatonin implants inserted at two different times after the winter solstice to restore reproductive activity in reduced seasonality ewes. Australian Journal of Agricultural Research. 2002;**53**:167-173. DOI: 10.1071/ar00172

[37] Abecia J, Forcada F, Zuñiga O. The effect of melatonin on the secretion of progesterone in sheep and on the development of ovine embryos in vitro. Veterinary Research Communications. 2002;**26**:151-158. DOI:10.1023/a:1014099719034

[38] Noël B, Mandiki S, Perrad B, Bister J, Paquay R. Terminal follicular growth, ovulation rate and hormonal secretion after melatonin pretreatment prior to FGA-PMSG synchronisation in Suffolk ewes at the onset of the breeding season. Small Ruminant Research. 1999;**32**:269-277. DOI:10.1016/s0921-4488(98)00187-4

[39] Caraty A, Locatelli A, Martin G. Biphasic response in the secretion of gonadotrophin releasing hormone in ovariectomized ewes injected with oestradiol. Journal of Endocrinology. 1989;**123**:375-382. DOI:10.1677/joe.0.1230375

[40] Smith JT, Li Q, Yap KS, Shahab M, Roseweir AK, et al. Kisspeptin is essential for the full preovulatory LH surge and stimulates GnRH release from the isolated ovine median eminence. Endocrinology. 2011;**152**:1001-1012. DOI: 10.1210/en.2007-0554

[41] Smith JT, Clay CM, Caraty A, Clarke IJ. KiSS-1 messenger ribonucleic acid expression in the hypothalamus of the ewe is regulated by sex steroids and season. Endocrinology. 2007;**148**:1150-1157. DOI: 10.1210/en.2006-1435

[42] Kumar A, Mehrotra S, Singh G, Maurya VP, Narayanan K, Mahla AS, Chaudhari RK, Singh M, Soni YK, Kumawat BL, Dabas SK, Srivastava N. Supplementation of slow-release melatonin improves recovery of ovarian cyclicity and conception in summer anoestrous buffaloes (*Bubalus bubalis*). Reproduction in Domestic Animals. 2016;**51**:10-17 DOI: 10.1111/rda.12639

[43] Ghuman SS, Singh J, Honparkhe M, Dadarwal D, Dhaliwal GS, Jain AK. Induction of ovulation of ovulatory size non-ovulatory follicles and initiation of ovarian cyclicity in summer anoestrous buffalo heifers (*Bubalus bubalis*) using melatonin implants. Reproduction in Domestic Animals. 2010;**45**:600-607. DOI: 10.1111/j.1439-0531.2008.01310.x

[44] Misztal T, Romanowicz K, Barcikowski B. Natural and melatonin stimulated changes in the circadian rhythm of prolactin secretion in the ewe during seasonal anestrus. Neuroendocrinology. 1997;**66**:360-367. DOI:10.1159/000127259

[45] Sheth A, Wadadekar K, Moodbidri S, Janakiraman K, Paramesh M. 1978. Seasonal alteration in the serum prolactin and LH levels in the water buffaloes. Current Science. 47:75-77.

[46] Arunji JTK. Non-invasive monitoring of buffalo estrous cycle. M.V. Sc. Thesis Submitted to Deemed to be University IVRI, Izatnagar 2008.

[47] Echternkamp SE, Hansel W. Concurrent changes in bovine plasma hormone levels prior to and during the first postpartum estrous cycle. Journal of Animal Science. 1973;**37**:1362-1370. DOI: 10.2527/jas1973.3761362x

[48] Vázquez M, Forcada F, Sosa C, Casao A, Sartore I, Fernández-Foren A, Meikle A, Abecia J. Effect of exogenous melatonin on embryo viability and uterine environment in undernourished ewes. Animal Reproduction Science. 2013;**141**:52-61. DOI:10.1016/j.anireprosci.2013.07.007

[49] Beard A, Lamming G. Oestradiol concentration and the development of the uterine oxytocin receptor and oxytocin-induced PGF2a release in ewes. Reproduction. 1994;**100**:469-475. DOI:10.1530/jrf.0.1000469

[50] Misztal T, Romanowicz K, Barcikowski B. Melatonin–a modulator of the GnRH/LH axis in sheep. Reproduction Biology. 2002a;**2**:267-275

[51] Rao LV, Pandey RS. Seasonal variations in oestradiol-17b and luteinizing hormone in blood of buffalo cows (Bubalus bubalis). Journal Endocrinology. 1983;**98**:251-255. DOI: 10.1677/joe.0.0980251

[52] Misztal T, Romanowicz K, Barcikowski B. Effect of melatonin on daily LH secretion in intact and ovariectomized ewes during the breeding season. Animal Reproduction Science. 2002b;**69**:187-198. DOI: 10.1016/s0378-4320(01)00194-4

[53] Palta P, Madan ML. Alterations in hypophysial responsiveness to synthetic GnRH at different postpartum intervals in Murrah buffalo (*Bubalus bubalis*). Theriogenology. 1995;**44**:403-411. DOI: 10.1016/0093-691x(95)00194-d

[54] Alam MGS, Dobson H. Pituitary responses to a challenge test of GnRH and oestradiol benzoate in postpartum and regularly cycling cows. Animal Reproduction Science. 1987;**14**:1-9. DOI: 10.1016/0378-4320(87)90071-6

[55] Dholpuria S, Vyas S, Purohit GN, Pathak KML. Sonographic monitoring of early follicle growth induced by melatonin implants in camels and the subsequent fertility. Journal of Ultrasound. 2012;**15**:135-141. DOI: 10.1016/j.jus.2012.02.008

[56] Singh J, Ghuman SPS, Dadarwal D, Honparkhe M, Dhaliwal GS, Jain AK. Estimations of blood plasma metabolites following melatonin implants treatment for initiation of ovarian cyclicity in true anestrus buffalo heifers. Indian Journal Animal Science. 2010;**80**:229-231

[57] Ramadan TA, Sharma RK, Phulia SK, Balhara AK, Ghuman SS, Singh I. Effects of melatonin and controlled internal drug release device treatment on blood metabolites of buffalo heifers during out-of-breeding season under tropical conditions. Egyptian Journal of Animal Production. 2015;**52**(Suppl Issue): 9-17

[58] Zieba DA, Klocek B, Williams GL, Romanowicz K, Boliglowa L, Wozniak M. In vitro evidence that leptin suppresses melatonin secretion during long days and stimulates its secretion during short days in seasonal breeding ewe. Domestic Animal Endocrinology. 2007;**33**:358-365. DOI: 10.1016/j.domaniend.2006.06.004

[59] Darul K, Kruczynska H. Effect of melatonin on biochemical variables of the blood in dairy cows. Acta Veterinaria Hungarica. 2004;**52**:361-370. DOI: 10.1556/avet.52.2004.3.11

[60] Himmelfarb J, Mcmonagle E. Albumin is the major plasma protein target of oxidant stress in uremia. Kidney International. 2001;**60**:358-363. DOI: 10.1046/j.1523-1755.2001.00807.x

[61] Rabiee AR, Lean IJ, Gooden JM, Miller BG, Scaramuzzi RJ. An evaluation of transovarian uptake of metabolites using arteriovenous differences methods in dairy cattle. Animal Reproduction Science. 1997;**48**:9-25. DOI: 10.1016/s0378-4320(97)00032-8

[62] Foster DL, Nagatani S. Physiological perspectives on leptin as a regulator of reproduction: Role in timing puberty. Biology of Reproduction. 1999;**60**:205-215. DOI: 10.1095/biolreprod60.2.205

[63] Randhawa SS, Uppal SK, Randhawa CS, Brar RS, Joshi BP. Haemato-biochemical profile of buffaloes (*Bubalus bubalis*) with leucoderma. Indian Journal Animal Science. 2009;**79**:12-14

[64] Wise T. Biochemical analysis of bovine follicular fluid: albumin, total protein, lysosomal enzymes, ions, steroids and ascorbic acid content in relation to follicular size, rank, atresia classification and day of estrous cycle. Journal of Animal Science. 1987;**64**:1153-1169. DOI: 10.2527/jas1987.6441153x

[65] Mishra OP, Pandey JN, Gawande PG. Study on biochemical constituents of caprine ovarian follicular fluid after superovulation. Asian Australian Journal Animal Science. 2003;**16**:1711-1715. DOI: 10.5713/ajas.2003.1711

[66] Tucker CB, Rogers AR, Schutz KE. Effect of solar radiation on dairy cattle behaviour, use of shade and body temperature in a pasture-based system. Applied Animal Behaviour Science. 2008;**109**:141-154. DOI: 10.1016/j.applanim.2007.03.015

[67] Shimamura K, Sugino N, Yoshida Y, Nakamura Y, Ogino K, Kate H. Changes in lipid peroxide and antioxidant enzyme activities in corpora lutea during pseudopregnancy in rats. Journal of Reproduction Fertility. 1995;**105**:253-257. DOI: 10.1530/jrf.0.1050253

[68] Khan FA, Das GK. Follicular characteristics and intrafollicular concentrations of nitric oxide and ascorbic acid during ovarian acyclicity in water buffalo (*Bubalus bubalis*). Tropical Animal Health and Production. 2012;**44**:125-131. DOI: 10.1007/s11250-011-9898-x

[69] Megahed GA, Alghandour SEM, Othman RH, El-Zohery FA. The relationship between oxidant/antioxidant imbalance and postpartum fertility in cattle. Assiut Veterinary Medical Journal. 2006;**52**:226-240

[70] Jan MH, Das GK, Khan FA, Singh J, Bashir ST, Khan S, et al. Evaluation of follicular oxidant-antioxidant balance and oxidative damage during reproductive acyclicity in water buffalo (*Bubalus bubalis*). Asian Pacific Journal of Reproduction. 2014;**3**:35-40. DOI: 10.1016/s2305-0500(13)60182-7

[71] Ahmed WM, Bashandy MM, Ibrahim AK, Shalaby SIA, El-Moez SIA, El-Moghazy FM, et al. Investigations on delayed puberty in Egyptian buffalo-heifers with emphasis on clinicopathological changes and treatment using GnRH (Receptal). Global Veterinaria. 2010;**4**:78-85

[72] Reiter J, Tan DX, Manchester LC, Qi W. Biochemical reactivity of melatonin with reactive oxygen and nitrogen species: A review of the evidence. Cell Biochemistry and Biophysics. 2001;**34**:247-256

[73] Rodriguez C, Mayo JC, Sainz RM, Antolin I, Herrera F, Martin V, et al. Regulation of antioxidant enzymes: a significant role for melatonin. Journal of Pineal Research. 2004;**36**:1-9. DOI: 10.1046/j.1600-079x.2003.00092.x

[74] Pieri C, Marra M, Moroni F, Recchioni R, Morcheselli F. Melatonin: a peroxyl radical scavenger more effective than vitamin E. Life Science. 1994;**55**: PL271-6. DOI: 10.1016/0024-3205(94)00666-0

[75] Reiter RJ, Manchester LC, Tan DX. Melatonin in walnuts: influence on levels of melatonin and total antioxidant capacity of blood. Nutrition. 2005;**21**:920-924. DOI: 10.1016/j.nut.2005.02.005

[76] Kumar A, Mehrotra S, Singh G, Mourya S, Narayanan K, Singh SK, Soni YK, Singh M, Mahla AS, Srivastava N, Verma MR. Sustained delivery of exogenous melatonin influences biomarkers of oxidative stress and total antioxidant capacity in summer stressed anoestrous water buffalo (*Bubalus bubalis*). Theriogenology. 2015;**83**:1402-1407. DOI: 10.1016/j.theriogenology.2014.12.023

[77] Ahmed WM, El-Khadrawy HH, El Hamed ABD, Amal R, Amer HA. Applied investigations on ovarian inactivity in buffalo heifers. International Journal of Academic Research. 2010;**2**:26

[78] Lucky HS, Gupta S, Kim Y, Agarwal A. Female infertility and antioxidants. Current Women's Health Reviews. 2010;**6**:84-95. DOI: 10.2174/157340410791321381

[79] Reynolds LP, Grazul-Bilska AT, Redmer DA. Angiogenesis in the female reproductive organs: pathological implications. International Journal of Experimental Pathology. 2002;**83**:151-164. DOI: 10.1046/j.1365-2613.2002.00277.x

[80] Rapoport R, Sklan D, Wolfenson D, Shaham-Albalancy A, Hanukoglu I. Antioxidant capacity is correlated with steroidogenic status of the corpus luteum during the bovine estrous cycle. Biochimica et Biophysica Acta. 1998;**1380**:133-140. DOI: 10.1016/s0304-4165(97)00136-0

[81] Sugino N, Takiguchi S, Kashida S, Karube A, Nakamura Y, Kato H. Superoxide dismutase expression in the human corpus luteum during the menstrual cycle and in early pregnancy. Molecular Human Reproduction. 2000;**6**:19-25. DOI: 10.1093/molehr/6.1.19

[82] Laloraya M, Kumar PG, Laloraya MM. Changes in the levels of superoxide anion radical and superoxide dismutase during the estrous cycle of Rattus norvegicus and induction of superoxide dismutase in rat ovary by lutropin. Biochemical and Biophysical Research Communications. 1988;**157**:146-153. DOI: 10.1016/s0006-291x(88)80025-1

[83] Singh J, Ghuman SPS, Cheema RS, Bansal AK. Melatonin implant induces estrus and alleviates oxidative stress in summer anestrus buffalo. Indian Journal of Animal Reproduction. 2016;**37**(2):28-32.

[84] Leon J, Acuna-Castroviejo D, Escames G, Tan DX, Reiter RJ. Melatonin mitigates mitochondrial malfunction. Journal of Pineal Research. 2005;**38**:1-9. DOI: 10.1111/j.1600-079x.2004.00181.x

[85] Rensis FD, Scaramuzzi RJ. Heat stress and seasonal effects on reproduction in the dairy cow—A review. Theriogenology. 2003;**60**:1139-1151. DOI: 10.1016/s0093-691x(03)00126-2

[86] Gimeno N, Landa A, Sterin-Speziale N, Cardinali D, Gimeno A. Melatonin blocks in vitro generation of prostaglandin by the uterus and hypothalamus. European Journal of Pharmacology. 1980;**62**:309-317. DOI:10.1016/0014-2999(80)90098-9

[87] Bojanowska E, Forsling M. The effects of melatonin on vasopressin secretion in vivo: interactions with acetylcholine and prostaglandins. Brain Research Bulletin. 1997;**42**:457-461. DOI: 10.1016/s0361-9230(96)00372-3

5

Melatonin in Childhood Epilepsy and in Child Neurology

Justyna Paprocka, Marek Kijonka and Maria Sokół

Abstract

Melatonin (MLT) was isolated as a hormone by Lerner in 1958, and since then, intense studies have been under way with respect to its action and possibilities of application in various fields of medicine. Despite the existence of multiple antiepileptic medications and progress that has taken place in neurosurgical treatment of epilepsy, drug-resistant epilepsy continues to be a phenomenon that occurs in 30–35% children treated for epileptic seizures. Reports presented in the study have shown that children with epilepsy suffer from sleep disorders. Sleep deprivation may cause seizures, and on the other hand, an increased frequency of seizures may lead to sleep disturbances.

Keywords: melatonin, children, epilepsy, autism, hypoxic-ischemic brain injury

1. Melatonin

The sleep/wake cycle, body temperature, and melatonin (MLT) rhythms have a stable internal phase relationship with maximum sleepiness coinciding with the melatonin excretion peak and the core body temperature nadir in humans and other diurnal species [1]. Several genes known as *clock genes* play a role of regulators of circadian rhythms generated by suprachiasmatic nucleus among them are *PER, NPAS2, BMAL1, and CLOCK* [2]. Also, *Period genes* (*Per1, Per2, Per3*) and *Cryptochrome gene* (*Cry 1, Cry 2*) are involved in auto-regulatory translation-transcription feedback loops [3].

Melatonin, as a hormone, is secreted by the pineal gland, and its production is regulated by light and retino-hypothalamic tract. Melatonin secretion depends on the age—the highest values of its concentration are detected between 1 and 7 years of age. In healthy subjects, the serum melatonin concentration peak occurs between 2 am and 4 am, and then it gradually declines; however, melatonin release may be shifted with time zone due to its day and night light dependence [3–5]. During the day, melatonin is not produced in measurable quantities.

Measurement of the whole 24-h rhythm of melatonin is considered to be the most robust sleep phase marker of various circadian rhythm sleep disorders [1–6]. Because melatonin secretion is suppressed by light, the melatonin levels should be measured in dim light conditions. Serial sampling of melatonin measured in the blood or saliva can be used to assess circadian timing by determining the dim light melatonin onset (DLMO), the parameter indicating the time point in which melatonin levels begin to rise in the evening above baseline [2]. Another useful circadian phase marker is dim light melatonin offset (DLMOff), the point in time when melatonin levels diminish in the morning. The melatonin secretion profile can also be analyzed in a more complex way—by approximation of the empirical or analytical models. The models of melatonin secretion can provide a set of parameters with biophysical and clinical significance that directly characterize melatonin cycle. Moreover, mathematical modeling facilitates statistical analysis of the patients' hormone levels, offering a set of parameters that enable the objectification of the secretion description.

Melatonin for many years remained the most mysterious and forgotten human hormone with not exactly understood role and suggested pleiotropic actions. It is well known that melatonin is released in a circadian pattern with a night peak. Endogenous melatonin production varies among individuals. Endogenous melatonin production varies among individuals. Melatonin is secreted mainly by pinealocytes from tryptophan through hydroxytryptophan and serotonin. Then, two enzymes, arylalkylamine-N-acetyltransferase (AA-NAT) and acetylserotonin-O-methyltransferase (ASMT), form melatonin from serotonin [1–6]. The organization of the sleep-wake rhythm is set around 6 months of age, but melatonin rhythm may be set earlier, from 3 months of age. At the age of 3, a stabilization of these rhythms is visible. Between 4 and 7 years, nocturnal melatonin secretion reaches the highest values [1–6].

Gender difference (a lower melatonin secretion in girls) and age-related decline have been described [7]. According to the latest Task Force of American Academy of Sleep Medicine, melatonin application is recommended in children with delayed sleep-wake phase disorders, children with neurological disorders, and with an irregular sleep cycle [5, 6].

Melatonin should be administered at a time related to DLMO—the onset of melatonin endogenous production [7–9]. Actually, prior to melatonin administration, DLMO should be measured to let for optimal treatment. In saliva, DLMO is defined as a melatonin range of 3–5 pg/ml [9, 10].

2. Sleep and epilepsy

A complex interaction between sleep and epilepsy is still a matter of debate. Sleep deprivation may activate epileptiform activity. Epilepsy *per se* and antiepileptic treatment may cause sleep deprivation or fragmentation causing the vicious circle.

Accumulating evidences suggest that melatonin modulates the electrical activity of neurons. Based on experimental studies, melatonin probably may mediate the GABA-ergic, 5HT-ergic, and NO/L-arginine pathways and glutamate neurotransmission [11]. On the contrary, Steward and Leung suggested that proconvulsive action of melatonin is connected with the suppression of the GABA A receptors in pyramidal cells [12, 13]. Antioxidant properties of melatonin may also have a positive effect on children with epilepsy [14]. Our knowledge about possible melatonin role in epilepsy has increased in recent years but still remains controversial. For some time, melatonin has been recommended for children with epilepsy due to its ability to promote sleep and to avoid sleep deprivation.

Sleep problems in children with developmental disabilities and epilepsy can be connected with an improper deranged circadian melatonin secretion, an insufficient melatonin production, or melatonin receptor insensitivity. Usually, falling asleep and maintain a sleep are the most frequently encountered problems of pediatric populations. The prevalence rates of sleep problems in childhood are estimated between 30 and 40% [15–20].

At the cellular level, sleep deprivation impairs synaptic plasticity, increases hippocampal oxidative stress, and facilitates neuronal loss, which can affect neurocognitive skills especially attention, behavioral, and emotional aspects of development.

In adults with epilepsy, 55% have insomnia, 34% have sleep-onset insomnia, and 52% have maintenance insomnia [15–20]. On nights with seizures, patients experience up to 50% reduction of REM sleep and an increased REM latency [15–20]. In specific childhood epilepsy syndromes, like juvenile myoclonic epilepsy, the sufficient amount of sleep may completely protect from seizures. In autosomal-dominant nocturnal frontal lobe epilepsy, the epileptic seizures dominate at night, while in juvenile myoclonic epilepsy after awakening in the morning.

The stage of sleep also matters. Seizures are rare in REM sleep, and indeed the rate of REM seizures' onset is low (0–5%) [21]. According to the studies conducted by Minecam et al. and Herman et al., most related to sleep seizures appear in stage 2 NREM sleep (61–68%), and lower rates are evident in stages 3 and 4 as 9–14% [19, 21, 22]. Some authors believe that the area of REM discharges could be an indicator of epileptic zone [17–22]. Jan et al. postulated that the occurrence of seizures may show a 24-rhythmicity and circadian occurrence pattern (**Table 1**) [23].

Sleep deprivation is one of the most frequent precipitating factors of seizures and interictal epileptiform discharges (IED). On the other hand, site epileptic seizures, epileptiform activity, or antiepileptic drugs (AEDs) may disrupt sleep pattern. The analysis of the questionnaires filled by the patients revealed that the most common sleep-related complaints are excessive daytime sleepiness (EDS), insomnia, and poor sleep quality. The other important remark is that more sleep abnormalities are concerned with focal than generalized epilepsies. Also, sudden unexpected death in epilepsy (SUDEP) is most frequent to appear between 6 am and noon [17–21]. Long-standing epilepsy can affect insula, anterior cingulated gyrus, ventromedial frontal cortex, and through their influence on cardiac rhythm may provoke SUDEP [16–22].

Antiepileptic drugs (AEDs) may affect sleep parameters. For example, a frequently administrated valproic acid, due to its interaction with GABA transmission at suprachiasmatic nucleus, may lower melatonin secretion [27]. However, Braam et al. [28, 29] compared the endogenous melatonin levels in children administered with valproate and those who did not use it, and

Seizures' occurrence pattern	Sleep	Wakefulness
Seizures' types	Tonic seizures, generalized tonic-clonic seizures, frontal lobe seizures	Clonic, absence, atonic, myoclonic seizures
Relation with sleep	78% of frontal lobe seizures 20% of temporal lobe seizures	
Epilepsy with generalized seizures	Generalized epilepsy • West syndrome: hypsarrhythmia most evident in early NREM sleep • Lennox-Gastaut syndrome: paroxysmal fast activity during sleep	Generalized epilepsy of unknown etiology: JME, GTCE (on EEG spike—waves discharges most prominent in stage 2 sleep)
Epilepsy with focal seizures	BECTS (interictal epileptiform discharges activated by light NREM) • Time peak of occurrence 6–9 am for frontal lobe seizures, NFLE: 23.00–5.00 (6–12 h after DLMO) EEG-stages 3 and 4 as effective facilitator of epileptiform discharges	• Time peak of occurrence 3–6 pm for temporal lobe seizures, TLE: 11.00–17.00 (6 h before DLMO)

Table 1. Seizures' circadian occurrence pattern [23–26].

Takaesu et al. [30] observed a minimal impact of sodium valproate on the low serum levels that do not have such supposition. Carbamazepine may increase slow-wave sleep, reduce REM, and reduce awakenings and arousals [31]. Similarly, lamotrigine and valproic acid appear to stabilize sleep (more REM and slow-wave sleep) [27–31]. Newer AEDs have little effect on sleep architecture (levetiracetam) or little is known about these effects (lacosamide, eliscarbazepine, and retigabine) [31]. The direct effect of AEDs on sleep is difficult to measure because of many confounding factors, with the leading one—polypharmacy. Antiepileptic treatment with more than one drug increases the risk of obstructive sleep apnea (OSA). The prevalence of OSA is significantly higher in the epilepsy group—35% versus healthy children—7.4%. In refractory epilepsy, 44% children have the diagnosis of OSA, in other form of epilepsy around 31% [32, 33]. It is especially important for clinicians, who frequently under-recognize and misinterpret sleep disorders in epilepsy patients.

3. Melatonin secretion in epilepsy

The dynamics of melatonin secretion in epileptic subjects is more complex compared to healthy subjects. Though it appears that human seizure occurrence may have 24-h rhythmicity (and such rhythmicity has also been shown in animals), but there is still no answer to the question on the relationship between the occurrence of seizures and the human circadian rhythm. Many studies on epilepsy have examined the processes that have circadian variation, like hormones secretion, body temperature changes, activity, sleep, and wakefulness, and it is obvious that circadian rhythm and epilepsy at least interact. Unfortunately, there are considerable gaps in the knowledge of such interaction, especially in humans [34].

In epilepsy, melatonin secretion may be disturbed: higher nocturnal melatonin concentrations, a higher melatonin concentration after seizures, or loss/shift of the characteristic diurnal rhythm of secretion are reported by some authors [35–40], while other authors found low baseline levels [41, 42]. Melatonin concentration in patients with epilepsy is sometimes claimed to be slightly increased or unchanged as compared to normal values [38, 43].

However, we observed a statistical dependence between melatonin release amplitude and the number of seizures in different time intervals in the epilepsy of children. Moreover, the time since last seizure has a significant effect on the secretion of melatonin. It should be noted that antiepileptic treatment itself may affect melatonin secretion, which, in fact, was seen in our studies [35, 42]. On the contrary, Dabak et al. showed lower post-seizure melatonin levels in the patients with febrile and afebrile seizures [43]. On the other hand, a normal plasma melatonin curve in epilepsy patients under dim-lit conditions [25] as well as in the study involving epileptic children was found [4].

There is also no agreement between the animal models and the results obtained in the human studies. In animal studies, the data suggest anticonvulsant properties of melatonin, whereas in human studies, it is difficult to reach unambiguous conclusions.

Having in mind the heterogeneity of melatonin secretion and the mode of action in children with epilepsy, Praninskiene et al. postulated that probably not only peripheral melatonin levels but also measurements of melatonin receptors in the brain and melatonin level in central components may be of value [44, 45].

4. Melatonin supplementation in epilepsy in randomized trials

Before the era of randomized trials with melatonin, we witnessed the add-on melatonin supplementation in a few described trials by Peled et al. (improvement in seizures' frequency in five of six children on 3-mg melatonin add-on therapy) [46], Ross et al. (clinical improvement in seizure control and sleep in 20 of 24 children treated with 2.5–7.5 mg of melatonin add-on therapy) [47], and Molina-Carballo et al. (clinical improvement of one child with refractory myoclonic epilepsy treated with melatonin add-on therapy of 200 mg daily) [48].

The first randomized, double-blind, placebo-controlled trial concerning melatonin in epilepsy was conducted in 2004 by Copolla et al. [49]. A total of 25 participants (with mental retardation and epilepsy) aged 3.6–26 years were randomized to oral synthetic fast release melatonin (an initial dose of 3 mg, possible tiltration to 9 mg). In 2 of 11 seizure-free patients, epileptic seizures appeared on melatonin supplementation [49]. Among seven patients with not adequately controlled epilepsy, the results were not promising (N = 1 seizure-free, N = 2 partial improvement, N = 2 unchanged, N = 2 increase of seizures) [49].

In the same year, Gupta et al. assessed the effect of melatonin add-on supplementation in children with epilepsy aged 3–12 years on carbamazepine or valproic acid monotherapy using the parental questionnaire (Sleep Behavior Questionnaire) [50–54]. In these studies, the children were seizure-free for at least 6 months before the first visit; that is why the authors could not report the influence of melatonin on seizures' frequency [50, 51].

In 2005, Hancock et al. in the next randomized, double-blind, crossover trial evaluated melatonin supplementation (two dose regimen: 5 or 10 mg) in 8 patients aged 18 months to 31 years with epilepsy and tuberous sclerosis complex [55, 56]. During the study period of 6 months, no change in seizure frequency was noted at either dose [55, 56].

Goldberg-Stern et al. conducted another trial investigating response to melatonin (10 mg) in 10 patients with a refractory epilepsy aged 9–32 years (N = generalized epilepsy, N = focal epilepsy) [57]. The mean seizure frequency was 7.75 per day on placebo and 4.6 on melatonin treatment [57]. The limitation of this study was the absence of dim light melatonin-onset measurement.

The randomized double-blind placebo-controlled trial performed by Jain et al. showed that a 9-mg sustained release melatonin formulation decreased sleep latency and wakefulness after sleep onset (WASO) as compared to placebo [58]. This group consisted of 10 children aged 6–11 years diagnosed with epilepsy (focal epilepsy N = 6, generalized epilepsy-childhood absence epilepsy N = 3, undetermined N = 1) with intelligence quotient (IQ) > 70 [58]. Melatonin was given for 30 min before bedtime for 9 weeks. Apart from melatonin, children received different antiepileptic drugs as monotherapy: zonisamide, lamotrigine, levetiracetam, oxcarbazepine, and carbamazepine. According to the authors of the study, no worsening in seizures frequency was observed. Eight participants remained seizure-free, and another two experienced 50% reduction in seizure frequency on melatonin treatment.

Elkhayat et al. in a group of 23 children with refractory epilepsy and in 14 children with controlled seizures (aged 2–15 years) measured melatonin level and assessed the sleep parameters before and after melatonin supplementation (melatonin dose of 1.5–3 mg daily) [59]. The most frequent antiepileptic drug was valproic acid (in intractable epilepsy in 78.2% of patients, in controlled seizures group—85.7%) [59]. After 3 months of melatonin therapy, children with intractable epilepsy experienced improvement in sleep continuity (bedtime resistance, sleep duration, sleep latency, frequent nocturnal arousals, and excessive daytime sleepiness), sleep apnea, nocturnal enuresis, sleep walking, forcible teeth grinding, and Epworth sleepiness score. Melatonin diurnal secretion and the frequency of seizures in controlled seizures group and refractory epilepsy did not differ significantly. Some children experience a decreased severity of seizures.

There are some significant limitation of the abovementioned studies like the small sample size and lack of the homogeneity of the sample: diversity of the epilepsy syndromes, different etiology of seizures, different seizure types, and short period of observation. But treating epilepsy with antiepileptic drugs may also improve sleep architecture and restore sleep cycle. The very limited number of randomized studies did not allow to draw definite conclusions about melatonin add-on therapy and influence of the treatment on epileptic seizures.

5. Melatonin in attention-deficit/hyperactivity disorder (ADHD)

About 25–50% of children with ADHD experience sleep problems [60]. The frequency of sleep problems is almost two-fold higher in a case of stimulant treatment. Sleep disturbances are included among diagnostic criteria for ADHD in the DSM third edition.

Miano et al. distinguished five sleep phenotypes in ADHD [61, 62]:

1. phenotype related to hypoarousal state, primary form of ADHD;
2. phenotype related to delayed sleep phase syndrome;
3. phenotype related to sleep-disordered breathing (SDB) from snoring to obstructive sleep apnea;
4. phenotype related to restless leg syndrome and/or periodic limb movements;
5. phenotype related to sleep epilepsy and/or EEG interictal epileptic discharges.

The most common complaint is sleep-onset insomnia, and rarely, sleep problems are related to a delayed sleep phase syndrome. Also, SDB is highly associated with disturbed attention and hyperactivity, and children with SDB are more sensitive to oxidative stress [61–63].

Based on trials conducted in this population, melatonin treatment in doses ranging between 3 and 6 mg/day may reduce sleep-onset delay and increased sleep duration time [61–63].

6. Melatonin in autism spectrum disorders (ASDs)

Autistic spectrum disorders are frequently connected with sleep disturbances (30–53% or up to 50–80%) [64, 65]. The most common medication used in sleep difficulties is melatonin, apart from behavioral interventions.

In children with autistic spectrum disorders, melatonin levels are lower [65–67] or within normal values [64, 68, 69]. Based on parental questionnaires and clinician completed forms of 1518 ASD children aged 4–10 years, Braam et al. informed about a much higher percentage of sleep problems in ASD (71%) and a higher necessity of drug intake (>46% children on more than one drug promoting sleep) [29]. In the latest double-blind study conducted by Gringras et al., 125 ASD children (among them 3.2% children with the diagnosis of Smith-Magenis syndrome (SMS)) received prolonged-release melatonin or placebo for 13 weeks [70]. Melatonin treatment prolonged the total sleep time (melatonin 57.5 min vs. placebo 9.14 min) and decreased sleep latency (melatonin 39.6 min vs. placebo 12.5 min) [70]. Veatch et al. studied the possible genetic background of sleep problems in ASD by evaluation of two melatonin pathway genes: acetylserotonin O-methyltransferase (ASMT) and cytochrome P450 1A2 (CYP1A2) [68]. The authors found a higher prevalence of variants responsible for a decreased expression of ASMT and a lower CYP1A2 enzyme activity [68]. On the other hand, a lower CYP1A2 enzyme activity may be responsible for slow metabolism and the possibility of lack of efficacy of exogenous melatonin with time. That is why some children may benefit from low melatonin dose like 0.5 mg rather than higher (exceeding 5–6 mg) [64, 65, 71, 72].

Some authors speculate that melatonin as a hormone derived from serotonin may be of a special interest in autism neurobiology [73]. Another interesting finding is that melatonin levels may be negatively correlated with the severity of autistic features. This assumption was made by the examination of sulfatoxymelatonin level in urine of 60 mothers of a child with ASD features and in control group.

A few RDBPC trials showed that melatonin may improve communication [74] and anxiety in children with ASD [75]. Based on the knowledge from placebo-controlled studies, long-acting melatonin preparations at bedtime improve the sleep latency and the total sleep time [67, 69, 70, 74, 76–80].

7. Melatonin in other neurodevelopmental disabilities (NDDs)

Reported prevalence of sleep disturbances in children with neurodevelopmental disabilities is up to 86% [81]. An interesting double-masked randomized placebo-controlled phase III trial was performed by Gringras et al. One hundred and forty-six children aged 3–15 years were treated with melatonin (0.5–12 mg) or placebo for 12 weeks [82]. In melatonin-treated group, the total sleep time increased by 23 min and sleep latency was reduced by around 38 min [82].

Melatonin may be affective in sleep problems in many genetic syndromes, especially in Angelman syndrome (AS), Smith-Magenis syndrome (SMS), Rett syndrome (RS), San Filippo syndrome, and tuberous sclerosis complex syndrome (TSCS) [83–90]. In these genetic conditions, sleep problems are one of the phenotype features. Sleep apnea is a frequent finding in children with Down syndrome and with Prader-Willi syndrome [83–91].

The results of Hancock et al. on the urinal 6-sulfatoxymelatonin excretion in seven TSCS patients revealed, however, no evidence of abnormal excretion of melatonin in patients with tuberous sclerosis complex and sleep disorder [55, 56, 83, 92]. All but one of the patients showed a normal circadian rhythm of melatonin secretion. However, the authors were aware that a small number of analyzed cases weakened their reasoning. Our investigations suggest that not only disordered sleep but also the shift of melatonin secretion may be expected in TSCS children with frequent seizures [88]. We also noticed that melatonin profiles are not homogeneous in TSCS patients [88]. Unfortunately, both researchers supposition are based on the results gathered from a small TSCS group.

Children with Angelman syndrome may present with sleep-onset insomnia as well as sleep maintenance problems, and low endogenous melatonin levels are often claimed to be an essential feature of melatonin secretion in their circadian rhythms [83–90]. Our studies with mathematical modeling of melatonin secretion showed that the phase parameters of melatonin cycle (DMLO parameters, phase or duration of melatonin amplitude) could be the key characteristic of AS children [87].

The recommended melatonin dose in Angelman syndrome is very small like 0.3–0.5 mg, because of the high prevalence of slow melatonin metabolizers [90]. In TSCS, a decreased sleep total time and multiple awakenings are evident; the recommended dose of melatonin is 5–10 mg. Melatonin may reduce the sleep problems (the frequent awakenings) in Rett syndrome in the daily dose of 2.5–7.5 mg [83–85, 92]. Children with SMS have an early sleep onset (19.30–20.30), repeated and prolonged walking at night, and an early sleep offset (04:00–05.00) [91].

Because of inverted melatonin circadian profile, a complex but promising treatment was found: a combination of acebutolol in the morning (10 mg/kg decrease melatonin level during the day) and melatonin in the evening [91].

During the conference in Rome in 2014, Bruni et al. postulated recommendation for melatonin treatment guidelines in children with neurodevelopmental disabilities and insomnia [15]:

1. no age limit (safe administration >6 months of age),
2. if used as a chronobiotic 3–4 hs before bedtime (if used as a sleep inductor 30 min before sleep time) with starting dose 0.2–0.5 mg (tiltrated by 0.2–0.5 mg every week till maximum dose of 3 (<40 kg) and 5 mg (>40 kg),
3. treatment duration should not be <1 month, therapy adjusted to the patient; if normal sleep cycle is restored 1 week without melatonin treatment, once a year is recommended (especially during summer).

8. Melatonin in hypoxic-ischemic brain injury

During the last decade, melatonin has started to be considered as an attractive option in order to minimize the neurological sequelae from hypoxic-ischemic brain injury [93–95]. The brain itself is particularly sensitive to free radicals damage due to its high utilization of oxygen, its relatively poorly developed antioxidant defense, and its high amount of easily oxidizable fatty acids. Melatonin may serve as a potential therapeutic free radical scavenger (hydroxyl radicals, hydrogen peroxide, singlet oxygen) and broad-spectrum antioxidant (upregulation of antioxidant pathways: superoxide dismutase, glutathione, catalase, glutathione peroxidase, glutathione reductase) [96–98]. Based on experimental studies, melatonin may increase the number of neurons in the CA1, CA2–CA3 areas and dentate gyrus of the hippocampus and parietal cortex, reduce the expression of the glial fibrillary acidic protein, and regulate the expression of myelin basic protein and oligodendrocytes' function (regulation of myelination process) [96–98].

Aly et al. examined the effect of melatonin on clinical, biochemical, neurophysiological, and radiological outcomes of neonates with hypoxic-ischemic encephalopathy (HIE) [99]. They performed a prospective trial involving 45 newborns randomized in the hypothermia alone and hypothermia and melatonin groups. All infants were studied with repeated EEG and brain MRI. In all patients, superoxide dismutase (SOD) and nitric oxide (NO) were measured. These examinations showed an increased melatonin and a decreased NO in the hypothermia-melatonin group [99]. Because of postulated unpredicted bioavailability of oral melatonin, Merchant et al. gave blood transfusion of 0.04–0.6 μg/kg melatonin to 18 preterm babies (less than 31 weeks gestation, less than 7 days old) for 2 h [100]. As a result they found melatonin concentration peak similar to adults. Another challenge might be the possibility to administer melatonin antenatally, in order to prevent or reduce brain hypoxic insult in preterm babies [94]. Denihan et al. employed untargeted metabolomics to identify metabolomic biomarkers of umbilical cord blood after hypoxic injury [101]. The analysis was performed using direct injection FT-ICR mass spectrometry. Some metabolites allowed for differentiation between children with perinatal asphyxia with recovery and children with perinatal asphyxia followed by hypoxic-ischemic encephalopathy like melatonin leucine, kynurenine, and 3-hydroxydodecanoic acid. HIE itself was associated with abnormalities in tryptophan and pyrimidine metabolism.

Children after hypoxia-ischemia brain injury often develop circadian rhythm disorders. Yang et al. documented that in experimental studies, mRNA and protein expression of pineal arylalkylamine N-acetyltransferase (AANAT) and melatonin are impaired after hypoxic damage [102]. They postulated that miR-325-3p (micro RNA) may play a role of potential down-regulator of AANAT-rate-limiting enzyme for melatonin synthesis [102].

9. Conclusions

Melatonin may be effective not only in primary sleep disorders but also in some above-mentioned neurological disorders in children. In adults, postulated antioxidative potential of melatonin may be of value in neurodegenerative diseases like Parkinson, Alzheimer, and Huntington's disease [98].

Because disturbed circadian rhythms and poor sleep quality are associated with increased risks of cardiovascular, metabolic, and cognitive diseases, poor quality of life, and even with mortality, exogenously administered melatonin is often claimed to be a remedy for all these problems. However, many conflicting results obtained in various areas of research on the functions and roles of melatonin require caution and the extension of basic research [103–108]. First of all further standardized studies of the human circadian rhythm and of its disturbances affecting melatonin rhythms by interfering with its production and secretion are necessary, as well as the studies of the interaction between circadian rhythm and seizures in animal models. Moreover, the melatonin role in epilepsy and the effects of antiepileptic drug treatment (in relation to the circadian rhythm phases) should be explored. As concerning exogenous melatonin application, larger study groups are required to identify proper therapeutic dosage regarding age, concrete disease, and to check the clinical efficacy of melatonin add-on therapy.

Filling up the gaps in the knowledge about the interactions of circadian rhythm, human epilepsy, and melatonin will improve our understanding of the undergoing processes and the patients' treatment quality.

Author details

Justyna Paprocka[1]*, Marek Kijonka[2] and Maria Sokół[2]

*Address all correspondence to: justyna.paprocka@interia.pl

1 Department of Child Neurology, School of Medicine in Katowice, Medical University of Silesia, Katowice, Poland

2 Department of Medical Physics, Maria Skłodowska-Curie Memorial Cancer Center and Institute of Oncology, Gliwice Branch, Poland

References

[1] Lack L, Wright HR. Chronobiology of sleep in humans. CMLS. 2007;**64**:1205-1215

[2] Barnard AR, Nolan PM. When clocks go bad: Neurobehavioural consequences of disrupted circadian timing. PLoS Genetics. 2008;**30**:1-8

[3] Tordjman S, Chokron S, Delorme R, Charrier A, Bellissant E, Jaafari N, Fougerou C. Melatonin: Pharmacology, functions and therapeutic benefits. Current Neuropharmacology. 2017;**15**:434-443

[4] Brzezinski A. Melatonin in humans. The New England Journal of Medicine. 1997;**3363**: 186-195

[5] Lewy AJ, Sack RL, Blood ML, Bauer VK, Cutler NL, Thomas KH. Melatonin marks circadian phase position and resets the endogenous circadian pacemaker in humans. Ciba Foundation Symposium. 1995;**183**:303e17 [discussion 317e21]

[6] Zisapel N. New perspectives on the role of melatonin in human sleep, circadian rhythms and their regulation. British Journal of Pharmacology. 2018. DOI: 10.1111/bph.14116

[7] Lewy AJ, Sack RL, Singer CM. Immediate and delayed effects of bright light on human melatonin production: Shifting "dawn" and "dusk" shifts the dim light melatonin onset (DLMO). Annals of the New York Academy of Sciences. 1985;**453**:253-259

[8] Lewy AJ, Sack RL. The dim light melatonin onset as a marker for circadian phase position. Chronobiology International. 1989;**6**:93-102

[9] Mandrell BN, Avent Y, Walker B, Loew M, Tynes BL, Crabtree VM. In home salivary melatonin collection: Methodology for children and adolescents. Developmental Psychobiology. 2018;**60**:118-122

[10] Keijzer H, Smits MG, Peeters T, Looman CW, Endenburg SC, Gunnewiek JM. Evaluation of salivary melatonin measurements for dim Light Melatonin onset calculations in patients with possible sleep-wake rhythm disorders. Clinica Chimica Acta. 2011;**17**:417-418

[11] Tchekalarova J, Moyanova S, De Fusco A, Ngomba RT. The role of the melatoninergic system in epilepsy and comorbid psychiatric disorders. Brain Research Bulletin. 2015; **119**:80-92

[12] Stewart LS. Endogeneous melatonin and epileptogenesis: Facts and hypothesis. The International Journal of Neuroscience. 2001;**107**:77-85

[13] Steward LS, Leung LS. Hippocampal melatonin receptors modulate the seizure threshold. Epilepsia. 2005;**46**:473-480

[14] Reiter R, Tan DX, Rosales-Corral S, Galano A, Zhou XJ, Xu B. Mitochondria: Central organelles for melatonin's antioxidant and anti-aging actions. Molecules. 2018;**23**:509. DOI: 10.3390/molecules23020509

[15] Bruni O, Alonso-Alconada D, Besag F, Biran V, Braam W, Cortese S, Mooavero R, Parisi P, Smits M, van der Heijden K, Curatolo P. Current role of melatonin in pediatric neurology: Clinical recommendations. European Journal of Paediatric Neurology. 2015;**19**:122-133

[16] Hofstra WAE, de Weerd AW. The circadian rhythm and its interaction with human epilepsy: a review of literature. Sleep Medicine Reviews. 2009;**13**:413-420

[17] Van Golde E, Gutter T, de Weerd AW. Sleep disturbances in people with epilepsy: Prevalence, impact and treatment. Sleep Medicine Reviews. 2011;**15**:357-368

[18] Derry CP, Duncan S. Sleep and epilepsy. Epilepsy & Behavior. 2013;**26**:394-404

[19] Minecan D, Natarajan A, Marzec M, Malow B. Relationship of epileptic seizures to sleep stage and sleep depth. Sleep. 2002;**25**:899-904

[20] Foldvary-Schaefer N, Grigg-Damberg M. Sleep and epilepsy: What we know, don't know, and need to know. Journal of Clinical Neurophysiology. 2006;**23**:4-20

[21] Herman JH. Circadian rhythm disorders in pediatrics. Pediatric Annals. 2008;**37**:488-495

[22] Herman ST, Walczak TS, Bazil CW. Distribution of partial seizures during the sleep-wake cycle: Differences by seizures onset site. Neurology. 2001;**56**:1453-1459

[23] Jain SV, Kothare SV. Sleep and epilepsy. Seminars in Pediatric Neurology. 2015;**22**:86-92

[24] Hofstra WA, Grootemarsink BE, Dieker R, van der Palen J, de Weerd AW. Temporal distribution of clinical seizures over 24-hour day: A retrospective observational study in tertiary epilepsy clinic. Epilepsia. 2009;**50**:2019-2026

[25] Pavlova MK, Shea SA, Scheer FAJL, Bromfield EB. Is there a circadian variation of epileptiform abnormalities in idiopathic generalized epilepsy? Epilepsy & Behavior. 2009;**16**: 461-467

[26] Gogou M, Haidopoulou K, Eboriadou M, Pavlidou E, Hatzistylianou M, Pavlou E. Sleep respiratory parameters in children with idiopathic epilepsy: A cross-sectional study. Epilepsy Research. 2016;**126**:10-15

[27] Monteleone P, Tortorella A, Borriello R, Natale M, Cassandro P, Maj M. Suppression of nocturnal plasma melatonin levels by evening administration of sodium valproate in healthy humans. Biological Psychiatry. 1997;**41**:336-341

[28] Braam W, Smits MG, Didden R, Korzilius H, Van Geijlswijk I, Curfs LMG. Exogenous melatonin for sleep problems in individuals with intellectual disability: a meta-analysis. Developmental Medicine and Child Neurology. 2009;**51**:340-349

[29] Braam W, Ehrhart F, Maas APHM, Smits MG, Curfs L. Low maternal melatonin level increases autism spectrum disorder risk in children. Research in Developmental Disabilities. 2018 Feb 28. DOI: 10.1016/j.ridd.2018.02.017

[30] Takaesu Y, Futenma K, Kobayashi M, Komada Y, Tanaka N, Yamashina A, Inoue Y. A preliminary study on the relationships between diurnal melatonin secretion profile and sleep variables in patients emergently admitted to the coronary care unit. Chronobiology International. 2015;**32**:875-879

[31] Bazil CW. Effects of antiepileptic drugs on sleep structure: Are the drugs equal? CNS Drugs. 2003;**17**:719-728

[32] Urquhart DS, Kehinde OO, Mclellan AE. Observational pilot study of reported symptoms of obstructive sleep apnoea in children with epilepsy. Developmental Medicine and Child Neurology. 2016;**58**:1063-1068

[33] Accardo JA, Malow BA. Sleep, epilepsy, and autism. Epilepsy & Behavior. 2015;**47**:202-206

[34] Wytske A, Hofstra WAE, de Weerd AW. How to access the circadian rhythm in humans: A review of the literature. Epilepsy & Behavior. 2008;**13**:438-444

[35] Paprocka J, Rec R, Marszał E. Melatonin and childhood refractory epilepsy- a pilot study. Medical Science Monitor. 2010;**16**:CR389-CR396

[36] Paprocka J, Marszał E. Melatonina w neurologii. Klinika Pediatryczna. 2007;**15**:432-437

[37] Schapel GJ, Beran RG, Kennaway DL, McLoughney J, Matthews CD. Melatonin response in active epilepsy. Epilepsia. 1995;**36**:75-78

[38] Molina-Carballo A, Munoz-Hoyos A, Rodrıguez-Cabezas T. Acuña-Castroviejo D. Day-night variations in melatonin secretion by the pineal gland during febrile and epileptic convulsions in children. Psychiatry Research. 1994;**52**:273-283

[39] Molina-Carballo A, Munoz-Hoyos A, Sanchez-Forte M, Uberoz-Fernandez J, Moreno-Madrid F, Acuna-Castroviejo D. Melatonin increases following convulsive seizures may be related to its anticonvulsant properties at physiological concentrations. Neuropediatrics. 2007;**38**:122-125

[40] Waldhauser F, Kovács J, Reiter E. Age-related changes in melatonin levels in humans and its potential consequences for sleep disorders. Experimental Gerontology. 1998;**33**:759-772

[41] Bazil CW, Short D, Crispin D, Zheng W. Patients with intractable epilepsy have low melatonin, which increases following seizures. Neurology. 2000;**55**:1746-1748

[42] Paprocka J, Kijonka M, Pęcka M, Sokół M. Melatonin in Epilepsy: A New Mathematical Model of Diurnal Secretion. International Journal of Endocrinology. 2016;**2016**:3861461. DOI: 10.1155/2016/3861461

[43] Dabak O, Altun D, Arslan M, Yaman H, Vurucu S, Yesilkaya E, Unay B. Evaluation of plasma melatonin levels in children with afebrile and febrile seizures. Pediatric Neurology. 2016;**57**:51-55

[44] Praninskiene R, Dumalakienie I, Kemezys R, Mauricas M, Jucaite A. Melatonin secretion in children with epilepsy. Epilepsy & Behavior. 2012;**25**:315-322

[45] Praninskiene R, Dumalakienie I, Kemezys R, Mauricas M, Jucaite A. Diurnal melatonin patterns in children: Ready to apply in clinical practice? Pediatric Neurology. 2012;**46**:70-76

[46] Peled N, Shorer Z, Peled R, Pillar G. Melatonin effect on seizures in children with severe neurologic deficit disorders. Epilepsia. 2001;**43**:1208-1210

[47] Ross C, Davies P, Whitehouse W. Ross Melatonin treatment for sleep disorders in children with neurodevelopmental disorders: An observational study. Developmental Medicine and Child Neurology. 2002;**44**:339-344

[48] Molina-Carballo A, Muñoz-Hoyos A, Reiter RJ, Sánchez-Forte M, Moreno-Madrid F, Rufo-Campos M, Molina-Font JA, Acuña-Castroviejo D. Utility of high doses of melatonin as adjunctive anticonvulsant therapy in a child with severe myoclonic epilepsy: Two years' experience. Journal of Pineal Research. 1997;**23**:97-105

[49] Coppola G, Iervolino G, Mastrosimone M, La Torre G, Ruiu F, Pascotto A. Melatonin in wake-sleep disorders in children, adolescents and young adults with mental retardation with or without epilepsy: A double-blind, crossover, placebo-controlled trial. Brain & Development. 2004;**26**:373-376

[50] Gupta M, Gupta YK, Anieja AS, Kohli K. Effects of add-on melatonin on sleep in epileptic children on carbamazepine monotherapy: A randomized placebo controlled trial. Sleep and Biological Rhythms. 2004;**2**:215-219

[51] Gupta M, Anieja S, Kohli K. Add-on melatonin improves quality of life in epileptic children on valproate monotheraphy: a randomized, double-blind, placebo-controlled trial. Epilepsy & Behavior. 2004;**5**:316-321

[52] Gupta M, Gupta YK, Agarwal S, Anieja S, Kalaivani M, Kohli K. Effects of add-on melatonin administration on antioxidant enzymes in children with epilepsy taking carbamazepine monotherapy: A randomized, double-blind, placebo-controlled trial. Epilepsia. 2004;**45**: 1636-1639

[53] Gupta M, Kohli K, Gupta YK. Modulation of serum concentrations of melatonin by carbamazepine and valproate. Indian Journal of Physiology and Pharmacology. 2006;**50**: 79-82

[54] Gupta M, Anieja S, Kohli K. Add-on melatonin improves sleep behavior in children with epilepsy: Randomized, double-blind, placebo-controlled trial. Journal of Child Neurology. 2005;**20**:112-115

[55] Hancock E, O'Callaghan F, English J, Osborne JP. Melatonin excretion in normal children and in tuberous sclerosis complex with sleep disorder responsive to melatonin. Journal of Child Neurology. 2005;**20**:21-25

[56] Hancock E, O'Callaghan F, Osborne JP. Effect of melatonin dosage on sleep disorder in tuberous sclerosis complex. Journal of Child Neurology. 2005;**20**:78-80

[57] Goldberg-Stern H, Oren H, Peled N, Garty BZ. Effect of melatonin of seizures frequency in intractable epilepsy: A pilot study. Journal of Child Neurology. 2012;**27**:1524-1528

[58] Jain SV, Horn PS, Simakajornboon N, Beebe DW, Holland K, Byars AW, Glauser TA. Melatonin improves sleep in children with epilepsy: A randomized, double-blind crossover study. Sleep Medicine. 2015;**16**:637-644

[59] Elkhayat HA, Hassanein SM, Tomoum HY, Abd-Elhamid IA, Asaad T, Elwakkad AS. Melatonin and sleep-related problems in children with intractable epilepsy. Pediatric Neurology. 2010;**42**:250-254

[60] Cortese S, Brown TE, Corkum P, Gruber R, O'Brien LM, Stein M, Weiss M, Owens J. Assessment and management of sleep problems in youths with attention-deficit/hyperactivity disorder. Journal of the American Academy of Child and Adolescent Psychiatry. 2013;**52**:784-796

[61] Miano S, Parisi P, Villa MP. The sleep phenotypes of attention deficit hyperactivity disorder: The role of arousal during sleep and implications for treatment. Medical Hypotheses. 2012;**79**:147-153

[62] Miano S, Esposito M, Foderaro G, Ramelli GP, Pezzoli V, Manconi M. Sleep-related disorders in children with attention-deficit hyperactivity disorder: Preliminary results of a full sleep assessment study. CNS Neuroscience & Therapeutics. 2016;**22**:906-914

[63] Um YH, Hong S-C, Jeong J-H. Sleep problems as predictors in attention-deficit hyperactivity disorders: Causal mechanisms, consequences and treatment. Clinical Psychopharmacology and Neuroscience. 2017;**15**:9-18

[64] Goldman SE, Adkins KW, Calcutt MW, Carter MD, Goodpaster RL, Wang L, Shi Y, Burgess HJ, Hachey DL, Malow BA. Melatonin in children with autism spectrum disorders, endogenous and pharmacokinetic profiles in relation to sleep. Journal of Autism and Developmental Disorders. 2014;**44**:2525-2535

[65] Liu X, Hubbard JA, Fabes RA, Adam JB. Sleep disturbances and correlates of children with autism spectrum problems. Child Psychiatry and Human Development. 2006;**37**: 179-1991

[66] Krakowiak P, Goodlin-Jones B, Hertz-Picciotto I, Croen LA, Hansen RI. Sleep problems in children with autism spectrum disorders, developmental delays, and typical development: A population-based study. Journal of Sleep Research. 2008;**17**:197-206

[67] Tordjman S, Najjar I, Bellissant E, Anderson GM, Barburoth M, Cohen D, Jaafari N, Schischmanoff O, et al. Advances in the research of melatonin in autism spectrum disorders. International Journal of Molecular Sciences. 2013;**14**:20508-20542

[68] Veatch OJ, Pendergast JS, Allen MJ, Leu RM, Johnson CH, Elsea SH, Malow BA. Genetic variation in melatonin pathway enzymes in children with autism spectrum disorder and comorbid sleep onset delay. Journal of Autism and Developmental Disorders. 2015;**45**: 100-110

[69] Veatch OJ, Goldman SE, Adkins KW, Malow BA. Melatonin in children with autism spectrum disorders: how does the evidence fit together? Journal of Natural Sciences. 2015;**1**:125

[70] Gringras P, Nir T, Breddy J, Frydman-Maron A, Findling RL. Efficacy and safety of pediatric prolonged-release melatonin form insomnia in children with autism spectrum disorder. Journal of the American Academy of Child and Adolescent Psychiatry. 2017;**56**: 948-957

[71] Malow BA. The interaction between sleep and epilepsy. Epilepsia. 2007;**48**:36-38

[72] Jones C, Huyton M, Hindley D. Melatonin and epilepsy. Archives of Disease in Childhood. 2005;**90**:1203

[73] Mazzone L, Postorino V, Siracusano M, Riccioni A, Curatolo P. The relationship between sleep problems, neurobiological alterations, core symptoms of autism spectrum disorder, and psychiatric comorbidities. Journal of Clinical Medicine. 2018;**7**:102. DOI: 10.3390/jcm7050102

[74] Wright B, Sims D, Smart S, Alwazeer A, Alderson-Day B, Allgar V, Whitton C, Tomlinson H, Bennett S, Jardine J, McCaffrey N, Leyland C, Jakeman C, Miles J. Wright Melatonin versus placebo in children with autism spectrum conditions and severe sleep problems not amenable to behaviour management strategies: A randomised controlled crossover trial. Journal of Autism and Developmental Disorders. 2001;**41**:175-184

[75] Wasdell MB, Jan JE, Bomben MM, Freeman RD, Rietveld WJ, Tai J, Hamilton D, Weiss MD. A randomized, placebo-controlled trial of controlled release melatonin treatment of delayed sleep phase syndrome and impaired sleep maintenance in children with neurodevelopmental disabilities. Journal of Pineal Research. 2008;**44**:57-64

[76] Guenole F, Godbout R, Nicolas A, Franco P, Claustrat B, Baleyte JM. Melatonin for disordered sleep in individuals with autism spectrum disorders: Systematic review and discussion. Sleep Medicine Reviews. 2011;**15**:379-387

[77] Hellmer K, Nystrom P. Infant acetylcholine, dopamine, and melatonin dysregulation: Neonatal biomarkers and causal factors for ASD and ADHD phenotypes. Medical Hypotheses. 2017;**100**:64-66

[78] Kotagal S, Broomall E. Sleep in children with autism spectrum disorder. Pediatric Neurology. 2012;**47**:242-251

[79] Andersen IM, Kaczmarska J, McGrew SG, Malow BA. Melatonin for insomnia in children with autism spectrum disorders. Journal of Child Neurology. 2008;**23**:482-485

[80] Cuomo BM, Vaz S, Lee EAL, Thompson C, Rogerson JM, Falkmer T. Effectiveness of sleep-based interventions for children with autism spectrum disorder: A meta-synthesis. Pharmacotherapy. 2017;**37**:555-578

[81] Robinson-Shelton A, Malow BA. Sleep disturbances in neurodevelopmental disorders. Current Psychiatry Reports. 2016;**18**:6

[82] Gringras P, Gamble C, Jones AP, Wiggs ML, Williamson PR, Sutcliffe A, Montgomery P, Whitehouse WP, Choonara I, Allport T, Edmond A, Appleton R, MENDS Study Group. Melatonin for sleep problems in children with neurodevelopmental disorders: Randomized double masked placebo controlled trial. BMJ. 2012;**345**:6664

[83] Schwichtenberg AJ, Malow BA. Melatonin treatment in children with developmental disabilities. Sleep Medicine Clinics. 2015;**10**:181-187

[84] Checa-Ros A, Munoz-Gallego A, Munoz-Gallego M, Molina-Carballo A, Narbona-Galdo S, Jerez-Calero A, Augustin-Morales MDC, Munoz-Hoyos A. Clinical considerations derived from the administration of melatonin to children with sleep disorders. Pediatric Neurology. 2018;**78**:61-69

[85] Appleton RE, Jones AP, Gamble C. The use of melatonin in children with neurodevelopmental disorders: Randomized double masked placebo controlled, parallel study (MENDS). Health and Technology Access. 2012;**16**:1-239

[86] Spruyt K, Braam W, Smits M, Curfs LMG. Sleep complaints and the 24-h melatonin level in individuals with Smith-Magenis syndrome: Assessment for effective intervention. CNS Neuroscience & Therapeutics. 2016;**22**:928-935

[87] Paprocka J, Kijonka M, Wojcieszek P, Pęcka M, Emich-Widera E, Sokół M. Melatonin and Angelman syndrome – implications and mathematical model of diurnal secretion. International Journal of Endocrinology. 2017;(**2017**), Article ID 5853167. DOI: 10.1155/2017/5853167

[88] Paprocka J, Kijonka M, Boguszewicz Ł, Sokół M. Melatonin in Tuberous Sclerosis Complex Analysis Using Modern Mathematical Modeling Methods. International Journal of Endocrinology. 2017;**2017**:8234502. DOI: 10.1155/2017/8234502

[89] Sheldon S. Proconvulsant effects of oral melatonin in neurologically disabled children. Lancet. 1988;**351**:1254

[90] Takaesu Y, Komada Y, Inoue Y. Melatonin profile and its relationship to circadian rhythm sleep disorders in Angelman syndrome patients. Sleep Medicine. 2002;**13**:1164-1170

[91] Spruyt K, Braam W, Smits M, Curfs LMG. Sleep complaints and the 24-h melatonin level in individuals with Smith-Magenis syndrome: Assessment for effective intervention. CNS Neuroscience & Therapeutics. 2016;**22**:928-935

[92] Bruni O, Angriman M, Calisti F, Comandini A, Esposito G, Cortese S, Ferri R. Practitioner review: Treatment of chronic insomnia in children and adolescent with neurodevelopmental disabilities. The Journal of Child Psychology and Psychiatry. 2018;**59**:489-508

[93] Alonso-Alconada D, Alvarez A, Martinez-Ibarguen A, Hilario E. Neuroprotective effect of melatonin: A novel therapy against perinatal hypoxia-ischemia. International Journal of Molecular Sciences. 2013;**14**:9379-9395

[94] Biran V, Phan Duy A, Decobert F, Bednarek N, Alberti C, Baud O. Is melatonin ready to be used in preterm infants as a neuroprotectant? Developmental Medicine and Child Neurology. 2014;**568**:717-723

[95] Hendaus M, Jamha FA, Alhammadi A. Melatonin in the management of perinatal hypoxic-ischemic encephalopathy: Light at the end of the tunnel? Neuropsychiatric Disease and Treatment. 2016;**12**:2473-2479

[96] Hassell KJ, Ezzati M, Alonso-Alconada D, Hausenloy D, Robertson NJ. New horizons for newborn brain protection: Enhancing endogeneous neuroprotection. Archives of Disease in Childhood. Fetal and Neonatal Edition. 2015;**100**:F541-F552

[97] Martinello K, Hart AR, Yap S, Mitra S, Robertson NJ. Management and investigation of neonatal encephalopathy: 2017 update. Archives of Disease in Childhood. Fetal and Neonatal Edition. 2017;**102**:F346-F358

[98] Muller AJ, Marks JD. Hypoxic ischemic brain injury: Potential therapeutic interventions for the future. NeoReviews. 2014;**15**:177-186

[99] Aly H, Elmahdy H, El-Dib M, Rowisha M, Awny M, El-Gohary T, Elbatch M, Hamisa M, El-Mashad AR. Melatonin use for neuroprotection in perinatal asphyxia: A randomized controlled pilot study. Journal of Perinatology. 2015;**35**:186-191

[100] Merchant NM, Azzopardi DV, Hawwa AF, McElnay JC, Middleton B, Arendt J, Arichi T, Gressens P, Edwards AD. Pharmacokinetics of melatonin in preterm infants. British Journal of Clinical Pharmacology. 2013;**76**:725-733

[101] Deniham NM, Kirwan JA, Walsh BH, Dunn WB, Broadhurst DI, Boylan B, Murray DM. Untargeted metabolomic analysis and pathway discovery in perinatal asphyxia and hypoxic-ischaemic encephalopathy. JCBFM. 2017:1-16

[102] Yang Y, Sun B, Huang J, Xu L, Pan J, Fang C, Li M, Li G, Tao J, Xang X, Wu Y, Miao P, Wang Y, Li H, Ren Y, Zhan M, Fang Y, Feng X, Ding X. Up-regulation of miR-325-3p suppresses pineal aralkylamine N-acetyltransferase (Aanat) after neonatal hypoxia-ischemia brain injury in rats. Brain Research. 1668;**2017**:28-35

[103] Yalyn O, Arman F, Erdogan F, Kula M. A comparison of the circadian rhythms and the levels of melatonin in patients with diurnal and nocturnal complex partial seizures. Epilepsy & Behavior. 2006;**8**:542-546

[104] Ardura J, Anders J, Garmendia JR, Ardura F. Melatonin in epilepsy and febrile seizures. Journal of Child Neurology. 2010;**25**:888-891

[105] Fauteck J, Schmidt H, Lerch A, Kurlemann G, Witkowski W. Melatonin in epilepsy: First results of replacement therapy and first clinical results. Biological Signals and Receptors. 1999;**8**:105-110

[106] Laakso MI, Leinonen L, Haltonen T, Alila A, Heiskala H. Melatonin, cortisol, and body temperature rhythm in Lennox-Gastaut patients with and without circadian rhythm sleep disorders. Journal of Neurology. 1993;**240**:410-416

[107] Rao ML, Stefan H, Bauer J. Epileptic but not psychogenic seizures are accompanied by simultaneous elevation of serum pituitary hormones and cortisol levels. Neuroendocrinology. 1989;**49**:33-39

[108] Uberos J, Augustin-Morales MC, Molina Carballo A, Florido J, Narbona E, Muñoz-Hoyos A. Normalization of the sleep-wake pattern and melatonin and 6-sulphatoxy-melatonin levels after a therapeutic trial with melatonin in children with severe epilepsy. Journal of Pineal Research. 2011;**50**:192-196

6

An Overview of Melatonin as an Antioxidant Molecule: A Biochemical Approach

Aysun Hacışevki and Burcu Baba

Abstract

Melatonin is an endogenous hormone derived from tryptophan that is mainly released from the pineal gland in the dark. Melatonin regulates many biological functions such as sleep, circadian rhythm, immunity, and reproduction. Melatonin has a free radical scavenger, anti-inflammatory, and antioxidant effects. It scavenges reactive oxygen and nitrogen species and increases antioxidant defenses, thus it prevents tissue damage and blocks transcriptional factors of pro-inflammatory cytokines. Due to its small size and amphiphilic nature, it increases the efficacy of mitochondrial electron transport chain and reduces electron leakage. Melatonin prevents degenerative changes in the central nervous system in models of Alzheimer's and Parkinson's disease and reduces free radical damage to DNA which may lead to cancer and many other situations. Consequently, melatonin has beneficial effects including stimulation of antioxidant enzymes, inhibition of lipid peroxidation, and so it contributes to protection from oxidative damages.

Keywords: melatonin, antioxidant, free radical, oxidative stress, anti-inflammatory, neurohormone, tryptophan, disease

1. Introduction

Melatonin, N-acetyl-5-methoxytryptamine, which was first isolated from bovine pineal glands [1], is an endogenous neurohormone derived from tryptophan [2]. Melatonin controls various physiologic processes, including circadian rhythms, mood regulation, anxiety, sleep, appetite, immune responses, and cardiac functions [3]. The sleep–wake cycle is the most overt circadian rhythm [4]. More or less sleep shows negative effects on biological and physiological processes including alterations in metabolic, endocrine, and immune pathways that lead to health problems involving obesity, diabetes, hypertension, and respiratory diseases [4–6]. Timing of melatonin secretion is closely associated with the timing of sleep propensity, and it also coincides with decreases in core body temperature, alertness, and performance [7]. Melatonin regulates memory formation by directly affecting hippocampal neurons. There are antinociceptive, antidepressant, anxiolytic, antineophobic, and locomotor activity regulating effects of melatonin [3, 8]. Melatonin plays important roles in neurogenesis, neuroprotection, maintenance of oxidant/antioxidant balance, modulation of cardiovascular and/or immune system, and diabetes control. It exerts a direct antioxidant effect on tissues/organs and antiapoptotic effects on cells [9]. Other actions of melatonin include inhibition of dopamine release in the hypothalamus and retina, involvement in the aging process and pubertal development, blood pressure control, and free radical scavenging [7]. Melatonin dysfunction may contribute to many divergent diseases, such as neurodegenerative diseases, circadian and mood disorders, insomnia, type 2 diabetes, and pain [3]. Low levels of melatonin have been shown in Parkinson's disease (PD), Alzheimer's disease (AD), insomnia, epilepsy, ischemic injury, and neuropsychiatric disorders; in addition, roles for melatonin in the development of cataracts, aging, and retinitis have also been reported [10]. Melatonin has been utilized in several countries for circadian rhythm disorders, sleep disturbances, jet lag, and sleep–wake cycle disturbances in blind people and shift workers [7, 11, 12].

Melatonin is secreted primarily by the pineal gland in response to darkness [2, 13, 14]. It was later found to be also present or synthesized in extrapineal sites such as retina, Harderian gland, lymphocytes, gastrointestinal tract, bone marrow cells, platelets and skin [13, 15–17]. The neurohormone melatonin is not stored in the pineal gland but rather is released into the bloodstream and can penetrate all body tissues [18]. The synthesis of melatonin shows a clear circadian rhythm with low levels during the daytime and its secretory peak at night [19, 20]. The nocturnal synthesis and release of melatonin by the pineal gland are strictly controlled by the suprachiasmatic nucleus (SCN) clock and inhibited by lighting conditions [19, 21]. In humans and other mammals, detection of light drives activity in retinal ganglion cells that project to the SCN in the hypothalamus, causing the release of inhibitory γ-amino butyric acid that suppresses the circuit controlling melatonin synthesis and release [22]. Serum melatonin reaches a peak value (80–150 pg/mL) between midnight and 3 a.m., while its concentration during the day is low (10–20 pg/mL) [23]. Both normal melatonin patterns and the influence of light can vary considerably between individuals, either in terms of personal characteristics or as a consequence of aging or a chronic disease [24]. Serum concentrations of melatonin vary considerably with age, and infants secrete very low levels of melatonin before 3 months of age. Amplitude of the nocturnal peak in melatonin secretion reaches the highest levels between the 4th and 7th year of age [15, 19]. Other factors that alter melatonin levels are nightwork, impaired light–dark cycles, and obesity. Additionally, some nutritional factors could change melatonin production [13].

Melatonin, hormone of darkness, is synthesized from tryptophan, which is an essential amino acid by the pineal gland. The synthesis of melatonin is a multistep process. Firstly, tryptophan is hydroxylated by tryptophan-5-hydroxylase (TPH) to form 5-hydroxytryptophan, which is subsequently decarboxylated to 5-hydroxytryptamine (serotonin) by L-aromatic amino acid decarboxylase (AADC). Serotonin is N-acetylated by arylalkylamine N-acetyltransferase (AA-NAT, also called "Timezyme," is the rate-limiting enzyme for melatonin synthesis), to form N-acetylserotonin, which is converted to N-acetyl-5-methoxytryptamine (melatonin) by N-acetylserotonin-O-methyltransferase (ASMT, also called hydroxyindole-O-methyltransferase or HIOMT). The last step is the rate-limiting step in the biosynthesis of melatonin (**Figure 1**) [18, 20, 25–28].

Melatonin synthesis depends on intact beta-adrenergic receptor function. Norepinephrine activates the N-acetyltransferase, and beta-receptor blockers depress melatonin secretion [29]. Both AA-NAT and ASMT activities are controlled by noradrenergic and neuropeptidergic projections to the pineal gland. The pineal gland receives input from postganglionic fibers, leading to the release of norepinephrine. Norepinephrine induces its $\alpha 1/\beta$-adrenoceptors that activate adenylate cyclase-cAMP system. Thus, intracellular levels of the second messengers include cAMP, Ca^{2+}, phosphatidylinositol, diacetylglycerol, and protein kinase C increase. These messengers induce the expression and activity of AA-NAT and HIOMT [7, 14, 15, 18, 30].

The pineal gland is located outside the blood brain barrier, and loses it connections with the central nervous system, having sympathetic innervation as its main source. This may explain for the pineal gland ability to have a large uptake of tryptophan leading to a high melatonin production and secretion in response to darkness [18]. Once synthesized, melatonin is quickly released into the systemic circulation to reach central and peripheral target tissues. The effects of melatonin depend on the localization and types of melatonin receptors [15]. Melatonin activates two high-affinity G-protein-coupled receptors, termed MT1 and MT2. The MT1 and MT2 lead to an inhibition of the adenylate cyclase in target cells and regulate a variety of cellular and physiological processes including neuronal firing, arterial vasoconstriction, cell proliferation, immune responses, and reproductive and metabolic functions [8, 16, 27, 31–33]. MT1 and MT2 receptors are 350 and 362 amino acids long, located on chromosome 4q35.1 and chromosome 11q21-q22, respectively. MT1 receptors are expressed in the brain, cardiovascular system, immune system, testes, ovary, skin, liver, kidney, adrenal cortex, placenta, breast, retina, pancreas, and spleen. MT2 has been found in the immune system, brain, retina, pituitary, blood vessels, testes, kidney, gastrointestinal tract, mammary glands, adipose tissue, and the skin [27, 31, 32]. The MT3 receptor has a low affinity, unlike MT1 and MT2; it is not coupled to G proteins; it has a nanomolar affinity for melatonin, and it is not sensitive

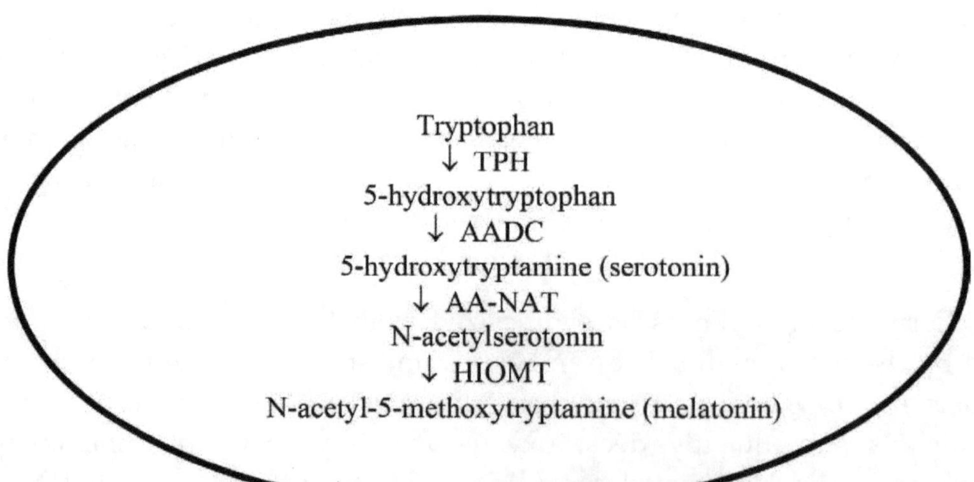

Figure 1. Biosynthesis of melatonin from tryptophan (TPH, tryptophan-5-hydroxylase; AADC, L-aromatic amino acid decarboxylase; AA-NAT, arylalkylamine N-acetyltransferase; HIOMT, hydroxyindole-O-methyltransferase).

to Na^{+2}, Mg^{+2}, and Ca^{+2}. The MT3 is equivalent to enzyme quinone reductase II [27]. The relationship between multiple physiological function of melatonin and this enzyme is possibly involved in the regulation of cellular redox status, although the exact role of this relationship remains unclear [16, 34]. Melatonin appears to be a natural ligand for the retinoid-related orphan nuclear hormone receptor family (RZR/ROR). RZR/RORα is expressed in a variety of organs, whereas RZRβ is specific for the brain and retina [35]. In addition, melatonin interacts with intracellular proteins such as calmodulin, calreticulin, or tubulin and antagonizes the binding of Ca^{2+} to calmodulin [7]. ROR/RZR has been proposed to work in coordination with the plasma membrane receptors MT1/MT2 to regulate gene expression. The low-affinity interaction between melatonin and calmodulin may be involved in its antioxidant action as well as other signaling processes [15, 16]. The membrane receptors have been defined in the central nervous system and in peripheral organs, such as liver, gastrointestinal tract, skin, kidney, heart, and adipose and lymphoid tissues in many mammalians [33]. Melatonin also acts through nonreceptor-mediated mechanisms, for example, serving as a scavenger for reactive oxygen species (ROS) and reactive nitrogen species (RNS) [27]. Melatonin and its metabolites have potent antioxidative and radioprotective properties [36]. Melatonin has been proven to be an efficient oxidant scavenger of a variety of radical and nonradical reactants [37].

In the circulation, melatonin is partially bound to albumin and can also bind to hemoglobin [38]. Melatonin metabolism is a rapid process, and its half-life in humans varies between 10 and 60 min following exogenous administration. It is deactivated mostly by the liver and excreted in the urine [13, 26]. There are three major pathways of melatonin degradation: (1) the classical hepatic degradation pathway that generates 6-hydroxymelatonin, (2) the alternative indolic pathway that produces 5-methoxyindole acetic acid (5-MIAA) or 5-methoxytryptophol (5-MTOL), and (3) the kynurenic pathway that produces the main brain metabolites of melatonin, N1-acetyl-N2-formyl-5-methoxykynuramine (AFMK), and its deformylated product N1-acetyl-5-methoxykynuramine (AMK). These metabolites are highly remarkable and are generated enzymatically, pseudoenzymatically, by free radical, and via photochemical processes. Recently, it was reported that AFMK and AMK detoxify reactive species and preserve tissues from damage by reactive intermediates [39]. This chapter summarizes effects of melatonin and its metabolites as antioxidants and their clinical significance in several diseases.

2. Free radicals

Free radicals are atoms or molecules that containing one or more unpaired electrons in the external orbitals of the molecules, usually unstable and highly reactive. The free radical chemical reactivity is directly associated with the damage that they can inflict to biological molecules. In biology system, oxygen-derived radicals and nitrogen-derived radicals are two types of free radicals. Oxygen-derived radicals, such as superoxide ($O_2^{\bullet -}$), hydroxyl radicals ($OH^{\bullet}$), alkoxyl radicals ($RO^{\bullet}$), as well as nonradicals such as hydrogen peroxide (H_2O_2), ozone and hypochlorous acid, are defined as reactive oxygen species (ROS). ROS are produced during the oxygen metabolism. Nitrogen-derived radicals and nonradicals, such as nitrogen dioxide (NO_2), nitric oxide radicals ($NO^{\bullet}$), and peroxynitrite (ONOO), are known as reactive nitrogen species (RNS) which are derived from nitric oxide and superoxide by inducible nitric oxide synthase (iNOS) and NADPH oxidase, respectively [16, 40–44]. Oxidants are produced as a result of normal intracellular metabolism in mitochondria and peroxisomes, as well as from diverse cytosolic enzyme systems such as lipoxygenases, NADPH oxidase, and cytochrome P450. Furthermore, various external agents including ionizing radiation, ultraviolet light, environmental toxins, inflammatory, and cytokines can trigger ROS production [16, 44]. Mitochondria are the major source of ROS and RNS production [45]. Generation of $O_2^{\bullet -}$ during oxidative phosphorylation takes place mainly in the mitochondria. $O_2^{\bullet -}$ is quickly converted to H_2O_2 enzymatically by superoxide dismutases (SODs). After that, H_2O_2 is converted into water or highly toxic hydroxyl radical [16]. Although hydroxyl radical formation can occur in several ways, by far the most important mechanism in vivo is likely to be the transition metal-catalyzed decomposition of superoxide anion and hydrogen peroxide [46]. Hydroxyl radicals are generated from hydrogen peroxide during cellular oxygen metabolism via the Fenton and Haber-Weiss reactions (**Figure 2**) [47], in the presence of free iron or copper ions [48]. The $OH^{\bullet}$ is formed during the Fenton reaction when H_2O_2 interacts with transition metals (Fe^{2+}, Cu^{1+}, etc.) [16, 40, 41]. It can also be produced by ultraviolet and ionizing radiations [41].

Alkoxyl radicals that are formed from the reduction of peroxides, are less reactive than $OH^{\bullet}$ and significantly more reactive than ROO radicals, provided that R is the same in both species. Therefore, they are suggested to be ideal candidates to evaluate the efficiency of antioxidants and also the reactivity of any species reacting with ROS. As regards RNS, the chemical reactivity and direct toxicity of $NO^{\bullet}$ are quite low. However, it reacts with $O_2^{\bullet -}$ forming peroxynitrite, which is a powerful oxidant. NO_2 is a mild oxidant, and its reactivity is between those of $NO^{\bullet}$ and $ONOO^-$ [41, 42, 44].

In healthy organisms, there is a delicate balance between the production and the removal of free radicals, which guarantees that they remain in low/moderate concentrations. Under such conditions, free radicals have beneficial effects [41]. ROS and RNS play important roles in regulation of a wide variety of physiology functions like gene expression, cellular growth, differentiation, modulation of chemical reactions, and induction of transcription factors such as nuclear factor-kappa B (NF-κB) and activator protein-1 (AP-1) and activation of signal transduction pathways. They also participate in blood pressure control, are mediators in the biosynthesis of prostaglandins, function in embryonic development, and act as signaling molecules within the individual cell and among cells during their life span [44–46]. The harmful and useful effects of ROS/RNS are associated with their concentrations, the cell type and the subcellular compartments that are produced, and their timing of production [16]. An imbalance between excessive ROS and RNS generation and rate of their elimination by the antioxidant capacity leads to oxidative stress [49, 50]. It has been shown that oxidative stress is involved in over 100 diseases, as their cause or consequence [51]. Oxidative stress results in macromolecular damage and is implicated in various disease states such as atherosclerosis, diabetes, cancer, neurodegeneration, and aging [52]. The cellular dysfunctions caused by excessive ROS and/or RNS might produce loss of energy metabolism, altered cell signaling

$$Fe^{2+} + H_2O_2 \text{ -> } Fe^{3+} + OH^- + OH^{\bullet -} \text{ (Fenton reaction)}$$

$$O_2^{\bullet -} + H_2O_2 \text{ -> } O_2 + OH^- + OH^{\bullet -} \text{ (Haber-Weiss reaction)}$$

Figure 2. Fenton and Haber-Weiss reactions.

and cell cycle, gene mutations, and impaired cellular transport mechanisms. The oxidative stress promotes decreased biological activities, immune activation, and inflammation [50]. It seems that both high levels of ROS (oxidative stress) and excessively low levels of ROS (reductive stress) are deleterious and apparently play a causative role in the pathologies caused by malfunctioning processes related to the dramatic change of redox environment [53].

3. Antioxidants

Based on the oxidative stress related to free radical theory, the antioxidants are the first line of choice to take care of the stress [45]. Antioxidants act as free radical scavengers and can prevent oxidative reactions that lead to various diseases [54]. The antioxidant defense system includes endogenous (enzymatic and nonenzymatic) and exogenous (dietary) antioxidants that interact in establishing redox homeostasis in the body [49]. Endogenous antioxidants, which are products of the body's metabolism, may be enzymatic or nonenzymatic compounds localized generally in the cytoplasm and diverse cell organelles [45, 49]. In eukaryotics, various antioxidant enzymes, for instance, SOD, catalase (CAT), and some peroxidases, transform ROS into more stable molecules (e.g., water and O_2) via complex cascade of reactions [45]. One of the most effective intracellular enzymatic antioxidants is SOD. In humans, there are three forms of SOD: cytosolic CuZn-SOD, mitochondrial Mn-SOD, and extracellular SOD. SOD catalyzes the dismutation of $O_2^{\bullet-}$ to H_2O_2, decreasing the amount of $O_2^{\bullet-}$ and thereby lowering the formation of $ONOO^-$ [44, 50]. Other important enzymatic antioxidants include CAT, glutathione peroxidase (GPx), glutathione reductase (GR), and peroxiredoxins (Prxs). These enzymes neutralize hydrogen peroxide, yielding water (CAT, GPx) and oxygen molecule (CAT) [45, 49]. CAT which is found in the peroxisomes and cytoplasm [55] presents a molecule of ferric ion at its active site and converts two molecules of H_2O_2 into one molecule each of water and diatomic oxygen [37]. Glutathione peroxidase can be found in many subcellular compartments including the mitochondria and nucleus depending on the family member [55]. Selenium, as a selenocysteine, is a component of the active site of GPx [37, 55, 56]. GPx uses reduced glutathione (GSH) as a substrate to transfer electrons to H_2O_2 (and other peroxides), thereby converting it into two molecules of water [37]. When hydrogen peroxide is metabolized by glutathione peroxidase, reduced glutathione is oxidized to glutathione disulfide (GSSG) which is converted back to GSH by the enzyme GR [57–59].

Small molecular nonenzymic antioxidants (e.g., GSH, NADPH, thioredoxin, vitamin E (α-tocopherol), vitamin C (ascorbic acid), and trace metals, such as selenium) also function as direct scavengers of ROS [45]. In particular, glutathione plays a central role in defense against oxidative stress [54]. The antioxidant properties of GSH which is a tripeptide, γ-L-glutamyl-L-cysteinyl-glycine, depend on the presence of a peptide bond between the amino group of cysteine and the alpha-carboxyl group, which provide an excellent protection against aminopeptidases, and the expression of the thiol group which derive from the cysteine residue. Complexation of metal ions, participation in the oxidation reactions, and formation of thiol radicals and disulfides are the most important functions of thiol groups in the biological systems [49]. Maintaining or reestablishment of redox homeostasis are ensured by endogenous and exogenous antioxidants that act synergistically [49, 60], such as during the regeneration of vitamin E by GSH or vitamin C to prevent lipid peroxidation, which can affect membrane fluidity and damage membrane proteins [60, 61]. Vitamin E and Vitamin C are the most frequently used antioxidant vitamins [62] that are thought to have a protective effect by either reducing or preventing oxidative damage [63]. Vitamin E belongs to the group of fat-soluble vitamins existing in eight different forms. The methylation pattern of the chroman ring determines the classification as α, β, γ, and δ tocopherols. These compounds have antioxidant properties. Vitamin E scavenges peroxyl radicals and hence acts to break the chain reaction of lipid peroxidation [64]. Besides its antioxidant role, vitamin E might also have a structural role in stabilizing membranes [46, 65, 66]. Vitamin C, which is readily water soluble, is an important antioxidant and thus works in aqueous environments of the body [46, 57, 67]. As an antioxidant, ascorbate is an efficient scavenger, or reducing antioxidant, capable of donating its electrons to ROS and eliminating them [44]. Loss of one electron generates the ascorbyl radical intermediate, and loss of two electrons generates dehydroascorbate (DHA, which can also be formed via dismutation of the ascorbyl radical) [61, 68]. It makes ascorbate a powerful important antioxidant [44]. Vitamin C serves as a co-antioxidant with vitamin E to regenerate α-tocopherol from α-tocopherol radicals in membranes and lipoproteins and protect protein thiol group against oxidation by increasing intracellular levels of GSH [46, 61, 69]. Vitamin C can also neutralize ROS (e.g., hydrogen peroxide) [46, 70]. Recently, toxicity of ascorbic acid has also been attributed to its autoxidation [45].

An efficient antioxidant should not only be ubiquitous but should also be present in adequate amounts in cells and easily reacts with a wide variety of free radicals which have short half-life due to high reactivity. A good antioxidant has the ability to cross physiologic barriers and to be quickly transported into the cells. Thus, it must be available to all cells. It is also important for an antioxidant to be available. Antioxidants should be available when needed. They should be easily acquired through the diet or produced in situ. Antioxidants should be suitable for regeneration. The reaction between an antioxidant and a free radical yields an oxidized form of the antioxidant which has less scavenging activity than the original compound. Therefore, many antioxidants have physiologically reducing mechanisms, or its oxidized forms can still efficiently react with new free radicals. An ideal antioxidant should be conserved by the kidneys. Otherwise, large urinary losses would occur and the half-life will be short. An important aspect to consider for evaluating the suitability of a compound as an antioxidant is its toxicity. It should be nontoxic prior to and after the free radical scavenging process takes place. In addition, it is also important to be aware of possible interactions with any drug that may be concurrently consumed [41, 71, 72].

Melatonin is a potent direct scavenger of free radicals. Unlike most of other radical scavengers, it is a multifunctional antioxidant. Melatonin can easily pass through cell membranes because of its high lipophilicity and hydrophilicity [73]. Melatonin is also widespread within cells. Its concentrations in human serum and cerebrospinal fluid vary widely. Melatonin is endogenously generated, and it is ingested in the food as it is widely available in fruits and vegetables. Hence, melatonin is produced internally and is also ingested in the diet. Only small amounts of melatonin are excreted into the urine in its unchanged form. It has minimal toxicity. Numerous in vivo studies on animals involving massive doses of melatonin have shown that acute and chronic toxicity of melatonin is extremely low [41, 74]. Unlike most small molecule biological antioxidants such as ascorbic acid, α-tocopherol, lipoic acid, etc., melatonin does not undergo redox cycling and, thus, does not promote oxidation. Melatonin can be considered a suicidal or terminal antioxidant. It undergoes molecular rearrangement, effectively removing the free electron from the system. Each of these products of rearrangement is also a potent antioxidant in its own right. Furthermore, most of these processes involve more than one ROS per step, so that one melatonin molecule has the capacity to scavenge up to 10 ROS versus the classic antioxidants that scavenge one or less ROS [17, 20, 70, 74]. It has been found that melatonin promotes the repair of oxidized DNA. This is probably due to the melatonin's capability of transforming guanosine radical to guanosine by electron transfer [42]. It was shown that melatonin reduced the formation of 8-hydroxy-2'-deoxyguanosine (8-OH-dG), a damaged DNA product, 60–70 times more effective than some classic antioxidants (ascorbate and α-tocopherol) [75]. Additionally, the relative position of melatonin and its metabolites in the antioxidant "pecking order" (electrochemical potential) may contribute greatly to its utility in biological systems [76]. Melatonin protects lipids, proteins, and nuclear DNA from oxidative damage suggests that its intracellular distribution is wide [17]. Melatonin turned out to be considerably more efficient than the majority of its naturally occurring structural analogs, indicating that the substituents of the indole moiety strongly influenced reactivity and selectivity [77].

4. Melatonin and its metabolites as antioxidants

Melatonin is an indoleamine with two side chains, a 5-methoxy group and 3-amide group. Its molecular weight is 232.2 g/mol [42]. Melatonin has multifunctional activities in addition to its function as a synchronizer of the biological clock and seasonal reproduction [78, 79]. One such activity is its antioxidant capacity. Melatonin and its metabolites were found to have important antioxidant properties owing to their direct and indirect antioxidant actions. Melatonin can easily cross cell membranes [80] and the blood brain barrier [78] and protects various biomolecules against damage caused by free radicals by acting as a direct scavenger to detoxify reactive oxygen and nitrogen species. In addition, melatonin can indirectly reduce oxidative stress by increasing the activities of antioxidative defense systems; stimulating the expression and function of a number of antioxidant enzymes, as well as glutathione, another very important nonenzymatic, low molecular weight antioxidant; interacting synergistically with other antioxidants; and increasing the efficiency of the mitochondrial electron transport chain [40, 78–82]. Also, melatonin has a chelating property which may contribute in reducing metal-induced toxicity [83]. Melatonin was shown to be much more specific than its structural analogs in undergoing reactions, which lead to the termination of the radical reaction chain and in avoiding prooxidant, C- or O-centered intermediates [33, 38]. Moreover, it has been shown that it has an ability to scavenge free radicals, including hydroxyl radicals, hydrogen peroxide, peroxyl radicals, singlet oxygen, nitric oxide, and peroxynitrite. It was demonstrated that melatonin inhibits the activity of NO synthase, beside it's NO and peroxynitrite scavenging activity [84].

Melatonin, an endogenously produced indoleamine, is a highly effective antioxidant and free radical scavenger [82]. Melatonin has been reported to neutralize the most toxic oxidizing agents, hydroxyl radical and the peroxynitrite anion, generated within the cells. Moreover, melatonin reportedly scavenges singlet oxygen ($^1O_2$), superoxide anion radical, hydrogen peroxide, nitric oxide, and hypochlorous acid (HClO) [17]. Due to the electron-deficient nature of halide ions, haloperoxyl radicals are significantly more reactive than the alkylperoxyl radical; accordingly, the trichloromethylperoxyl radical ($CCl_3OO^•$) was found to be potently trapped by melatonin [85]. Not only melatonin but also several of its metabolites that are formed when it functions as a direct free radical scavenger, i.e., cyclic 3-hydroxymelatonin (c3OHM), AFMK, AMK, etc., are also radical scavengers [57, 86]. Melatonin and its metabolites work in a "task-division" way, with some of them acting mainly as free radical scavengers, while others act as metal chelating agents and inhibitors of the hydroxyl radical ($OH^•$) production [87]. The sequential scavenging of ROS by melatonin and its metabolites is known as melatonin's antioxidant cascade [16]. The efficiency of AMK for scavenging ROS and preventing protein oxidation has been reported to be higher than that of AFMK. Therefore, it seems that at least in general, their protective activities against oxidative stress follow the order AMK > melatonin > AFMK [88] (**Table 1**).

4.1. Effects of melatonin and its metabolites on reactive oxygen species

Electron donation is the principal mechanism by which melatonin detoxifies the free radicals [17]. While melatonin has the capability of donating one or more electrons to free radicals resulting in their detoxification, the metabolites that are formed during this process, i.e., c3OHM, AFMK, and AMK, also have similar capabilities [90]. After donating an electron to $OH^•$, melatonin becomes a free radical itself, the indolyl radical cation. However, its reactivity is very low, and, therefore, it is not toxic to cells [41]. Oxidation of melatonin by hydroxyl radicals leads to several hydroxylated products which can be explained by interaction of melatonin with two hydroxyl radicals, one acting by hydrogen abstraction and the other by combining with the reaction partner especially, at the sides C2, C3, C6, and C7 [91].

6-Hydroxymelatonin (6OHM) is the major hepatic metabolite and photodegradation product of melatonin. It is an efficient metabolite for protecting against oxidative damage induced by UV irradiation. Due to its capability of scavenging $^1O_2$ and $O_2^{•-}$, 6OHM can reduce neurotoxicity induced by quinolinic acid. It also lowers Fe(II)-induced neurotoxicity and iron-induced lipid peroxidation. It also inhibits the oxidative damage induced by this metal, UV radiation, thiobarbituric acid, and cyanide. It may be more efficient than melatonin in this capacity. Moreover, it inhibits oxidative stress induced by Cu^{+2}-ascorbate mixtures and $OH^•$ production by sequestering Cu^{+2} ions. 6OHM also protects DNA damage induced by Fenton reagents and UV radiation [84, 92].

It was showed that the main hydroxylated metabolite of melatonin interaction with hypochlorous acid is 2-hydroxymelatonin (2OHM). Subsequently, 2OHM and its keto tautomer, melatonin 2-indolinone, were the oxidative products of melatonin's interaction with oxoferryl hemoglobin or $OH^•$ [93]. 4-Hydroxymelatonin (4OHM) is an excellent peroxyl radical scavenger and also a preventing antioxidant by inhibiting Cu(II). This effect would reduce the Cu(I) availability, which is the redox state required for the $OH^•$ to be formed, via Fenton-like reactions. 4OHM terminates the oxidant effects of copper-ascorbate mixtures. The key structural feature in the antioxidant activity of 4OHM is the presence of phenolic group, unlike 2OHM which has a relative low antioxidant protection [94]. 4OHM and 2OHM are generated during the UV-induced metabolism of melatonin. Further investigation needs to understand the antioxidant activity of these two compounds, as well as their potential role in protecting biomolecules against oxidative damage [87].

ROS/RNS neutralized by melatonin and its metabolites	Antioxidative enzymes that are stimulated by melatonin
Hydroxyl radical	Superoxide dismutase
Hydrogen peroxide	Glutathione peroxidase
Superoxide anion radical	Catalase
Nitric oxide	Glutathione reductase
Alkoxyl radical	Glutamyl-cysteine ligase
Peroxynitrite	Cyclooxygenase
Singlet oxygen	Heme oxygenase
Hydrogen peroxide	Nitric oxide synthase
Hypochlorous acid	Paraoxonase
Others	Myeloperoxidase
	Lipoxygenase

Table 1. Antioxidant effects of melatonin and its metabolites [89].

7-Hydroxymelatonin has been rarely considered, although the calculated activation energy for the respective reaction is as low as that for 6-hydroxylation. 3-Hydroxylation leads to an unusual compound cyclic 3-hydroxymelatonin (c3-OHM) [91]. c3-OHM is an intermediate metabolite of melatonin [16]. c3-OHM effectively scavenges $OH^{\bullet}$, $ABTS^{\bullet+}$ (2,20-azino-bis(3-ethylbenzthiazoline-6-sulphonic acid)) [95], and peroxyl radicals [96] and can also chelate Cu(II), preventing its reduction and the consequent $OH^{\bullet}$ production via Fenton-like reactions [93, 97]. It is demonstrated that c3-OHM inhibits oxidative DNA damage and 8-OHdG lesions, induced by Fenton reagents, under in vitro conditions [98]. Indeed, c3-OHM is considered a footprint molecule, excreted in small amounts in the urine, and evidence of the in vivo scavenging activity of melatonin [41]. c3-OHM also undergoes oxidation resulting in the formation of AFMK [16, 77, 99].

AFMK is one of the metabolites of melatonin and can be formed by both enzymatic or pseudoenzymatic and nonenzymatic metabolic pathways [10, 88]. Pyrole ring cleavage of melatonin by varied enzymes including indoleamine 2,3-dioxygenase (IDO), myeloperoxidase (MPO), and hemoperoxidases, varied pseudoenzymatic catalysts such as oxoferryl hemoglobin and in varied reactions with ROS involving free radicals and singlet oxygen, generates AFMK [39, 88, 100]. Melatonin oxidation by MPO and IDO generally requires $O_2^{\bullet-}$ that produced in large amounts in inflammatory circumstances [100]. Besides, there are also multiple hydroxylations, which are formed in the peroxidase and peroxidase-like reactions and in the conversion of c3-OHM to AFMK [39]. Nonenzymatically, direct reaction of melatonin with highly reactive oxygen species (e.g., hydroxyl radical and singlet oxygen) formed AFMK [100]. The formation of AFMK by singlet oxygen deserves attention, as this reactive oxygen species is formed under the influence of UV light [101]. In light of these findings, it appears that AFMK is a product common to several interactions of melatonin with oxygen-based reactants [85]. The generation of AMK occurs via deformylation of AFMK [10, 16, 77]. These compounds are also major melatonin metabolites in detoxifying ROS and reducing oxidative stress

[10, 16]. AFMK is obviously more stable than many other oxidative metabolites or its secondary product, AMK [39]. AFMK reduces lipid peroxidation and oxidative DNA damage induced by a variety of oxidative stressors under various conditions [16]. It protects neuronal cell from injuries caused by hydrogen peroxide and amyloid-β (Aβ) peptide [85, 88, 93]. It has been suggested that neuroprotection of AFMK against radiation-induced oxidative damage to the brain is due to its free radical scavenging function [88].

Lipid peroxidation is a natural metabolic process under normal aerobic conditions, and it is one of the most investigated consequences of ROS action on membrane structure and function [44]. Alterations in the fluidity of membranes result in negative effects on their functions such as signal transduction processes and implicate in aging as well as in diseases [102]. Melatonin is known to be a stabilizer or protector of cell and organelle membranes because of its inhibitory effects on lipid peroxidation. Melatonin and its metabolites scavenge free radicals and thus terminate the initiation and propagation of lipid peroxidation [103]. Although melatonin and its metabolites, AFMK and AMK, are peroxyl radical scavengers, it is indicated that melatonin's ability to resist lipid peroxidation may also involve its metabolite, c3-OHM [104]. For the reaction with the peroxyl radical, c3-OHM was several orders of magnitude faster than melatonin, AFMK and AMK, and it was roughly 100-fold faster than water soluble vitamin E (Trolox) [96, 105]. Melatonin also directly scavenges the alkoxyl radical, a product resulting from the transition metal-catalyzed degradation of lipid peroxides. This is important for the control of lipid peroxidation since the alkoxyl radical can abstract a hydrogen atom from a polyunsaturated fatty acids; the resulting peroxyl radical can obviously continue the propagation of lipid degradation [104, 106].

4.2. Effects of melatonin and its metabolites on reactive nitrogen species

Reactive nitrogen species represent another category of potentially destructive substances, which react with melatonin [77]. $ONOO^{\bullet}$ itself is a very damaging species able to react with proteins, lipids, and DNA. Therefore, the reaction between two rather innocuous free radicals produces a much more reactive one [41]. Melatonin readily combines with a superoxide releasing NO, thus preventing the formation of peroxynitrite, a free radical even more harmful than NO. It has been described as a direct peroxynitrite scavenger [40].

Scavenging of nitric oxide by melatonin in a nitrosation reaction is well documented. Whether this can be regarded as a detoxification reaction keeping NO from forming, the more dangerous peroxynitrite is uncertain because nitrosomelatonin easily decomposes, thereby releasing NO. Melatonin also scavenges peroxynitrite, but it is difficult to discriminate direct reactions with peroxynitrite and with hydroxyl radicals generated by decomposition of peroxynitrous acid. The interaction with products from the peroxynitrite-CO_2 adduct ($ONOOCO_2^-$) which carbonate radicals ($CO_3^{\bullet -}$) and $NO_2^{\bullet}$ seems to be more important than direct scavenging of peroxynitrite [33, 77]. There is evidence for the formation of cyclic 2-hydroxymelatonin, cyclic 3-hydroxymelatonin, and 6-hydroxymelatonin about the reaction of melatonin with $ONOO^-$. It was suggested that one electron is transferred from melatonin to $ONOO^-$ in the melatonin $+ONOO^-$ reaction and/or nitrated intermediates occur in the oxidation. In addition, the 6-hydroxymelatonin is not generated in the presence of CO_2. Therefore, it was suggested that formation of 6-hydroxymelatonin required an activated peroxynitrite that can only exist in the absence of bicarbonate [41, 107, 108]. AFMK has the ability to interact with the ABTS cation radical as well as with ROS/RNS to form AMK. When AMK interacts with the ABTS cation radical or with $ONOO^-$, it forms products that may also be ROS and RNS scavengers [59]. AMK was described as better a NO scavenger than melatonin or AFMK [88]. AMK effectively inhibits neuronal nitric oxide synthase activity and reduces intracellular NO levels [93].

4.3. Effects of melatonin and its metabolites on antioxidant enzymes

Cells are protected against oxidative stress by an interacting network of antioxidant enzymes [70]. Antioxidative enzymes provide a major defense mechanism against free radical damage either by metabolizing them to less reactive species or to nontoxic by-products [85]. The activities of antioxidative enzymes depend on the duration and severity of oxidative stress. Under prolonged oxidative stress conditions, free radicals directly damage the antioxidant enzymes or reduce enzyme activities [90, 109]. Besides its ability to directly neutralize a number of free radicals and reactive oxygen and nitrogen species, melatonin stimulates several antioxidative enzymes which increase its efficiency as an antioxidant [58]. The major antioxidative enzymes such as intracellular superoxide dismutases (CuZn-SOD and Mn-SOD), the selenium-containing glutathione peroxidases and catalase, are stimulated by melatonin under basal conditions [43, 75, 110]. Melatonin plays a significant role in maintaining indirect protection versus free radical injury by stimulating gene expression of antioxidant enzymes including those for SOD and GSH-Px [43, 58, 62, 111]. Melatonin affects both antioxidant enzyme activity and cellular mRNA levels for these enzymes under physiological circumstances and during increased oxidative stress, presumably through epigenetic mechanisms. These properties in a single molecule are unique for an antioxidant, and both actions protect against pathologically generated free radicals [43, 62].

The concentration of the intracellular antioxidant, glutathione, is very high in many cells. During high oxidative stress conditions total glutathione levels can be reduced [90]. Melatonin maintains the activities of enzymes that enhance intracellular levels of reduced GSH. The recycling of GSH may well be a major effect of melatonin in reducing oxidative stress. GSH is oxidized to its disulfide, GSSG, which is then quickly reduced back to GSH by GR, an enzyme which has been demonstrated to be stimulated by melatonin. The ability of melatonin to regulate the GSH/GSSG balance by modulating enzyme activities seems to involve an action of melatonin at a nuclear binding site [85, 112]. The other GSH-metabolizing enzyme, i.e., CAT, also increases its activity in response to melatonin [85]. Furthermore, one of the melatonin actions is stimulation of gamma-glutamylcysteine synthetase that is the rate-limiting enzyme in glutathione production, thus glutathione levels do not drop significantly [36, 43, 58, 75, 77, 85, 86, 90, 110, 112, 113].

There are a number of prooxidative enzymes in multicellular organisms which generate free radicals [90]. Melatonin not only upregulates the expression of genes involved in detoxifying free radicals, but it also suppresses the activity or expression of genes involved in the generation of free radicals [16, 113]. Melatonin inhibits the prooxidative enzyme nitric oxide synthase which generates $NO^\bullet$ and lipoxygenase which result in the formation of the superoxide anion [90, 113, 114]. Although $NO^\bullet$ is not a strong free radical, when it couples with $O_2^{\bullet-}$, it forms the peroxynitrite anion which is potently reactive and damaging [90]. Lipoxygenase reaction is another possible source of ROS and other radicals. It catalyzes the hydroperoxidation of polyunsaturated fatty acids [115]. The prooxidative enzymes inhibited by melatonin also include myeloperoxidase and eosinophil peroxidase [110]. As a result, free radical and/or toxic reactant generation is alleviated [90, 114]. In addition, AFMK and AMK also have the ability to downregulate prooxidative and pro-inflammatory enzymes including iNOS [102] and cyclooxygenase-2 (COX-2) and to carry out free radical avoidance functions [93].

4.4. Effects of melatonin and its metabolites on the mitochondria

Mitochondria are critical in the control of metabolism and responsible for orchestrating cellular energy production. Therefore, they are central to the maintenance of life and the gatekeepers of cell death [116]. The production of energy in the form of ATP is crucial to optimal cell function, including aiding in repairing any cellular damage that has occurred and in improving survivability of the cell, of the tissue, and of the organism [90]. Up to 95% of the ATP produced in aerobic cells is a result of mitochondrial oxidative phosphorylation [59]. The ETC which is coupled to oxidative phosphorylation [59] is a system of oxidoreductase protein complexes (complexes I, II, III, and IV) [85]. Deficiencies in the ETC can result in the leakage of electrons which thereafter generate free radicals and other toxic reactants which leads to molecular damage in mitochondria; this damage culminates in and promotes what are referred to as mitochondria-related diseases [85]. Mitochondria are the primary source of free radicals [44, 45]. Increased free radical generation, enhanced mitochondrial iNOS activity, enhanced NO production, decreased respiratory complex activity, impaired electron transport system, and opening of mitochondrial permeability transition pores have all been suggested as factors responsible for impaired mitochondrial function [117].

Melatonin has important actions at the level of mitochondria [85]. Melatonin exhibits remarkable functional versatility to protect the morphological and functional aspects of the cell membrane scavenging free radicals, enhancing the activity of the antioxidant enzymes, and optimizing the transfer of electrons through the ETC in the inner mitochondrial membrane [118]. Melatonin increases the efficiency of the ETC and thus reduces electron leakage and free radical generation [38, 75, 105] that is a consequence of the respiratory process by stimulating complex I and complex IV of the mitochondrial respiratory chain that are involved in oxidative phosphorylation [38, 58, 59, 118]. By directly detoxifying ROS/RNS, melatonin enhances ATP production via maintaining high levels of mitochondrial GSH, protects mitochondrial proteins and DNA from oxidative damage, and improves ETC activity [16, 90, 118]. Moreover, AMK, like its precursor melatonin, promotes mitochondrial complex I activity to elevate ATP production by lowering electron leakage and inhibiting the opening of the mitochondrial permeability transition pore [93].

4.5. Effects of melatonin and its metabolites on transition metals

Heavy metals are known to cause oxidative deterioration of biomolecules by initiating free radical-mediated chain reaction resulting in lipid peroxidation, protein oxidation, and oxidation of nucleic acid like DNA and RNA [119]. The ability of antioxidants to chelate and deactivate transition metals prevents such metals from participating in the initiation of lipid peroxidation and oxidative stress through metal-catalyzed reaction [120]. Chemical mean of inhibiting metal-induced oxidation is chelation. This particular process is directly involved in the $OH^{\bullet}$-inactivating ligand (OIL) behavior of antioxidants. There are two different ways of action in the protection exerted by OIL species against $OH^{\bullet}$-induced oxidative damage: (i) inhibiting the reduction of metal ions; thus, their reduced forms are not available for Fenton-like reactions or (ii) deactivating $OH^{\bullet}$ after being produced by Fenton-like reactions [87].

Melatonin is able to prevent the oxidative actions of metals by neutralizing the produced ROS and capturing such metals to form chelates [83]. It was demonstrated that the interplay of melatonin with metals such as aluminum, cadmium, copper, iron, lead, and zinc depended on concentration. Melatonin chelates both iron(III) and iron(II), which is the form that attends the Fenton reaction. If iron is bound to a protein (e.g., hemoglobin), melatonin restores the highly covalent iron such as oxyferryl (Fe^{IV}-O) hemoglobin back to iron(III), thereby reestablishing the biological activity of the protein [89]. It is suggested that, under physiological circumstances, direct chelation mechanism would be the major chelation route for Cu(II). It was demonstrated that melatonin and its metabolites, 3OHM, AFMK, and AMK, fully inhibited the oxidative stress induced by Cu(II)-ascorbate mixtures, via Cu(II) chelation [97]. Melatonin decreases the Cu(II)/H_2O_2-induced damage to proteins and protects against copper-mediated lipid peroxidation, which led to the suggestion that the antioxidant and neuroprotective effects of melatonin may involve removing toxic metals from the central nervous system [42].

5. Melatonin and its metabolites as anti-inflammatory agents

Inflammation is an essential response to tissue injuries induced by physical, chemical, or biological insults [17]. The production of inflammatory cytokines including TNF-α (tumor necrosis factor-α), IL-1β (interleukin-1β), or IL-6 attenuates by melatonin in numerous experimental models of inflammation [2]. Melatonin has several additional anti-inflammatory effects, which are probably related to a direct interaction with specific binding sites located in lymphocytes and macrophages [103]. Anti-inflammatory activity of melatonin includes inhibition of the activation of COX-2 and iNOS, as well as blocking of the transcriptional factors that triggers pro-inflammatory cytokine production. These include not only NF-κB but also HIF, Nrf2, cAMP, CREB, STAT, PPARs, and AP-1 [2, 43, 121]. Melatonin may be useful for the treatment of inflammatory disease, as it reduces inflammatory injury by blocking transcription factors and NF-κB, thereby decreasing further ROS formation within cells [43]. In peripheral monocytes, melatonin and, even more, AFMK suppressed TNF-α and IL-8 production and, in macrophages, COX-2 and iNOS expression. Moreover, melatonin was found to be efficiently oxidized to AFMK by macrophages [91]. AMK was reported to downregulate COX-2—but not COX-1—expression in macrophages, an effect shared by its precursors AFMK and melatonin [122].

6. The clinical significance of melatonin

Melatonin plays important roles in neurogenesis, neuroprotection, maintenance of oxidant/antioxidant balance, and modulation of cardiovascular and/or immune system. It also exerts a direct antioxidant effect on tissues/organs and antiapoptotic effects on cells [9]. Melatonin has been investigated in a wide range of diseases, such as neurodegenerative, cardiovascular, liver, and kidney diseases, cancer, and diabetes [43].

Melatonin is a ubiquitously acting direct free radical scavenger and also an indirect antioxidant. Melatonin and its metabolites are efficient in scavenging ROS and RNS. It plays an effective role in regulating mitochondrial homeostasis [33, 38]. Mitochondrial dysfunction, i.e., cell energy impairment, apoptosis, and overproduction of ROS, is a final common pathogenic mechanism in aging and in neurodegenerative disease [43, 123]. Melatonin may be possible to treat neurodegenerative disorders by inhibiting mitochondrial cell death pathways. It may easily protect brain mitochondrial membranes from free radical attack, stabilizing them. The ability of melatonin to prevent GSH loss probably reflects its effect on the activities of the GSH redox cycle enzymes [33, 38, 83, 103]. Moreover, several neurological diseases including Alzheimer's disease, Parkinson's disease, Huntington's disease, and Wilson's disease (hepatolenticular degeneration) are characterized by an overload of copper and/or other metals. Melatonin and its metabolites, c3OHM, AFMK, and AMK, have the copper sequestering ability [89].

Excessive and/or sustained increase in ROS generation plays a pivotal role in the initiation, progression, and clinical consequences of cardiovascular diseases (CVDs) [64, 124]. Clinically, melatonin is being increasingly recognized in the pathophysiology of CVD. Low levels of serum melatonin as well as its urinary metabolite, 6-sulphatoxymelatonin, have been reported in various CVDs including coronary heart disease, angina, congestive heart failure, and myocardial infarcts [125]. Melatonin plays an important role in the regulation of several parameters of the cardiovascular system, including blood pressure, and is considered to be a putative antihypertensive agent [126]. It may have cardio-protective properties via its direct free radical scavenger activity and its indirect antioxidant activity together with its significant anti-inflammatory properties [127, 128]. Mitochondrial respiration, mainly at the level of complex I and complex III, is an important source of ROS generation and hence a potential contributor of cardiac reperfusion injury [129]. Most of the beneficial actions of melatonin at the heart level may depend on its effect on mitochondrial bioenergetics mediated through various mechanisms including general antioxidant actions at the level of ETC dysfunction, electron leakage, and mitochondrial oxidative damage and also through a direct action of melatonin on mitochondrial permeability transition pore opening [127]. It was reported that melatonin protects against mitochondrial dysfunction associated with cardiac ischemia reperfusion, by preventing alterations to several parameters involved in mitochondrial bioenergetics [17].

Melatonin may also exhibit anticancer and protective oncostatic activity through several mechanisms, including inhibition of cancer cell proliferation, decrease in oxidative stress, and increase in immune system activity [130, 131]. Oxidative stress has complex and different effects on each type of cancer development [132]. Oxidation of cellular lipids and proteins can adversely affect several steps of the carcinogenic process through changes in a variety of cell regulatory functions, including signal transduction and gene expression. ROS are postulated to be involved in carcinogenesis process, especially in the stages of initiation and promotion [133]. It appears that the DNA damage is predominantly linked with the initiation process [132]. Free radicals and ROS generated by environmental carcinogens, or by metabolic alterations, cause DNA damage and genetic instability [134]. Furthermore, DNA damage, apoptosis resistance, enhanced proliferation, mutation, COX-2 upregulation, oxidative stress, tumor vascularity, and metastatic potential may be caused by nitric oxide synthase overexpression and increased nitric oxide and other RNS productions [132]. A growing body of evidence implicates melatonin's antioxidant/free radical scavenging actions in the inhibition of cancer development and growth [75]. Melatonin is a powerful scavenger of ROS, such as hydroxyl radical, peroxyl radical, singlet oxygen, and nitric oxide, as well as a stimulator of the antioxidant enzymes, SOD, GPx, and CAT, all leading to a decrease in DNA damage [135]. Additionally, this indole stimulates antioxidant enzymes that remove ROS before they can inflict damage and aids in the repair of damaged DNA [136]. Melatonin could be an excellent candidate for the prevention and treatment of several cancers, such as breast cancer, prostate cancer, gastric cancer, and colorectal cancer [137].

A variety of antioxidants protect the liver from free radical-mediated damage, one of the best of which is melatonin. Clinical studies have confirmed that melatonin protects the liver from nonalcoholic liver disease and also during the surgical procedure of partial liver resection [138]. Melatonin is a well-known natural antioxidant and has many bioactivities. Melatonin exerts antioxidant effects in hepatocytes and epithelium of the liver by reducing lipid peroxidation and increasing the level of reduced liver glutathione. Melatonin is a highly valuable OH and H_2O_2 scavenger, during its metabolism to AFMK. It also induces several antioxidative enzymes such as glutathione peroxidase, glutathione reductase, and SOD and increases the synthesis of GSH [2, 88]. Melatonin exhibits potent anti-inflammatory, antioxidant, and fibrosuppressive activities against thioacetamide-induced hepatic fibrogenesis via the suppression of oxidative stress, DNA damage, pro-inflammatory cytokines, and fibrogenic gene transcripts [139]. Melatonin protects against lipid-induced mitochondrial dysfunction in hepatocytes and inhibits stellate cell activation during hepatic fibrosis in mice [140].

Inflammation and increased oxidative stress are also common features in chronic kidney disease patients [130, 141]. Oxidative stress and inflammation promote renal injury via damage to molecular components of the kidney by different mechanisms of action. ROS lead to the loss of significant functional properties, lipid peroxidation of cell membrane, decrease membrane viability, and cleavage, and cross-linking of renal DNA occurs leading to harmful mutations by oxidizing amino acids in the nephron. Furthermore, other ROS interactions in the nephron increase secondary radical production [130, 142]. Diabetes-associated hyperglycemia leads to mitochondrial ETC dysfunction culminating in a rise in ROS production [143]. Experimental evidence suggests that the indoleamine hormone melatonin is capable of influencing in development of diabetic complications by neutralizing the unnecessary ROS generation and protection of beta cells, as they possess low antioxidant potential and normalize redox state in the cell [144]. Melatonin acts as a cell survival agent by modulating autophagy in various cell types and under different conditions through amelioration of oxidative stress, ER stress, and inflammation [143].

7. Conclusion

Melatonin is a circulating neurohormone secreted predominantly at night, thereby called as hormone of darkness. It can cross all physiological barriers to exert widespread regulatory effects on body tissues. Melatonin is a universal antioxidant with multifunctional activities such as anti-inflammatory, antiapoptotic, and antioxidant effects in addition to its function as a synchronizer of the biological clock and seasonal reproduction. Melatonin and its derivatives have been shown to be powerful direct free radical scavengers. Besides direct scavenging of ROS/RNS, melatonin also stimulates antioxidant enzymes; suppresses prooxidant enzymes; improves mitochondrial function, hence reducing radical formation; and reduces metal-induced toxicity. Results from previous studies support these effects on several diseases including cancer, diabetes, neurodegenerative, cardiovascular, liver; and kidney diseases.

Author details

Aysun Hacışevki* and Burcu Baba

*Address all correspondence to: aysunsevki@gmail.com

Department of Biochemistry, Faculty of Pharmacy, Gazi University, Etiler, Ankara, Turkey

References

[1] Lerner AB, Case JD, Takahashi Y. Isolation of melatonin, a pineal factor that lightens melanocytes. Journal of the American Chemical Society. 1958;**80**:2587

[2] Eghbal MA, Eftekhari A, Ahmadian E, Yadollah Azarmi Y, Parvizpur A. A review of biological and pharmacological actions of melatonin: Oxidant and prooxidant properties. Pharmaceutical Bioprocessing. 2016;**4**(4):069-081

[3] Comai S, Gobbi G. Unveiling the role of melatonin MT2 receptors in sleep, anxiety and other neuropsychiatric diseases: A novel target in psychopharmacology. Journal of Psychiatry & Neuroscience. 2014;**39**(1):6-21

[4] Yin J, Jin X, Shan Z, Li S, Huang H, Li P, Peng X, Peng Z, Yu K, Bao W, Yang W, Chen X, Liu L. Relationship of sleep duration with all-cause mortality and cardiovascular events: A systematic review and dose-response meta-analysis of prospective cohort studies. Journal of the American Heart Association. 2017;**6**(9):1-15

[5] Altman NG, Izci-Balserak B, Schopfer E, Jackson N, Rattanaumpawan P, Gehrman PR, Patel NP, Grandner MA. Sleep duration versus sleep insufficiency as predictors of cardiometabolic health outcomes. Sleep Medicine. 2012;**13**(10):1261-1270

[6] Cappuccio FP, Cooper D, D'Elia L, Strazzullo P, Miller MA. Sleep duration predicts cardiovascular outcomes: A systematic review and meta-analysis of prospective studies. European Heart Journal. 2011;**32**(12):1484-1492

[7] Pandi-Perumal SR, Trakht I, Srinivasan V, Spence DW, Maestroni GJ, Zisapel N, Cardinali DP. Physiological effects of melatonin: Role of melatonin receptors and signal transduction pathways. Progress in Neurobiology. 2008;**85**(3):335-353

[8] Emet M, Ozcan H, Ozel L, Yayla M, Halici Z, Hacimuftuoglu A. A review of melatonin, its receptors and drugs. Eurasian Journal of Medicine. 2016;**48**:135-141

[9] Onaolapo OJ, Onaolapo AY. Melatonin, adolescence, and the brain: An insight into the period-specific influences of a multifunctional signaling molecule. Birth Defects Research. 2017;**109**(20):1659-1671

[10] Singh M, Jadhav HR. Melatonin: Functions and ligands. Drug Discovery Today. 2014;**19**(9):1410-1418

[11] Kubatka P, Zubor P, Busselberg D, Kwon TK, Adamek M, Petrovic D, Opatrilova R, Gazdikova K, Caprnda M, Rodrigo L, Danko J, Kruzliak P. Melatonin and breast cancer: Evidences from preclinical and human studies. Critical Reviews in Oncology/Hematology. 2018;**122**:133-143

[12] Rios ER, Venâncio ET, Rocha NF, Woods DJ, Vasconcelos S, Macedo D, Sousa FC, Fonteles MM. Melatonin: Pharmacological aspects and clinical trends. The International Journal of Neuroscience. 2010;**120**(9):583-590

[13] Peuhkuri K, Sihvola N, Korpela R. Dietary factors and fluctuating levels of melatonin. Food & Nutrition Research. 2012;**56**:1-9

[14] Konturek SJ1, Konturek PC, Brzozowska I, Pawlik M, Sliwowski Z, Cześnikiewicz-Guzik M, Kwiecień S, Brzozowski T, Bubenik GA, Pawlik WW. Localization and biological activities of melatonin in intact and diseased gastrointestinal tract (GIT). Journal of Physiology and Pharmacology. 2007;**58**(3):381-405

[15] Tordjman S, Chokron S, Delorme R, Charrier A, Bellissant E, Jaafari N; Fougerou C. Melatonin: Pharmacology, functions and therapeutic benefits. Current Neuropharmacology. 2017;**15**(3):434-443

[16] Zhang HM, Zhang Y. Melatonin: A well-documented antioxidant with conditional pro-oxidant actions. Journal of Pineal Research. 2014;**57**(2):131-146

[17] Anwar MJ, Muhammad BY, Bader AA, Abdulghani M, Mahmood D, Haider M. An insight into the scientific background and future perspectives for the potential uses of melatonin. Egyptian Journal of Basic and Applied Sciences. 2015;**2**:139-152

[18] Masters A, Pandi-Perumal SR, Seixas A, Girardin JL, McFarlane SI. Melatonin, the hormone of darkness: From sleep promotion to ebola treatment. Brain Disorders and Therapy. 2014;**4**(1):1-10

[19] Karasek M, Winczyk K. Melatonin in humans. Journal of Physiology and Pharmacology. 2006;**57**(5):19-39

[20] Tan DX, Manchester LC, Esteban-Zubero E, Zhou Z, Reiter RJ. Melatonin as a potent and inducible endogenous antioxidant: Synthesis and metabolism. Molecules. 2015;**20** (10):18886-18906

[21] Pevet P, Challet E. Melatonin: Both master clock output and internal time-giver in the circadian clocks network. Journal of Physiology, Paris. 2011;**105**(4-6):170-182

[22] Bedrosian TA, Herring KL, Walton JC, Fonken LK, Weil ZM, Nelson RJ. Evidence for feedback control of pineal melatonin secretion. Neuroscience Letters. 2013;**542**:123-125

[23] Maitra S, Baidya DK, Khanna P. Melatonin in perioperative medicine: Current perspective. Saudi Journal of Anaesthesia. 2013;**7**(3):315-321

[24] De Almeida EA, Di Mascio P, Harumi T, Spence DW, Moscovitch A, Hardeland R, Cardinali DP, Brown GM, Pandi-Perumal SR. Measurement of melatonin in body fluids: Standards, protocols and procedures. Child's Nervous System. 2011;**27**(6):879-891

[25] Ren W, Liu G, Chen S, Yin J, Wang J, Tan B, Wu G, Bazer FW, Peng Y, Li T, Reiter RJ, Yin Y. Melatonin signaling in T cells: Functions and applications. Journal of Pineal Research. 2017;**62**(3):1-15

[26] Zawilska JB, Skene DJ, Arendt J. Physiology and pharmacology of melatonin in relation to biological rhythms. Pharmacological Reports. 2009;**61**(3):383-410

[27] Slominski RM, Reiter RJ, Schlabritz-Loutsevitch N, Ostrom RS, Slominski AT. Melatonin membrane receptors in peripheral tissues: Distribution and functions. Molecular and Cellular Endocrinology. 2012;**351**(2):152-166

[28] Chattoraj A, Liu T, Zhang LS, Huang Z, Borjigin J. Melatonin formation in mammals: In vivo perspectives. Reviews in Endocrine & Metabolic Disorders. 2009;**10**(4):237-243

[29] Malhotra S, Sawhney G, Pandhi P. The therapeutic potential of melatonin: A review of the science. Medscape General Medicine. 2004;**6**(2):1-45

[30] Mahmood D, Muhammad BY, Alghani M, Anwar J, el-Lebban N, Haider M. Advancing role of melatonin in the treatment of neuropsychiatric disorders. Egyptian journal of basic and applied sciences. 2016;**3**:203-218

[31] Liu J, Clough SJ, Hutchinson AJ, Adamah-Biassi EB, Popovska-Gorevski M, Dubocovich ML. MT1 and MT2 melatonin receptors: A therapeutic perspective. Annual Review of Pharmacology and Toxicology. 2016;**56**:361-383

[32] Jockers R, Delagrange P, Dubocovich ML, Markus RP, Renault N, Tosini G, Cecon E, Zlotos DP. Update on melatonin receptors: IUPHAR review 20. British Journal of Pharmacology. 2016;**173**(18):2702-2725

[33] Hardeland R, Cardinali DP, Srinivasan V, Spence DW, Brown GM, Pandi-Perumal SR. Melatonin—A pleiotropic, orchestrating regulator molecule. Progress in Neurobiology. 2011;**93**(3):350-384

[34] Mailliet F, Ferry G, Vella F, Berger S, Cogé F, Chomarat P, Mallet C, Guénin SP, Guillaumet G, Viaud-Massuard MC, Yous S, Delagrange P, Boutin JA. Characterization of the melatoninergic MT3 binding site on the NRH:Quinone oxidoreductase 2 enzyme. Biochemical Pharmacology. 2005;**71**(1-2):74-88

[35] Ekmekcioglu C. Melatonin receptors in humans: Biological role and clinical relevance. Biomedicine & Pharmacotherapy. 2006;**60**:97-108

[36] Najafi M, Shirazi A, Motevaseli E, Geraily G, Norouzi F, Heidari M, Rezapoor S. The melatonin immunomodulatory actions in radiotherapy. Biophysical Reviews. 2017;**9**(2):139-148

[37] Rodriguez C, Mayo JC, Sainz RM, Antolín I, Herrera F, Martín V, Reiter RJ. Regulation of antioxidant enzymes: A significant role for melatonin. Journal of Pineal Research. 2004;**36**(1):1-9

[38] Srinivasan V, Spence DW, Pandi-Perumal SR, Brown GM, Cardinali DP. Melatonin in mitochondrial dysfunction and related disorders. International Journal of Alzheimer's Disease. 2011;**2011**:326320

[39] Hardeland R, Tan DX, Reiter RJ. Kynuramines, metabolites of melatonin and other indoles: The resurrection of an almost forgotten class of biogenic amines. Journal of Pineal Research. 2009;**47**(2):109-126

[40] Loren P, Sánchez R, Arias ME, Felmer R, Risopatrón J, Cheuquemán C. Melatonin scavenger properties against oxidative and Nitrosative stress: Impact on gamete handling and in vitro embryo production in humans and other mammals. International Journal of Molecular Sciences. 2017;**18**(6):1-17

[41] Galano A, Tan DX, Reiter RJ. Melatonin as a natural ally against oxidative stress: A physicochemical examination. Journal of Pineal Research. 2011;**51**:1-16

[42] Galano A, Castañeda-Arriaga R, Pérez-González A, Tan DX, Reiter RJ. Phenolic melatonin-related compounds: Their role as chemical protectors against oxidative stress. Molecules. 2016;**21**(11):1-42

[43] Bonnefont-Rousselot D, Collin F. Melatonin: Action as antioxidant and potential applications in human disease and aging. Toxicology. 2010;**278**(1):55-67

[44] Kohen R, Nyska A. Oxidation of biological systems: Oxidative stress phenomena, antioxidants, redox reactions, and methods for their quantification. Toxicologic Pathology. 2002;**30**(6):620-650

[45] Rahal A, Kumar A, Singh V, Yadav B, Tiwari R, Chakraborty S, Dhama K. Oxidative stress, prooxidants, and antioxidants: The interplay. BioMed Research International. 2014;**2014**:761264

[46] Kurutas EB. The importance of antioxidants which play the role in cellular response against oxidative/nitrosative stress: Current state. Nutrition Journal. 2016;**15**(71):1-22

[47] Patel M, Ramavataram DV. Non transferrin bound iron: Nature, manifestations and analytical approaches for estimation. Indian Journal of Clinical Biochemistry Indian. 2012;**27**(4):322-332

[48] Łuczaj W, Gęgotek A1, Skrzydlewska E. Antioxidants and HNE in redox homeostasis. Free Radical Biology & Medicine. 2017;**111**:87-101

[49] Mirończuk-Chodakowska I, Witkowska AM, Zujko ME. Endogenous non-enzymatic antioxidants in the human body. Advances in Medical Sciences. 2018;**63**(1):68-78

[50] Peyrot F, Ducrocq C. Potential role of tryptophan derivatives in stress responses characterized by the generation of reactive oxygen and nitrogen species. Journal of Pineal Research. 2008;**45**(3):235-246

[51] Poljsak B, Šuput D, Milisav I. Achieving the balance between ROS and antioxidants: When to use the synthetic antioxidants. Oxidative Medicine and Cellular Longevity. 2013;**2013**(956792):1-11

[52] Ray PD, Huang BW, Tsuji Y. Reactive oxygen species (ROS) homeostasis and redox regulation in cellular signaling. Cellular Signalling. 2012;**24**(5):981-990

[53] Zorov DB, Juhaszova M, Sollott SJ. Mitochondrial reactive oxygen species (ROS) and ROS-induced ROS release. Physiological Reviews. 2014;**94**(3):909-950

[54] Sarangarajan R, Meera S, Rukkumani R, Sankar P, Anuradha G. Antioxidants: Friend or foe? Asian Pacific Journal of Tropical Medicine. 2017;**10**(12):1111-1116

[55] Weydert CJ, Cullen JJ. Measurement of superoxide dismutase, catalase and glutathione peroxidase in cultured cells and tissue. Nature Protocols. 2010;**5**(1):51-66

[56] Wołonciej M, Milewska E, Roszkowska-Jakimiec W. Trace elements as an activator of antioxidant enzymes. Postępy Higieny i Medycyny Doświadczalnej. 2016;**70**:1483-1498

[57] Reiter RJ, Tan DX, Gitto E, Sainz RM, Mayo JC, Leon J, Manchester LC, Vijayalaxmi KE, Kilic U. Pharmacological utility of melatonin in reducing oxidative cellular and molecular damage. Polish Journal of Pharmacology. 2004;**56**(2):159-170

[58] Reiter RJ, Tan DX, Osuna C, Gitto E. Actions of melatonin in the reduction of oxidative stress. A review. Journal of Biomedical Science. 2000;**7**(6):444-458

[59] Reiter RJ, Paredes SD, Korkmaz A, Jou MJ, Tan DX. Melatonin combats molecular terrorism at the mitochondrial level. Interdisciplinary Toxicology. 2008;**1**(2):137-149

[60] Bouayed J, Bohn T. Exogenous antioxidants–Double-edged swords in cellular redox state: Health beneficial effects at physiologic doses versus deleterious effects at high doses. Oxidative Medicine and Cellular Longevity. 2010;**3**(4):228-237

[61] Hacışevki A. An overview of ascorbic acid biochemistry. Journal of Faculty of Pharmacy of Ankara University. 2009;**38**(3):235-257

[62] Korkmaz A, Reiter RJ, Topal T, Manchester LC, Oter S, Tan DX. Melatonin: An established antioxidant worthy of use in clinical trials. Molecular Medicine. 2009;**15**(1-2):43-50

[63] Ryan MJ, Dudash HJ, Docherty M, Geronilla KB, Baker BA, Haff GG, Cutlip RG, Alway SE. Vitamin E and C supplementation reduces oxidative stress, improves antioxidant enzymes and positive muscle work in chronically loaded muscles of aged rats. Experimental Gerontology. 2010;**45**(11):882-895

[64] Hacışevki A, Torun M, Çengel A. Effect of short-term α-tocopherol supplementation on biomarkers of oxidative stress and antioxidant defence in subject with angina pectoris. Oxidation Communications. 2012;**35**(1):128-137

[65] Schmölz L, Birringer M, Lorkowski S, Wallert M. Complexity of vitamin E metabolism. World Journal of Biological Chemistry. 2016;**7**(1):14-43

[66] Schubert M, Kluge S, Schmölz L, Wallert M, Galli F, Birringer M, Lorkowski S. Long-chain metabolites of vitamin E: Metabolic activation as a general concept for lipid-soluble vitamins? Antioxidants (Basel). 2018;**7**(1):1-54

[67] Bozkır A, Şimşek B, Güngör A, Torun M. Ascorbic acid and uric acid levels in lung cancer patients. Journal of Clinical Pharmacy and Therapeutics. 1999;**24**:43-47

[68] Pullar JM, Bayer S, Carr AC. Appropriate handling, processing and analysis of blood samples is essential to avoid oxidation of vitamin C to dehydroascorbic acid. Antioxidants (Basel). 2018;**7**(2):1-26

[69] Rahman K. Studies on free radicals, antioxidants, and co-factors. Clinical Interventions in Aging. 2007;**2**(2):219-236

[70] Lobo V, Patil A, Phatak A, Chandra N. Free radicals, antioxidants and functional foods: Impact on human health. Pharmacognosy Reviews. 2010;**4**(8):118-126

[71] Galano A. Free radicals induced oxidative stress at a molecular level: The current status, challenges and perspectives of computational chemistry based protocols. Journal of the Mexican Chemical Society. 2015;**59**(4):231-262

[72] Rose RC, Bode AM. Biology of free radical scavengers: An evaluation of ascorbate. The FASEB Journal 1993;**7**(12):1135-1142

[73] Tamura H, Takasaki A, Taketani T, Tanabe M, Kizuka F, Lee L, Tamura I, Maekawa R, Aasada H, Yamagata Y, Sugino N. The role of melatonin as an antioxidant in the follicle. Journal of Ovarian Research. 2012;**5**:1-9

[74] Tan DX, Manchester LC, Reiter RJ, Qi WB, Karbownik M, Calvo JR. Significance of melatonin in antioxidative defense system: Reactions and products. Biological Signals and Receptors. 2000;**9**(3-4):137-159

[75] Anisimov VN, Popovich IG, Zabezhinski MA, Anisimov SV, Vesnushkin GM, Vinogradova IA. Melatonin as antioxidant, geroprotector and anticarcinogen. Biochimica et Biophysica Acta. 2006;**1757**(5-6):573-589

[76] Johns JR, Platts JA. Theoretical insight into the antioxidant properties of melatonin and derivatives. Organic & Biomolecular Chemistry. 2014;**12**(39):7820-7827

[77] Hardeland R, Pandi-Perumal SR. Melatonin, a potent agent in antioxidative defense: Actions as a natural food constituent, gastrointestinal factor, drug and prodrug. Nutrition & Metabolism (London). 2005;**2**(22):1-42

[78] Swarnakar S, Paul S, Singh LP, Reiter RJ. Matrix metalloproteinases in health and disease: Regulation by melatonin. Journal of Pineal Research. 2011;**50**(1):8-20

[79] Vázquez J, González B, Sempere V, Mas A, Torija MJ, Beltran G. Melatonin reduces oxidative stress damage induced by hydrogen peroxide in *Saccharomyces cerevisiae*. Frontiers in Microbiology. 2017;**8**:1066, 1-14

[80] Kratz EM, Piwowar A. Melatonin, advanced oxidation protein products and total antioxidant capacity as seminal parameters of prooxidant-antioxidant balance and their connection with expression of metalloproteinases in context of male fertility. Journal of Physiology and Pharmacology. 2017;**68**(5):659-668

[81] Bisquert R, Muñiz-Calvo S, Guillamón JM. Protective role of intracellular melatonin against oxidative stress and UV radiation in *Saccharomyces cerevisiae*. Frontiers in Microbiology. 2018;**9**(318):1-11

[82] Gitto E, Aversa S, Reiter RJ, Barberi I, Pellegrino S. Update on the use of melatonin in pediatrics. Journal of Pineal Research. 2011;**50**:21-28

[83] Romero A, Ramos E, de Los Ríos C, Egea J, Del Pino J, Reiter RJ. A review of metal-catalyzed molecular damage: Protection by melatonin. Journal of Pineal Research. 2014;**56**(4):343-370

[84] Aydogan S, Yerer MB, Goktas A. Melatonin and nitric oxide. Journal of Endocrinological Investigation 2006;**29**(3):281-287

[85] Reiter RJ, Tan DX, Mayo JC, Sainz RM, Leon J, Czarnocki Z. Melatonin as an antioxidant: Biochemical mechanisms and pathophysiological implications in humans. Acta Biochimica Polonica. 2003;**50**(4):1129-1146

[86] Reiter RJ, Tan DX, Korkmaz A, Rosales-Corral SA. Melatonin and stable circadian rhythms optimize maternal, placental and fetal physiology. Human Reproduction Update. 2014;**20**(2):293-307

[87] Galano A, Tan DX, Reiter RJ. Melatonin: A versatile protector against oxidative DNA damage. Molecules. 2018;**23**(3):1-36

[88] Galano A, Tan DX, Reiter RJ. On the free radical scavenging activities of melatonin's metabolites, AFMK and AMK. Journal of Pineal Research. 2013;**54**(3):245-257

[89] Reiter RJ, Mayo JC, Tan DX, Sainz RM, Alatorre-Jimenez M, Qin L. Melatonin as an antioxidant: Under promises but over delivers. Journal of Pineal Research. 2016;**61**(3):253-278

[90] Reiter RJ, Tan DX, Manchester LC, Pilar Terron M, Flores LJ, Koppisepi S. Medical implications of melatonin: Receptor-mediated and receptor-independent actions. Advances in Medical Sciences. 2007;**52**:11-28

[91] Hardeland R. Melatonin metabolism in the central nervous system. Current Neuropharmacology. 2010;**8**(3):168-181

[92] Álvarez-Diduk R, Galano A, Tan DX, Reiter RJ. N-acetylserotonin and 6-hydroxymelatonin against oxidative stress: Implications for the overall protection exerted by melatonin. The Journal of Physical Chemistry. 2015;**119**(27):8535-8543

[93] Tan DX, Manchester LC, Terron MP, Flores LJ, Reiter RJ. One molecule, many derivatives: A never-ending interaction of melatonin with reactive oxygen and nitrogen species? Journal of Pineal Research. 2007;**42**(1):28-42

[94] Pérez-González A, Galano A, Alvarez-Idaboy JR, Tan DX, Reiter RJ. Radical-trapping and preventive antioxidant effects of 2-hydroxymelatonin and 4-hydroxymelatonin: Contributions to the melatonin protection against oxidative stress. Biochimica et Biophysica Acta. 2017;**1861**(9):2206-2217

[95] Tan DX, Hardeland R, Manchester LC, Poeggeler B, Lopez-Burillo S, Mayo JC, Sainz RM, Reiter RJ. Mechanistic and comparative studies of melatonin and classic antioxidants in terms of their interactions with the ABTS cation radical. Journal of Pineal Research. 2003;**34**(4):249-259

[96] Galano A, Tan DX, Reiter RJ. Cyclic 3-hydroxymelatonin, a key metabolite enhancing the peroxyl radical scavenging activity of melatonin. RSC Advances. 2014;**4**:5220-5227

[97] Galano A, Medina ME, Tan DX, Reiter RJ. Melatonin and its metabolites as copper chelating agents and their role in inhibiting oxidative stress: A physicochemical analysis. Journal of Pineal Research. 2015;**58**(1):107-116

[98] López-Burillo S, Tan DX, Rodriguez-Gallego V, Manchester LC, Mayo JC, Sainz RM, Reiter RJ. Melatonin and its derivatives cyclic 3-hydroxymelatonin, N1-acetyl-N2-formyl-5-methoxykynuramine and 6-methoxymelatonin reduce oxidative DNA damage induced by Fenton reagents. Journal of Pineal Research. 2003;**34**:178-184

[99] Paredes Royano SD, Reiter RJ. Melatonin: Helping cells cope with oxidative disaster. Cell Membranes and Free Radical Research. 2010;**2**(3):99-111

[100] Silva SO, Ximenes VF, Livramento JA, Catalani LH, Campa A. High concentrations of the melatonin metabolite, N1-acetyl-N2-formyl-5-methoxykynuramine, in cerebrospinal fluid of patients with meningitis: A possible immunomodulatory mechanism. Journal of Pineal Research. 2005;**39**(3):302-306

[101] Hardeland R. Taxon- and site-specific melatonin catabolism. Molecules. 2017;**22**(11):1-23

[102] Reiter RJ, Fuentes-Broto L, Paredes SD, Tan DX, Garcia JJ. Melatonin and the pathophysiology of cellular membranes. Marmara Pharmaceutical Journal. 2010;**14**:1-9

[103] Esposito E, Cuzzocrea S. Antiinflammatory activity of melatonin in central nervous system. Current Neuropharmacology. 2010;**8**(3):228-242

[104] Reiter RJ, Tan DX, Galano A. Melatonin reduces lipid peroxidation and membrane viscosity. Frontiers in Physiology. 2014;**5**(377):1-4

[105] Manchester LC, Coto-Montes A, Boga JA, Andersen LP, Zhou Z, Galano A, Vriend J, Tan DX, Reiter RJ. Melatonin: An ancient molecule that makes oxygen metabolically tolerable. Journal of Pineal Research. 2015;**59**(4):403-419

[106] Zavodnik IB, Domanski AV, Lapshina EA, Bryszewska M, Reiter RJ. Melatonin directly scavenges free radicals generated in red blood cells and a cell-free system: Chemiluminescence measurements and theoretical calculations. Life Sciences. 2006;**79**(4):391-400

[107] Zhang H, Squadrito GL, Pryor WA. The reaction of melatonin with peroxynitrite: Formation of melatonin radical cation and absence of stable nitrated products. Biochemical and Biophysical Research Communications. 1998;**251**(1):83-87

[108] Zhang H, Squadrito GL, Uppu R, Pryor WA. Reaction of peroxynitrite with melatonin: A mechanistic study. Chemical Research in Toxicology. 1999;**12**:526-534

[109] Gönenç A, Hacışevki A, Tavil Y, Çengel A, Torun M. Oxidative stress in patients with essential hypertension: A comparison of dippers and non-dippers. European Journal of Internal Medicine. 2013;**24**:139-144

[110] Reiter RJ, Tan DX, Galano A. Melatonin: Exceeding expectations. Physiology (Bethesda, Md.). 2014;**29**(5):325-333

[111] Kotler M, Rodríguez C, Sáinz RM, Antolín I, Menéndez-Peláez A. Melatonin increases gene expression for antioxidant enzymes in rat brain cortex. Journal of Pineal Research. 1998;**24**(2):83-89

[112] Bhatti GK, IPS S, Bhatti JS. Protective effect of melatonin against malathion induced alterations in antioxidant defense system and morphology of erythrocytes in Wistar rats. Journal of Basic & Applied Sciences. 2013;**9**:438-446

[113] Hardeland R. Neuroprotection by radical avoidance: Search for suitable agents. Molecules. 2009;**14**(12):5054-5102

[114] Reiter RJ, Acuña-Castroviejo D, Tan DX, Burkhardt S. Free radical-mediated molecular damage: Mechanisms for the protective actions of melatonin in the central nervous system. Annals of the New York Academy of Sciences. 2001;**939**:200-215

[115] Blokhina O, Virolainen E, Fagerstedt KV. Antioxidants, oxidative damage and oxygen deprivation stress: A review. Annals of Botany. 2003;**91**:179-194

[116] Osellame LD, Blacker TS, Duchen MR. Cellular and molecular mechanisms of mitochondrial function. Best Practice & Research. Clinical Endocrinology & Metabolism. 2012;**26**(6):711-723

[117] Ganie SA, Dar TA, Bhat AH, Dar KB, Anees S, Zargar MA, Masood A. Melatonin: A potential anti-oxidant therapeutic agent for mitochondrial dysfunctions and related disorders. Rejuvenation Research. 2016;**19**(1):21-40

[118] García JJ, López-Pingarrón L, Almeida-Souza P, Tres A, Escudero P, García-Gil FA, Tan DX, Reiter RJ, Ramírez JM, Bernal-Pérez M. Protective effects of melatonin in reducing oxidative stress and in preserving the fluidity of biological membranes: A review. Journal of Pineal Research. 2014;**56**(3):225-237

[119] Flora SJ, Shrivastava R, Mittal M. Chemistry and pharmacological properties of some natural and synthetic antioxidants for heavy metal toxicity. Current Medicinal Chemistry. 2013;**20**(36):4540-4574

[120] Adefegha SA, Oboh G. Water extractable phytochemicals from some Nigerian spices inhibit Fe^{2+}-induced lipid peroxidation in Rat's brain–in vitro. Journal of Food Processing and Technology. 2011;**2**(1):1-6

[121] Cardinali DP, Vigo DE, Olivar N, Vidal MF, Brusco LI. Melatonin therapy in patients with Alzheimer's disease. Antioxidants (Basel). 2014;**3**(2):245-277

[122] Hardeland R. Melatonin, hormone of darkness and more: Occurrence, control mechanisms, actions and bioactive metabolites. Cellular and Molecular Life Sciences. 2008;**65**(13):2001-2018

[123] Gonenc A, Hacisevki A, Erdemoglu AK, Dagkiran ME, Torun M. Evaluation of oxidative stress markers and antioxidant status in Alzheimer disease, vascular dementia and the Parkinson disease. Oxidation Communications. 2013;**36**(1):235-245

[124] Csányi G, Miller FJ Jr. Oxidative stress in cardiovascular disease. International Journal of Molecular Sciences. 2014;**15**:6002-6008

[125] Baker J, Kimpinski K. Role of melatonin in blood pressure regulation: An adjunct antihypertensive agent. Clinical and Experimental Pharmacology & Physiology. 2018:1-12. DOI: 10.1111/1440-1681.12942. [Epub ahead of print]

[126] Pechanova O, Paulis L, Simko F. Peripheral and central effects of melatonin on blood pressure regulation. International Journal of Molecular Sciences. 2014;**15**(10):17920-17937

[127] Favero G, Franceschetti L, Buffoli B, Moghadasian MH, Reiter RJ, Rodella LF, Rezzani R. Melatonin: Protection against age-related cardiac pathology. Ageing Research Reviews. 2017;**35**:1-366

[128] Dominguez-Rodriguez A, Abreu-Gonzalez P, Sanchez-Sanchez JJ, Kaski JC, Reiter RJ. Melatonin and circadian biology in human cardiovascular disease. Journal of Pineal Research. 2010;**49**(1):14-22

[129] Petrosillo G, Di Venosa N, Pistolese M, Casanova G, Tiravanti E, Colantuono G, Federici A, Paradies G, Ruggiero FM. Protective effect of melatonin against mitochondrial dysfunction associated with cardiac ischemia- reperfusion: Role of cardiolipin. The FASEB Journal. 2006;**20**(2):269-276

[130] Sánchez A, Calpena AC, Clares B. Evaluating the oxidative stress in inflammation: Role of melatonin. International Journal of Molecular Sciences. 2015;**16**(8):16981-17004

[131] Bukowska A. Anticarcinogenic role of melatonin--potential mechanisms. Medycyna Pracy. 2011;**62**(4):425-434

[132] Matés JM, Segura JA, Alonso FJ, Márquez J. Intracellular redox status and oxidative stress: Implications for cell proliferation, apoptosis, and carcinogenesis. Archives of Toxicology. 2008;**82**:273-299

[133] Hacışevki A, Baba B, Gönenç A, Aslan S. Protein carbonyl content as the most general and well-used biomarker of severe oxidative stress, oxidation. Communication. 2012;**35**(2):413-422

[134] Srinivasan V, Spence DW, Pandi-Perumal SR, Trakht I, Cardinali DP. Therapeutic actions of melatonin in cancer: Possible mechanisms. Integrative Cancer Therapies. 2008;**7**(3):189-203

[135] Jung B, Ahmad N. Melatonin in cancer management: Progress and promise. Cancer Research. 2006;**66**(20):9789-9793

[136] Reiter RJ, Rosales-Corral SA, Tan DX, Acuna-Castroviejo D, Qin L, Yang SF, Xu K. Melatonin, a full service anti-cancer agent: Inhibition of initiation, progression and metastasis. International Journal of Molecular Sciences. 2017;**18**(4):1-47

[137] Li Y, Li S, Zhou Y, Meng X, Zhang JJ, Xu DP, Li HB. Melatonin for the prevention and treatment of cancer. Oncotarget. 2017;**8**(24):39896-39921

[138] Chojnacki C, Walecka-Kapica E, Romanowski M, Chojnacki J, Klupinska G. Protective role of melatonin in liver damage. Current Pharmaceutical Design. 2014;**20**(30):4828-4833

[139] Lebda MA, Sadek KM, Abouzed TK, Tohamy HG, El-Sayed YS. Melatonin mitigates thioacetamide-induced hepatic fibrosis via antioxidant activity and modulation of pro-inflammatory cytokines and fibrogenic genes. Life Sciences. 2018;**192**:136-143

[140] Das N, Mandala A Naaz S, Giri S, Jain M, Bandyopadhyay D, Reiter RJ, Roy SS. Melatonin protects against lipid-induced mitochondrial dysfunction in hepatocytes and inhibits stellate cell activation during hepatic fibrosis in mice. Journal of Pineal Research. 2017;**62**(4):1-21. DOI: 10.1111/jpi.12404

[141] Hacışevki A, Baba B, Sezer S, Özkan Y. Increased kynurenine/tryptophan and neopterin levels in hemodialysis. Oxidation Communications. 2013;**36**(1):246-253

[142] Hacışevki A, Gönenç A, Sezer S, Karakan Ş, Şimşek B, Torun M. Accumulation of an endogenous inhibitor of nitric oxide synthesis and oxidative DNA damage in end-stage renal disease. Clinical Laboratory. 2013;**59**:1353-1361

[143] Dehdashtian E, Mehrzadi S, Yousefi B, Hosseinzadeh A, Reiter RJ, Safa M, Ghaznavi H, Naseripour M. Diabetic retinopathy pathogenesis and the ameliorating effects of melatonin; involvement of autophagy, inflammation and oxidative stress. Life Sciences. 2018;**193**:20-33

[144] Zephy D, Ahmad J. Type 2 diabetes mellitus: Role of melatonin and oxidative stress. Diabetes and Metabolic Syndrome: Clinical Research and Reviews. 2015;**9**(2):127-131

7

Melatonin and its Indisputable Effects on the Health State

Hanan Farouk Aly and Maha Zaki Rizk

Abstract

Melatonin is a hormone synthesized from the amino acid tryptophan produced especially at night in the pineal gland and helps induce sleep. It is reported to play a role in preventing the production of free radicals and is thus a potent antioxidant. It can also enhance the function of the immune system and appears to have an antitumor effect. Melatonin secretion, mediated by photoperiod, directly influences reproductive function and dopamine which moves into frontal lobe regulating flow of information coming in from other areas of the brain. Additional side effects may be produced from treatment with melatonin and include stomach cramps, dizziness, headache, irritability, breast enlargement in men (called gynecomastia), and decreased sperm count. For clinical trials, the direct effect of exogenous melatonin administration on patients manifested with cancer should be studied to find its oncostatic effects on some cancers and provide information on its dosage and long-term safety. Moreover, mechanisms of action should be further investigated.

Keywords: melatonin, anti-aging, anticancer antiproliferative effect, geroprotector

1. Hormone description

Melatonin is a hormone (N-acetyl-5 methoxytryptamine) produced especially at night in the pineal gland which helps in the maintenance of the body's hormone balance and regulation, in immune system integrity, and in circadian rhythm (daily metabolic balance). This gland functions as a biological clock and time keeper of the brain by secreting melatonin and many other neuropeptides at night, helps to govern the sleep-wake cycle and, in animals, seasonal rhythms of migration, mating, and hibernation. Secretion of melatonin is stimulated by the dark and inhibited by light. Melatonin levels start to be released at sunsets, where neural signals are triggered which stimulate the pineal gland to begin releasing the hormone.

Melatonin is synthesized from the amino acid tryptophan. Tryptophan (l-tryptophan) is an essential amino acid formed from proteins during digestion by the action of proteolytic enzymes. Tryptophan is converted to serotonin, a brain chemical involved with mood during the day and the latter finally converted to the indole melatonin (**Figures 1** and **2**). Melatonin occurs naturally in some foods but in fairly small amounts. Of all the plant-based foods, oats, sweet corn and rice are the richest source in melatonin, containing between 1000 and 1800 picograms while ginger, tomatoes, bananas and barley levels amount to 500 picograms per gram. In the human population, melatonin levels are highest in children and middle-aged adults and usually about 5–25 micrograms of melatonin are secreted each night. This amount tends to decline with age, a possible link with an age-related rise in difficulty sleeping and in the production of free radicals [1]. Synthetic melatonin and melatonin derived from bovine pineal glands are available as dietary supplements over-the-counter.

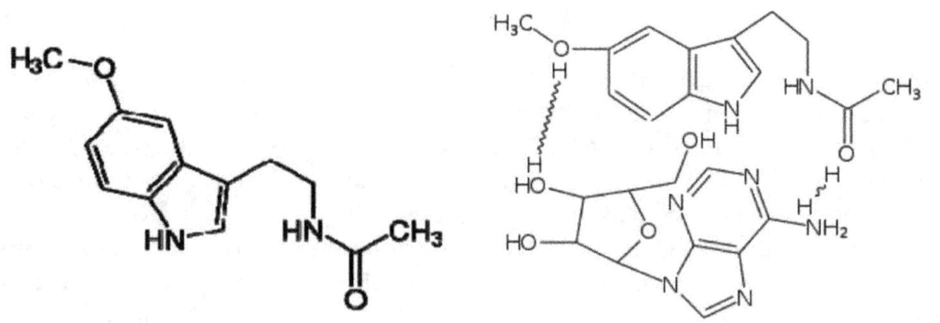

(A) (B)

Figure 1. Chemical structure of Tryptophan (A) and Melatonin (B).

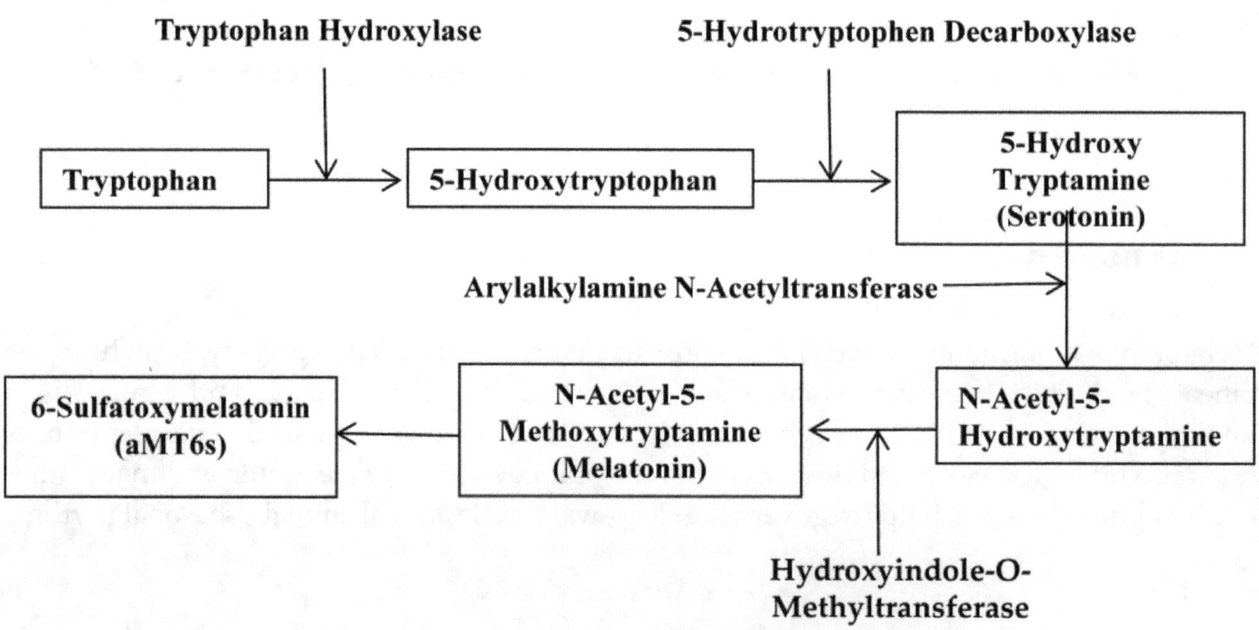

Figure 2. The biosynthesis and metabolism process of melatonin. www.impactjournals.com/oncotarget.

2. Biological functions

Melatonin, stimulated by darkness and inhibited by light, is involved in synchronizing the body's hormone secretions and in regulating their levels, setting the brain's internal biological clock and hence controlling circadian rhythms (daily biorhythms) or sleep-wake. Melatonin regulates many neuroendocrine functions and can inhibit secretion of luteinizing hormone (LH) and follicle stimulating hormone (FSH) from the anterior pituitary gland. When the timing or intensity of melatonin peak is disrupted (as in aging, stress, jet-lag, or artificial jet-lag syndromes), the biological clock is upset and many physiological and mental functions are adversely affected including the ability to think, remember, and make sound decisions can be profoundly hampered. Melatonin is also controls the timing and release of female reproductive hormones and hence helps determine when menstruation begins and ends (menopause), and the frequency and duration of menstrual cycles [1].

In addition to its hormone actions, melatonin also has strong antioxidant properties and may scavenge and eliminate cell-damaging free radicals. The latter are chemical constituents that have an unpaired electron and cause lipid peroxidation, DNA damage and protein oxidation. Besides, it inhibits nitric oxide synthetase enzyme leading to reduction in the formation of peroxynitrite in tissues of brain. Melatonin stimulates the activities of antioxidant enzymes; glutathione peroxidase, superoxide dismutase and catalase. Melatonin is twice as effective at protecting cell membranes from lipid peroxidation as vitamin E and is five times more effective than glutathione for neutralizing hydroxyl radicals. As an antioxidant, it possibly helps to control or delay the development of heart disease, cancer and other conditions and may be effective in destroying malignant cells when combined with certain anticancer drugs. Since glutathione concentrations are not very high in the brain, both melatonin and adenosine may be particularly important in protecting brain cells [1].

3. Melatonin as an activity enhancer of antioxidative enzymes

Two decades ago, melatonin was found to be a free radical scavenger [2]. However, abundant data ascertaining its ability to reduce oxidative stress have rapidly accumulated [3, 4]. The efficacy of melatonin in functioning in this subject is related to its direct free radical scavenging actions. Owing to its chemical formula, melatonin can interact with various forms of free radicals such as H_2O_2, $\bullet OH$, singlet oxygen ($^1O_2$), superoxide anion ($\bullet O_2^-$), peroxynitrite anion ($ONOO^-$) and peroxyl radical ($LOO\bullet$) [4]. The main photoproduct metabolites of melatonin degradation are potent antioxidants such as *N*1-acetyl-5-methoxykynuramine (AMK) or *N*1-acetyl-*N*2-formyl-5-methoxykynuramine (AFMK) [4]. Moreover, investigations on free radicals produced as a result of UV exposure, showed that by using cell-free melatonin-containing systems exposed to UV radiation (UVB: 60%, UVA: 30%) four metabolites were identified by HPLC and LC–MS: 2-OH-melatonin, 4-OH-melatonin, 6-OH-melatonin and AFMK [5]. Since these metabolites are potent antioxidants, this may suggest that, unlike other classic antioxidants, they do not induce prooxidant reactions. In addition, melatonin acts as a potent antioxidant through enhancing activity of antioxidant enzymes [6]. It should be noted that not only enzyme activity, but also gene transcription of antioxidant enzymes such as manganese superoxide dismutase (Mn-SOD), copper-zinc superoxide dismutase (Cu/Zn-SOD), glutathione peroxidase (GPx) and gamma-glutamyl cysteine synthetase (γ-GCS) were maintained by melatonin n brain of rat [4]. This continuing enhancement proposed a possible role of activation of melatonin receptors to modulate antioxidant enzymes regulation following stress signals [7]. Actually, there are some suggestions that melatonin-modified antioxidant enzymes expression following signal pathways of membrane, cytosolic and nuclear receptors [8].

4. The melatoninergic antioxidative system (MAS) of the skin

It should be mentioned that synthesis of melatonin is not only confined to the pineal gland, but also extends to various other organs including the skin [4]. After exposure to UV, melatonin is metabolized in the skin and in turn causes production of antioxidant melatonin metabolites in human keratinocytes. This antioxidant cascade can be suggested for the skin, the same as in several described melatonin-related antioxidant cascades in chemical or other tissue homogenate systems [9]. This cascade has been defined as the melatoninergic antioxidative system (MAS) of the skin (**Figure 2**) forming an important barrier organ and protecting it against UV-induced oxidative stress-mediated damaging events on the nuclear, subcellular, protein and cell morphology level [5]. Melatonin forms a defense mechanism against the multifaceted threats of environmental stress, especially UV, to which the skin is life-long exposed. Owing to its chemical structure, melatonin as well as its metabolites are strongly lipophilic, which renders them easily diffusible in every skin and cell compartment, therefore penetrating beyond the epidermis, namely to the dermis and the hair follicle [10]. When the skin is exposed to UV irradiation, the reactive hydroxyl radical is generated in the skin and reacts directly with melatonin [11]. The scavenging effect of melatonin to hydroxyl radicals causes decrease in the lipid peroxides, oxidation of protein and damage of mitochondrial DNA. Thus, the cascade of melatoninergic antioxidative is significant in decreasing the free radicals emerging from radiation of UV and subsequently performs, a very hopeful strategy to keep the skin versus stressor factor of environmental condition as well as causative agent for aging of skin and promotion of tumor.

5. Anti-aging

Another functional importance of melatonin is its potency to enhance, augment or neutralize the negative effects that stress, drugs and infections have on the body's immune system. The decrease in melatonin secretion by age is so reliable that blood melatonin levels have been proposed as a measurement of biological age.

Melatonin is critical for the regulation of circadian and seasonal changes in various aspects of physiology and neuroendocrine functions [12]. The reduction in life span was detected in rats as a result of a pinealectomy [12], whereas prolongation in the life span occurs upon transfer of pineal gland grafting from young mice into thymus of old mice or into pinealectomized old mice which reveals the ability of melatonin to extend life span [12]. Analysis of available data on the effect of melatonin on longevity supports its geroprotective effect. We believe that melatonin biosafety is important for the study of it's the long-term effects at different doses and in different strains and species (e.g., in rats). In adequately designed work (50 rats in each group), small doses of melatonin were supplemented at the night (2.5–3 mg/kg), slow the starting of age-associated disorders in function of estrous and elevated the animals survival. There are multiple evident on the melatonin suppressive effect on the growth of impulsive mammary carcinogenesis and that initiated in mice and rats as a results of chemicals and radiation [13–15], carcinogenesis induced in colon of rats by 1,2-dimethyl hydrazine [16], while, carcinogenesis induced in uterine cervix and vagina of mice by DMBA [16] and liver cancer induced in rats by N-nitrosodiethylamine [17]. In these cases, it was observed that melatonin exerted a positive effect in the treatment of advanced cancer patients [18]. Melatonin has a dual effect: it is potent geroprotector, suppressor of tumor growth in vivo and in vitro. There are no discrepancies between results of the carcinogenic and anticarcinogenic potential of melatonin since previous reports showed that other antioxidants, such as α-tocopherol has geroprotector and tumorigenic effects and could be powerful anticarcinogens as well. The data of melatonin supplementation to perimenopausal women are hopeful [19]. Simultaneously, there are actual results on the unfavorable impacts of melatonin [12] such as melatonin may produce infertility, damage of retina and hypothermia, it stimulates high blood pressure, diabetes, and cancer by suppressing sex drive in males. It was remark that melatonin may be harmful for people with cardiovascular risk factors and it should not be obtain by individuals who have immune-system or mental disorders, or by people administered steroids.

6. Melatonin as a protector against UV-induced skin aging

Because of its properties as wide antioxidant and scavenger of free radical, melatonin may act as a preventative factor against damage induced by UV in the skin [5]. Clinically melatonin is worthy to protect damage of sun when it is taken before irradiation of UV [20]. These effects of melatonin as a protective agent versus damage induced by UV have in vitro studies powerful support [20, 21]. Melatonin counteracting the formation of polyamine levels so it enhances cell viability in UV-irradiated fibroblasts, and malondialdehyde accumulation while inhibited apoptosis cells [21].

Regarding to Ryoo et al. [22] study in fibroblasts exposed to UV, only 56% of the cells survived (140 mJ/cm^2), while the survival rate of cells reached to 92.50% when preincubated with 1 nM melatonin which was paralleled with marked decrease in malondialdehyde and death of cells. Other experimental comparative study using fibroblasts treated by UV declared identical correlation in viability of cells using 100 nM melatonin [21]. Additionally, melatonin is considered as a powerful anti-apoptotic compound that inhibited caspase 9 and caspase 3 by suppresses mitochondria-dependent (intrinsic) apoptosis however, it does not inhibit receptor-dependent (extrinsic) pathway of apoptosis mediated by caspase 8 "[23]. UV irradiation is considered an immediate agent acted directly on skin, the oxidative stress resulting in all known successive, destruction events in the skin can distinctly, only be antagonized by antioxidants, melatonin which is already found at the target sites and at the same time of exposure to UV ([23]. Besides, there is clear evidence that the preventive actions of melatonin against photobiological distraction are ameliorated by the powerful antioxidative characteristic of this compound. Photodamage, is tightly connected with UV-induced generation of ROS and it was shown that melatonin is a markedly powerful free radicals scavenger compared with vitamin C or Trolox, a vitamin E analog [21].

7. Anti-cancer, immunity and reproduction

Tumor growth is showed to be inhibited by melatonin. Melatonin may be of a great value in patients with untreatable metastatic cancer, especially in ameliorating their life quality. Several experiments showed that the levels of melatonin may be connected with risk of breast cancer. Some chemotherapy drugs used to treat breast cancer may be enhanced also by melatonin. Supplementation of melatonin reduces luteinizing hormone concentrations leading to inhibition of ovulation in humans. Further, melatonin administration may aid menopausal women by eliciting and sustaining sleep. Levels of melatonin may have a role in the anorexia symptoms. It was found that melatonin was used in seasonal affective disorder (SAD), due to the disorder is considered to be produced by melatonin release at an inadequate time [1].

Melatonin immunopharmacological activity has been indicated in different models. Melatonin treatment elevates antibodies production of sheep erythrocytes and immune response to primary immunization with T-dependent antigens [24]. Melatonin is involved in complicated relationships between the endocrine and nervous systems [25]. There are membrane receptors of melatonin on helper (Th). Melatonin receptors activation results to an elevate the production of Th1 cytokines, such as γ-interferon, interleukin-1, and opioid cytokines (interleukin-4 and dinorphine) [25]. At physiological concentrations of melatonin, it induces release of interleukins-1, -6 and -12 in monocytes of human. These mediators can protect stress-stimulated immunodepression maintaining mice from virus- and bacteria caused lethal diseases [25]. It is useful noticing that γ-interferon and colony-inducing factors (CSFs) can stimulate melatonin release in the pineal gland [25].

It is well accepted that melatonin is considered not only a hormone, but also protector for cells [26], implicated in modulation of immune system, processes of antioxidant and hematopoiesis [27]. Moreover, melatonin has a powerful oncostatic characters, through receptor-dependent and -independent mechanisms [28]. The melatonin receptors MT1 (encoded by *MTNR1A*) and MT2 (encoded by *MTNR1B*) are associated with the G-protein-coupled receptor (GPCR) group [26], and are mainly responsible for mediating melatonin downstream effects [29]. The antiproliferative effects melatonin may be due to melatonin–stimulated suppression in the uptake of linoleic acid [26]. Melatonin also demonstrated the probability to be used as adjuvant in therapies of cancer, through augmentation the effects of therapeutic drugs and decreased chemotherapies or radiation side effects [26].

Some studies recommended an inverse association between circadian melatonin level and breast cancer incidence. In addition, it was demonstrated high melatonin level up to ≤39.5 pg/mL in female showed high risk for breast cancer than females had high melatonin level > 39.5 pg/mL in a case–control study. Besides, in another five prospective case control, an inverse relationship was demonstrated between risk of breast cancer and the highest levels of aMT6s in urine [30, 31]. In controversy, in case–control study declared that high aMT6s level in urine level was markedly linked with a low breast cancer risk [26]. However, it was demonstrated that, no confirmation was detected between level of melatonin and its association with risk of breast cancer in four case–control studies. Regardless of menopausal status, there is no statistically significant differences was detected in urinary aMT6s level between British women with breast cancer and healthy one in a prospective nested case–control [26]. In postmenopausal women, there was no suggestion that high melatonin levels in urine were inversely associated with risk of breast cancer [32]. In the study of Brown et al. [33], did not document an overall correlation between melatonin levels in urine and the onset risk of breast cancer [33]. Simultaneously, no markedly relation was detected between level of aMT6s and risk of breast cancer (either totally or by status of menopausal) [34].

In other types of cancer, it was found that, the men with low level of aMT6s in the urine below the median first morning connected with a four time increase in risk of in comparison with those with levels above the median. In addition, a case–control study showed that patients with high melatonin-sulfate levels or a high melatonin-sulfate/cortisol ratio were less likely to have prostate cancer or advanced stage prostate. It was found that the serum melatonin levels in women with ovarian cancer were significantly lower compared with control subjects ($p < 0.05$), demonstrating that decline in circulating melatonin level might contribute to the pathogenesis of ovarian cancer in a retrospective study [35].

It is worth mentioning that, the assessment melatonin levels are not equals, since concentrations of melatonin were determined in various sample as urine, plasma or serum. Also, the concentration of melatonin in human modifies with circadian rhythm; however, it has not been demonstrated which the best time for the sample collection could demonstrate the effects of melatonin. These variations might incorporate in the discrepancy of researches.

Research relating melatonin's effects on breast cancer is the serious, may be due to that melatonin has reported to attenuate various endocrine physiological biomarkers. Novel works showed that melatonin exhibited antiproliferative action against *in vitro* cell line of breast cancer [26], and suppressed mammary tumors development in rats [26]. Several melatonin mechanisms as anticancer were identified as it is apoptosis inducer [36], antiestrogenic effect through signaling pathway of ERα and decreased activity of aromatase enzyme [36], attenuation of receptors of melatonin [26], suppression on invasion [37] and angiogenesis [38].

Prostate cancer is the second most cancer type recorded and the fifth leading cause of cancer mortality in men [26]. It was found that melatonin at pharmacological concentrations could inhibit cell growth of both androgen-dependent and androgen-independent prostate cancer [26], through a range of mechanisms.

One of the leading causes of death among women with genital tract disorders is ovarian cancer [39]. Even though various surgical techniques and chemotherapies have been useful for treatment of ovarian carcinoma, the prognosis remains lacking [40]. In recent years, a few studies have reported the anticancer effect of melatonin on cancer of ovary.

Cervical cancer is considered the principle leading reason of female tumor worldwide, [41]. The melatonin effect on cervical cancer has been detected in insufficient works.

Visceral obesity is a risk factor of endometrial cancer, as it is associated with chronic inflammatory process [42]. Ciortea *et al.* [42] reported that the combinational treatment of melatonin and estrogen in ovariectomized rats was linked with lower body weight, less intra-retroperitoneal fat, reduction in endometrial proliferation, and less appearance of cellular atypia compared with estrogen replacement treatment. These results show that melatonin supplementation could be used in the prophylaxis of endometrial cancer in menopause women [42].

8. Oral cancer

Oral cancer is a common type of human head and neck cancers, and the majority of the cases involve oral squamous cell carcinoma [26]. In several *in vitro* studies, melatonin has shown remarkable effect on oral cancer.

It was reported that melatonin presented effect on oral cancer cell lines as an anti-metastatic action (HSC-3 and OECM-1), through modulation of expression and activity of MMP-9, which was occurred by decreasing acetylation of histone [26]. Also, melatonin could minimize SCC9 and SCC25 cell lines viabilities (both tongue carcinoma), and exhibit suppressive effect on the pro-metastatic *ROCK- 1*gene expression and *HIF-1α* pro-angiogenic genes as well as *VEGF* in SCC9 cell line [43]. Overall, inhibitory effect of melatonin was demonstrated on some oral cancer cells, and its mechanisms of action mainly involved inhibitory effect on metastasis and its related angiogenesis.

Cancer of liver is considered the common reason of death globally, and hepatocellular carcinoma (HCC) is contributed to the most common type of cancer (70–80%), occurrence in developing countries [44]. Treatment with surgery still remains the most pronounced way for HCC patients, however it is only occurs in a few cases, thus it is necessary to find efficient chemotherapeutic drug [45]. Hence, several studies pointed out to the effects of melatonin on hepatocellular carcinoma. Melatonin modulates the changes produced by N-nitrosodiethylamine-initiated cancer of liver and ameliorates biomarkers of liver enzymes (ALT, AST), levels of antioxidant, as well as the disturbance in circadian clock in mice [46, 47].

SO, melatonin exerts its anti-liver cancer effects mainly due to its anti- pro-apoptotic activity (via COX-2/PI3K/AKT pathway attenuation, modulates the ratio of Bcl-2/Bax, as well as it activates ER stress), anti-angiogenesis and anti-invasive effects.

Renal cancer is considered the third high cancer accounts for 3% with predominance of a male (3 male/1 female) [26].

Lung cancer is a principal cause of cancer-related death. For instance, lung cancer is the second most frequent type of cancer in males with approximately 17,330 new cases identified in 2016 in Brazil [26]. Non-small-cell lung cancer (NSCLC) is a main form of cancer of lung [26], and the literatures have suggested that the disturbance of rhythm of melatonin could elevate the incidence of NSCLC [26]. In different researches, melatonin due to mainly because melatonin showed to enhance the effects of it enhances radiotherapy and chemotherapeutic drugs.

Gastric cancer causes a mortality rate ranking second among malignant tumors worldwide one of the most frequent forms of cancer worldwide [26]. It was recorded that there were

951,600 new cases and 723,100 deaths from gastric cancer in 2012 worldwide [26]. Melatonin has been reported to inhibit gastric cancer through various mechanisms in numerous studies.

Pancreatic cancer is a highly fatal disease with a relatively low 5-year survival rate [48]. It responds poorly to radiotherapy and chemotherapy because the tumor cells are challenging to apoptosis [49].

Colorectal cancer is one of the major causes responsible for cancer death worldwide [26], and in several studies, melatonin recorded anticancer potency for various colorectal cancers. Overall, melatonin could be a new tempting therapeutic strategy for colorectal cancer, since it could regulate carcinogenesis, development, and progression of colorectal cancer. The underlying mechanisms involve multiple signaling pathways, including regulation of Ca MKII, ET-1, Nrf2 signaling pathways, and induction of aberrant crypt foci (ACF).

9. Effect of melatonin on gene expression

The presenting results on the melatonin genomic effect is rather few. In a study of cytogenecity, it was found that a decrease in the gene activity of ribosomes as a result of a pinealectomy in rats [12]. Menendez-Pelaez et al. [50] declared that melatonin treatment reduces mRNA level in the synthesis porphyrin, and 5- aminolevulinate synthase, in the Syrian hamsters Harderian glands. Melatonin declines mRNA levels of histone H4 and stopped age-attributed mRNA Bcl-2 reduction, in mice thymocytes [12]. Also, melatonin elevated some antioxidant enzymes mRNA (Mn-SOD, Cu,Zn-SOD) in Syrian hamsters Harderian gland [12]. Supplementation of melatonin produced significant enhancement in relative levels of mRNA for Mn-SOD, Cu,Zn-SOD and glutathione peroxidase in cerebral cortexes of rat [12]. Melatonin (1 nM) markedly modulates the mRNA of gonadotropin-releasing hormone. It was observed that melatonin regulate transforming growth factor-α gene expression level, macrophage-colony stimulating factor (M-CSF), tumor necrosis factor-α (TNFα) the stem cell factor in PEC, and interleukin-1β, M-CSF, TNFα, interferon-γ, and the stem cell factor in splenocytes [12]. These results are appropriate with results that the SCN is the main site for the exogenous melatonin effect on the amplitude rhythm of the endogenous melatonin [51]. Medication with melatonin suppressed the development of mammary tumor and regulated *HER-2/neu* onco gene in transgenic *HER-2/neu* mice [52].

Marked melatonin effect was noticed on some oncogenesis- associated genes expression [12]. Further, myeloblastosis oncogene-like 1 (Mybl1) expression was adjusted by melatonin. On the other hand, melatonin showed a great effect on a large number of genes attributed to exchange of calcium, as cullins, Kcnn4 and Dcamkl1, calmodulin, calbindin, Kcnn2 and Kcnn4. Meanwhile, cullin-1 expression in the heart of mouse is down regulated, that of cullin-5 is significantly upregulated, and cullins-2 and -3 expression are significantly not deformed. Six members of cullin family are included, and are implicated in ubiquinone-mediated protein destruction necessary for cell-cycle through the G1 and S phases. Nevertheless, cullin-1, but not other members of the cullin family, is responsible for cell proliferation and differentiation [53]. It is believe that melatonin may effect on expansion of tumor by intermediating with binding of calcium and preventing the MAPs/calmodulin and tubulin/calmodulin complexes formation to stop degradation of cytoskeletal [54]. Peutz-Jeghers syndrome, which is associated with high risk of tumor development in multiple localizations is associated with at least one of these, Stk11 kinase with an unclear function, has anticarcinogenic effects and mutations [55]. Eventually, these data present undeviating evidence for the different effect of melatonin on the expression of different genes *in vivo*. Specific gene expression profiles are connected with the aging process in animals and humans [12]. Lund et al. [56] have detected a reduction in gene expression of heat shock protein while an elevation in the insulin-like genes expression, resulting in a decline in gene expression of insulin signaling during aging. Pletscher et al. [57], showed that down regulation of a large number of genes implicated in cell growth and maintenance following caloric restriction. Weindruch et al. [58], declared that in mice, the process of aging is describe by the high level of reactive oxygen species in both the skeletal muscle and brain, inhibition in the genes expression of biosynthetic enzyme and genes implicated in turnover of protein. Hence, caloric restriction stimulated genes are implicated in the metabolism of fatty acid, glycolysis, and gluconeogenesis. Presented results on the melatonin effects on gene expression, mainly genes of mitochondria, suggest that some of them may be accountable for the hormone capacity to block disorders resulting from aging. Further studies are need in this direction.

10. Melatonin and reproduction

Pattern of melatonin secretion, mediated by photoperiod, directly affect reproductive function which was recorded in several evidence-based researches. The daily light/dark (LD) cycle is considered the main physiological melatonin role, so, the variation in the duration of signal of melatonin occurs in attribution to the night length. The variation in melatonin signal duration is used to synchronize neuroendocrine rhythms with the annual variation in day-length in seasonal mammals. In addition, fetal and newborn animals use the maternal signal of melatonin to entrain endogenous circadian rhythms before direct photic information is presented. It was found that, very marked effect for exogenous melatonin was detected in modulating reproductive function in different organisms, depending on the animal age, melatonin supplementation time [59].

The data presented above exhibited that the antigonadal effects of melatonin in humans are apparently much less significant than in some seasonally breeding mammalian species. This is due to humans are not 'seasonally breeding'. Recently, accumulated evidences declared the efficacy of melatonin in attenuation the reproductive function in human. The suppressive effect of melatonin at the level of CNS have decreased daring growth. During development of human, such suppressive action of melatonin on GnRH function gradually reduced due to a down regulation in the functional of melatonin receptors expression. In other adult rodents, melatonin does not have noticeable action on the functioning of pituitary, whereas the association between the release of melatonin release and the functions of hypothalamic, involving the release of GnRH, are right. These actions are markedly significant in coinciding the external photoperiods and functions of reproduction through well not characterized mechanisms. The circadian rhythm regulated genes are considered seriously players in regulation of gene throughout different organism, especially for regulatory genes of cell-cycle and apoptotic genes. Melatonin may have also ameliorating effectiveness against human disorders attributed to reproductive function. Such as illumination intensity during the night actually decreases circulating levels of melatonin and reconstruct the suprachiasmatic nuclei circadian pacemaker, leading to the elevation in risk of breast cancer, which may be due to down-regulating gonadal synthesis of steroids, by acting on receptor sites within the neuro-endocrine reproductive axis or altered estrogen receptor function [59]. Consequently, in the right circumstances, melatonin may be quite beneficial for reproductive health.

11. Dopamine and psychosis

Disorder in the system of dopamine has also been noticeably associated with psychosis and schizophrenia. Dopamine proceeds in the frontal lobe and regulating the information coming in from other parts of the brain. Normalization in the dopamine flow may produce interrupted or discontinuous cogitation as in schizophrenia. Schizophrenia is described by both 'positive '(additional experience and behavior) and 'negative symptoms' (lack in experience or behavior). Symptoms of positive response are classifying under the psychosis term and identically involve disorders of illusions, deliriums, and intellect. Symptoms of negative response may involve unsuitable emotional manifestation, lack of speech and stimulus. Some drugs, as cocaine, prevent dopamine return into the brain, coherently, dopamine buildup in the synapse, producing drug-initiated psychosis or schizophrenia [1].

12. Contraindications, interactions, precautions and side effects

Melatonin can produce sleepiness if given during the day. Additional, side effects that have been documented upon melatonin supplementation including cramps of stomach, vertigo, a continuous pain in the head, touchiness, moodiness, reduced sexual desire, enlargement of breast in the men and reduction in the count of sperm.

So, melatonin should not take during operating machine or drive. Further, melatonin could interrupt with human fertility and also melatonin should be not used for pregnant or nursing women. Utilization of melatonin by person who already have an augmentation level of melatonin as children, teenagers, pregnant and lactating women can result in melatonin overdose. MAOI drugs inhibit melatonin breakdown from the body, so people should not take melatonin with these drugs to prevent melatonin overdose.

Melatonin causes drug–drug interaction with antidepressants, such as Prozac (inhibitor of serotonin) or Nardil (inhibitor of monoamine oxidase). Melatonin Interaction with these kinds of drugs can produce heart attack, confusion, sweating, shaking, and fever, lack of coordination, elevated blood pressure, diarrhea, and convulsions [1].

13. Discussion and conclusion

Melatonin is considered as a potent geroprotector, anticarcinogen, and inhibitor of tumor growth *in vivo* and *in vitro*, and in some models it may induce tumors and promote tumor growth. An important mechanism of melatonin is its impact on hemopoiesis involves the stimulation of melatonin on opioid receptors of bone marrow. Hence, we confirm further experimental studies and clinical trials which are necessary to estimate both the effectiveness and the safety for humans. Some antioxidants, including natural ones (e.g., α-tocopherol), have both geroprotector and tumorigenic potential and could be potent anticarcinogens as well. The results of administration of melatonin to perimenopausal women are promising. There are no contradictions between data on the carcinogenic and anticarcinogenic potential of melatonin but there are real data on the adverse effects of melatonin. Melatonin might own some ameliorating actions on human disorders that are contributed to the reproductive func-tion. Such as lighting intensity during the night decreased the levels of circulating melatonin resulting in high risk of breast cancer [60]. Therefore, in the optimum condition, melatonin may have significant beneficial reproductive effects.

Epidemiological studies concerning the association between body circadian melatonin levels and cancer incidence led to controversial results, which were either significant association or no association at all. The effects of melatonin on cancers have been investigated, with a focus on hormone-dependent cancers. Different experimental works have suggested the ameliorative effect of melatonin in numerous types of metastatic tumors, including breast, ovarian, prostate, oral, gastric, and colorectal cancers. The mechanisms contributed with this improvement role of melatonin include various pathways of molecular origin, which are implicated with the activity of antioxidant enzymes, attenuation of MT1 and MT2 melatonin receptors, apoptosis regulation, metabolism of tumor, angiogenesis inhibition, invasion and metasta-sis, and initiation of epigenetic alteration.

In different clinical trials, melatonin exhibited the capability to augment the treatment effect of chemotherapeutic drugs, and might help in enhancing the cancer patient's life quality. Collectively, melatonin is considered a promising hormone for cancers prevention and treatment. So, it could be concluded that extensive future work may be occur which involves the effect of melatonin on autophagy and mitophagy, other mechanisms of molecular origin implicated in its anticancer effect. Melatonin improves also chemotherapeutic drugs, which should be further determined on a large scale of drugs. The oncostatic effects of melatonin on some type of cancers, dosage and safety of long-term supplementation of melatonin must be also further elucidated.

Author details

Hanan Farouk Aly* and Maha Zaki Rizk

*Address all correspondence to: hanan_abdallah@yahoo.com

Therapeutic Chemistry Department, National Research Centre, Giza-Dokki, Egypt

References

[1] Available from: http://www.Vitamins and Health

[2] Bartsch H, Buchberger A, Franz H, Bartsch C, Maidonis I, Mecke D, Bayer E. Effect of melatonin and pineal extracts on human ovarian and mammary tumor cells in a chemosensitivity assay. Life Sciences. 2000;**67**:2953-2960

[3] Lissoni P, Barni S, Mandala M, Ardizzoia A, Paolorossi F, Vaghi M, Longarini R, Malugani F, Tancini G. Decreased toxicity and increased efficacy of cancer chemotherapy using the pineal hormone melatonin in metastatic solid tumor patients with poor clinical status. European Journal of Cancer. 1999;**35**:1688-1692

[4] Di Bella G, Mascia F, Gualano L, Di Bella L. Melatonin anticancer effects: Review. International Journal of Molecular Sciences. 2013;**14**:2410-2430. DOI: 10.3390/ijms14022410

[5] Lissoni P, Bolis S, Brivio F, Fumagalli L. A phase II study of neuroimmunotherapy with subcutaneous low-dose IL-2 plus the pineal hormone melatonin in untreatable advanced hematologic malignancies. Anticancer Research. 2000;**20**:2103-2105

[6] Eck-Enriquez K, Kiefer TL, Spriggs LL, Hill SM. Pathways through which a regimen of melatonin and retinoic acid induces apoptosis in MCF-7 human breast cancer cells. Breast Cancer Research and Treatment. 2000;**61**:229-239

[7] Hill SM, Blask DE, Xiang S, Yuan L, Mao L, Dauchy RT, Dauchy EM, Frasch T, Duplesis T. Melatonin and associated signaling pathways that control normal breast epithelium and breast cancer. Journal of Mammary Gland Biology and Neoplasia. 2011;**16**:235-245

[8] SoybIr G, Topuzlu C, Odaba SO, Dolay K, BIlIr A, Koksoy F. The effects of melatonin on angiogenesis and wound healing. Surgery Today. 2003;**33**:896-901

[9] García-Pergañeda A, Pozo D, Guerrero JM, Calvo JR. Signal transduction for melatonin in human lymphocytes: Involvement of a pertussis toxin-sensitive G protein. Journal of Immunology. 1997;**159**:3774-3781

[10] Dong C, Yuan L, Dai J, Lai L, Mao L, Xiang S, Rowan B, Hill SM. Melatonin inhibits mitogenic cross-talk between retinoic acid-related orphan receptor alpha (RORalpha) and ERalphain MCF-7 human breast cancer cells. Steroids. 2010;**75**:944-951

[11] Soto-Vega E, Meza I, Ramírez-Rodríguez G, Benitez-King G. Melatonin stimulates calmodulin phosphorylation by protein kinase C. Journal of Pineal Research. 2004;**37**: 98-106

[12] Anisimov VN. Effects of exogenous melatonin—A review. Toxicologic Pathology. 2003; **31**:589-603

[13] Freedman DA, Zeizel H. From mouse—To man: The quantitative assessment of cancer risks. Statistical Science. 1988;**3**:3-56

[14] Warner HR, Ingram D, Miller RA, Nadon NL, Richardson AG. Program for testing biological interventions to promote healthy aging. Mechanisms of Ageing and Development. 2000;**55**:199-208

[15] Deerberg F, Bartsch C, Pohlmeyer G, Bartsch H. Effect of melatonin and physiological epiphysectomy on the developmet of spontaneous endometrial carcinoma in BDII/HAN rats. Cancer Biotherapy and Radiopharmaceuticals. 1997;**12**:420

[16] Anisimov VN. Melatonin and colon carcinogenesis. In: Bartsch C, Bartsch H, Blask DE, Cardinali DP, Hrushesky WJM, Mecke D, editors. The Pineal Gland and Cancer. Neuroimmunoendocrine Mechanisms in Malignancy. Berlin: Springer; 2001. pp. 240-258

[17] Imaida K, Hagiwara A, Yoshino H, Tamano S, Sano M, Futakuchi M, Ogawa K, Asamoto M, Shirai T. Inhibitory effects of low doses of melatonin on induction of preneoplastic liver lesions in a medium-term liver bioassay in F344 rats: Relation to the influence of electromagnetic near field exposure. Cancer Letters. 2000;**155**:105-114

[18] Lissoni P. Is there a role for melatonin in supportive care? Supportive Care in Cancer. 2002;**10**:110-116

[19] Bellipanni G, Bianchi P, Pierpaoli W, Bulian D, Ilyia E. Effects of melatonin in perimenopausal and menopausal women: A randomized and placebo controlled study. Experimental Gerontology. 2001;**36**:297-310

[20] Park SY, Jang WJ, Yi EY, Jang JY, Jung Y, Jeong JW, Kim YJ. Melatonin suppresses tumor angiogenesis by inhibiting HIF-1alpha stabilization under hypoxia. Journal of Pineal Research. 2010;**48**:178-184

[21] Kleszczynski K, Fischer TW. Melatonin and human skin aging. Dermato-Endocrinology. 2012;**4**(3):245-252

[22] Ryoo YW, Suh SI, Mun KC, Kim BC, Lee KS. The effects of the melatonin on ultraviolet-B irradiated cultured dermal fibroblasts. Journal of Dermatological Science. 2001;**27**: 162-169. DOI: 10.1016/ S0923-1811(01)00133-5

[23] Fischer TW, Zmijewski MA, Wortsman J, Slominski A. Melatonin maintains mitochondrial membrane potential and attenuates activation of initiator (casp-9) and effector caspases (casp-3/casp-7) and PARP in UVR-exposed HaCaT keratinocytes. Journal of Pineal Research. 2008;**44**:397-407. DOI: 10.1111/j.1600-079X.2007.00542.x

[24] Mao LL, Dauchy RT, Blask DE, Slakey LM, Xiang SL, Yuan L, Dauchy EM, Shan B, Brainard GC, Hanifin JP, Frasch T, Duplessis TT, Hill SM. Circadian gating of epithelial-to-mesenchymal transition in breast cancer cells via melatonin-regulation of GSK3. Molecular Endocrinology. 2012;**26**:1808-1820

[25] Kassayova M, Bobrov N, Strojny L, Orendas P, Demeckova V, Jendzelovsky R, Kubatka P, Kiskova T, Kruzliak P, Adamkov M, Bomba A, Fedorocko P. Anticancer and immunomodulatory effects of lactobacillus plantarum LS/07, inulin and melatonin in NMU-induced rat model of breast cancer. Anticancer Research. 2016;**36**:2719-2728

[26] Li Y, Li S, Zhou Y, X M, Zhang JJ, Xu DP, Li HB. Melatonin for the prevention and treatment of cancer. Oncotarget. 2017;**8**:39896-39921

[27] Cutando A, Lopez-Valverde A, Arias-Santiago S, De Vicente J, De Diego RG. Role of melatonin in cancer treatment. Anticancer Research. 2012;**32**:2747-2753

[28] Srinivasan V, Spence DW, Pandi-Perumal SR, Trakht I, Cardinali DP. Therapeutic actions of melatonin in cancer: Possible mechanisms. Integrative Cancer Therapies. 2008;**7**: 189-203

[29] Deming SL, Lu W, Beeghly-Fadiel A, Zheng Y, Cai QY, Long JR, Shu XO, Gao YT, Zheng W. Melatonin pathway genes and breast cancer risk among Chinese women. Breast Cancer Research and Treatment. 2012;**132**:693-699

[30] Abd El Moneim NA, El Masry H, Sorial MM. A molecular case-control study on the association of melatonin hormone and rs#10830963 single nucleotide polymorphism in its receptor MTNR1B gene with breast cancer. Middle East Journal of Cancer. 2015;**6**:11-20

[31] Basler M, Jetter A, Fink D, Seifert B, Kullak-Ublick GA, Trojan A. Urinary excretion of melatonin and association with breast cancer: Meta-analysis and review of the literature. Breast Care. 2014;**9**:182-187

[32] Sturgeon SR, Doherty A, Reeves KW, Bigelow C, Stanczyk FZ, Ockene JK, Liu S, Manson JE, Neuhouser ML. Urinary levels of melatonin and risk of postmenopausal breast cancer: Women's health initiative observational cohort. Cancer Epidemiology Biomarkers & Prevention. 2014;**23**:629-637

[33] Brown SB, Hankinson SE, Eliassen AH, Reeves KW, Qian J, Arcaro KF, Wegrzyn LR, Willett WC, Schernhammer ES. Urinary melatonin concentration and the risk of breast cancer in nurses' health study II. American Journal of Epidemiology. 2015;**181**:155-162

[34] Wang XS, Tipper S, Appleby PN, Allen NE, Key TJ, Travis RC. First-morning urinary melatonin and breast cancer risk in the Guernsey study. American Journal of Epidemiology. 2014;**179**:584-593

[35] Zhao M, Wan JY, Zeng K, Tong M, Lee AC, Ding JX, Chen Q. The reduction in circulating melatonin level may contribute to the pathogenesis of ovarian cancer: A retrospective study. Journal of Cancer. 2016;**7**:831-836

[36] Cos S, Martinez-Campa C, Mediavilla MD, Sanchez- Barcelo EJ. Melatonin modulates aromatase activity in MCF-7 human breast cancer cells. Journal of Pineal Research. 2005;**38**:136-142

[37] Lai L, Yuan L, Cheng Q, Dong CM, Mao LL, Hill SM. Alteration of the MT1 melatonin receptor gene and its expression in primary human breast tumors and breast cancer cell lines. Breast Cancer Research and Treatment. 2009;**118**:293-305

[38] Jardim-Perassi BV, Lourenco MR, Doho GM, Grigolo IH, Gelaleti GB, Ferreira LC, Borin TF, Moschetta MG, Zuccari D. Melatonin regulates angiogenic factors under hypoxia in breast cancer cell lines. Anti-Cancer Agents in Medicinal Chemistry. 2016;**16**:347-358

[39] Jablonska K, Pula B, Zemla A, Kobierzycki C, Kedzia W, Nowak-Markwitz E, Spaczynski M, Zabel M, Podhorska-Okolow M, Dziegiel P. Expression of the MT1 melatonin receptor in ovarian cancer cells. International Journal of Molecular Sciences. 2014;**15**:23074-23089

[40] Koshiyama M, Matsumura N, Konishi I. Recent concepts of ovarian carcinogenesis: Type I and type II. BioMed Research International. 2014;**2014**:1-11

[41] Scarinci IC, Garcia FAR, Kobetz E, Partridge EE, Brandt HM, Bell MC, Dignan M, Ma GX, Daye JL, Castle PE. Cervical cancer prevention. Cancer. 2010;**116**:2531-2542

[42] Ciortea R, Costin N, Braicu I, Haragas D, Hudacsko A, Bondor C, Mihu D, Mihu CM. Effect of melatonin on intra-abdominal fat in correlation with endometrial proliferation in ovariectomized rats. Anticancer Research. 2011;**31**:2637-2643

[43] Goncalves ND, Rodrigues RV, Jardim-Perassi BV, Moschetta MG, Lopes JR, Colombo J, Zuccari D. Molecular markers of angiogenesis and metastasis in lines of oral carcinoma after treatment with melatonin. Anti-Cancer Agents in Medicinal Chemistry. 2014;**14**:1302-1311

[44] Zhou Y, Li Y, Zhou T, Zheng J, Li S, Li H. Dietary natural products for prevention and treatment of liver cancer. Nutrients. 2016;**8**:156

[45] Kapitanov T, Neumann UP, Schmeding M. Hepatocellular carcinoma in liver cirrhosis: Surgical resection versus transarterial chemoembolization—A meta-analysis. Gastroenterology Research and Practice. 2015;**2015**:1-8

[46] Verma D, Hashim OH, Jayapalan JJ, Subramanian P. Effect of melatonin on antioxidant status and circadian activity rhythm during hepatocarcinogenesis in mice. Journal of Cancer Research and Therapeutics. 2014;**10**:1040-1044

[47] Moreira AJ, Ordonez R, Cerski CT, Picada JN, Garcia-Palomo A, Marroni NP, Mauriz JL, Gonzalez-Gallego J. Melatonin activates endoplasmic reticulum stress and apoptosis in rats with diethylnitrosamine-induced hepatocarcinogenesis. PLoS One. 2015;**10**: e014451712

[48] Leja-Szpak A, Jaworek J, Pierzchalski P, Reiter RJ. Melatonin induces pro-apoptotic signaling pathway in human pancreatic carcinoma cells (PANC-1). Journal of Pineal Research. 2010;**49**:248-255

[49] Talar-Wojnarowska R, Malecka-Panas E. Molecular pathogenesis of pancreatic adenocarcinoma: Potential clinical implications. Medical Science Monitor. 2006;**12**:RA186-RA193

[50] Menendez-Pelaez A, Rodriguez C, Dominguez D. 5-Aminolevulinate synthase mRNA levels in the Harderian gland of Syrian hamsters: Correlation with porphyrin concentrations and regulation by androgens and melatonin. Molecular and Cellular Endocrinology. 1991;**80**:177-182

[51] Bothorel B, Barassin S, Saboureau M, Perreau S, Vivien-Roels B, Malan A, Pevet P. In the rat, exogenous melatonin increases the amplitude of pineal melatonin secretion by a direct action on the circadian clock. European Journal of Neuroscience. 2002;**16**:1090-1098

[52] Baturin DA, Alimova IA, Anisimov VN, Popovich IG, Zabezhinski MA, Provinciali M, Mancini R, Franceschi C. The effect of light regimen and melatonin on the development of spontaneous mammary tumors in HER-2/neu transgenic mice is related to a down regulation of HER-2/neugene expression. Neuroendocrinology Letters. 2001;**22**:439-445

[53] Krek W. Proteolysis and the G1-S transition: The SCF connection. Current Opinion in Genetics & Development. 1998;**8**:36-42

[54] Blask DE, Sauer LA, Dauchy RT. Melatonin as a chronobiotic/ anticancer agent: Cellular, biochemical, and molecular mechanisms of action and their implications for circadian-based cancer therapy. Current Topics in Medicinal Chemistry. 2002;**2**:113-132

[55] Hemminki A. The molecular basis and clinical aspects of Peutz-Jeghers syndrome. Cellular and Molecular Life Sciences. 1999;**55**:735-750

[56] Lund J, Tedesco P, Duke K, Wang J, Kim SK, Johnson TE. Transcriptional profile of aging in *C. elegans*. Current Biology. 2002;**12**:1566-1573

[57] Pletscher SD, Macdonald SJ, Marguerie R, Certa U, Stearns SC, Goldstein DB, Patridge L. Genome-wide transcript profiles in aging and calorically restricted Drosophila melanogaster. Current Biology. 2002;**12**:712-723

[58] Weindruch R, Kayo T, Lee CK, Prolla TA. Gene expression profiling of aging using DNA microarrays. Mechanisms of Ageing and Development. 2000;**123**:177-193

[59] Srinivasan V, Spence WD, Pandi-Perumal SR, Zakharia R, Bhatnagar KP, Brzezinski A. Melatonin and human reproduction: Shedding light on the darkness hormone. Gynecological Endocrinology. 2009;**25**:779-785

[60] Stevens RG. Circadian disruption and breast cancer: From melatonin to clock genes. Epidemiology. 2005;**16**:254-258

8

Salivary Melatonin at Night: Responding to the Night Lighting and Cow's Milk Consumption at Breakfast in Japanese Junior High and University Students

Hitomi Takeuchi and Tetsuo Harada

Abstract

(1) In junior high school students aged 14–15 years old, the salivary melatonin level increased rapidly from 3.00 pg/ml at 21:45 to 9.18 pg/ml at 23:40 under orange light from light bulb, whereas it remained at less than 1.3 pg/ml under white light from fluorescent lamp. (2) In 3 weeks of intervention on university athlete students, the salivary melatonin concentration at 23:00 of G3 (protein-rich breakfast and following sunlight exposure and orange light from the light bulb at night) after intervention was significantly higher than that of G1 (protein-poor breakfast and not following exposure to sunlight and white light from the fluorescent lamp at night) and G2 (protein-rich breakfast and following exposure to sunlight and white lights from the fluorescent lamp at night). (3) This study evaluates the effects of cow's milk intake (Group 1: G1) for 20 days at breakfast on saliva melatonin concentration at 22:00 and 23:00 on 0, 10, and 21 days of the intervention period in Japanese university male athletes attending a university soccer club. In the intervention group (G1), salivary melatonin concentration increased at 22:00 in comparison with that before intervention, but there was no significant change in the control group (Group 2: G2). On the other hand, there were no significant differences in the melatonin at 23:00 between the both groups just after 21 days of intervention. Intake of cow's milk at breakfast might make the circadian phase in advance in the soccer athletes.

Keywords: junior high-school students, university soccer club students, salivary melatonin concentration in 22:00–23:00, orange or white lighting at night, cows' milk at breakfast

1. Background

Night sleep duration of Japanese children aged 10–18 years has become shorter by 1 hour during 1970–2000 in Japan [1]. In 2016, sleep hours in Japanese infants were reported to be only 9 hours (ideal hours, 12–13 hours) on average [2], while it ranged mainly in 7–10 hours for 8–11 years old of Japanese children (ideal hours, 10–11 hours) [3]. The so-called 24-hour society, which is currently in progress in Japan, seems to change environmental conditions surrounding the children. For example, mobile phones are used by more than 90% in 2000 and more than 98% in 2017 of university students, and more than 30% in 2000 and 95% in 2017 of junior high school students living in the urban area of Kochi city (33°N) had their own mobile phone (currently, most ones have smart phones) [4, 5]. Students can communicate with their colleagues even in the middle of the night with mobile phones. Frequent or long-time (more than 30 min) usage of the mobile phone makes university and junior high school students more evening-typed [4, 5]. At least for Japanese students in junior and senior high schools and universities, convenience stores have critical items for usual life, and these provide many kinds of foods and other goods for usual life. The total number of convenience stores by the main eight Japanese companies is 55,395 in 24 April 2018 all over Japan (http://mitok.info/?p=75099). Convenience stores are very bright places with luminance of 2000 Lux or more at the level of the eye height. Such bright light inside convenience stores may function as a merchandising technology which has been used all over the world for at least 75 years. Unconscious effects of using bright lights with higher color temperature in the evening or at night could be very serious for phase-delaying the circadian clock of students who had been exposed to bright lights [6].

Honma and Honma [6] reported an evidence that phase-delay effects were shown by light pulse exposure with higher color temperature from fluorescent lamp made only in the first half of the subjective night (about 19:00–24:00) in the circadian phase. On the other hand, phase advance of the circadian clock could be caused by the light exposure during 3 hours from the bottom point (about 4:00–5:00) of core body temperature rhythm. The effects of the night or evening use of convenience store was studied and showed that it was possible to make the diurnal rhythms of Japanese children mainly aged 12–15 years old become more evening-typed and take shorter sleep [7, 8]. Younger children attending kinder gardens and students attending elementary school were more sensitive to "light conditions" in normal life than university students, according to an epidemiological study [4].

Melatonin is synthesized in the pineal body of the hypothalamic area and secreted at night. It is well known as a key substance which may be effective in promoting the falling into night sleep by humans [9]. During daytime, the concentration of plasma melatonin was reported to be extremely low, whereas it increased rapidly during 22:00–23:00 as much as 10 or 20 times of daytime values [10, 11]. The melatonin intake caused higher EEG power density in the range of relatively low frequency of 5.25–9.0 Hz rather than that of placebo [12]. The melatonin level in the serum can be well and positively correlated with that in the saliva [13–16]. Secretion of melatonin exhibits circadian rhythms and is suppressed by bright light at night [17, 18]. Moreover, the plasma melatonin level at night was suppressed by the exposure of lights with 400 Lux for more than 4 min (or 300 Lux for more than 2 hours), whereas such suppression was not seen under dim lights [19, 20]. Even room lights such as fluorescent lamps can attenuate melatonin excretion duration at night [21]. Especially, blue lights with 460 nm as peak wave length in the evening can be well absorbed by melanopsin in the neuro-ganglia cells in the retina [22, 23]. Evening lighting conditions are also said to affect circadian rhythms [24, 25] and mental health in mice [26]. Tryptophan intake at breakfast is effective for the onset and offset of sleep in young children [27]. Moreover, questionnaire surveys showed that young children exposed to sunlight for more than 30 min after having sources of protein at breakfast are more morning-typed than those exposed for less than 30 min [28] and that the more young children take in vitamin B6 at breakfast, the more they exhibit morning typology [29]. These findings can lead to appear the following hypothesis. It would be that morning tryptophan and vitamin B6 intake and following exposure to sunlight in the morning can induce serotonin synthesis in the daytime especially in the morning at pineal, and the following metabolism from serotonin to melatonin synthesis at night also at pineal can be promoted. However, it is impossible to test this hypothesis by a simple questionnaire study. Moreover, this melatonin synthesis could be inhibited by the night exposure to shortwave length (blue light, high color temperature) lights emitted from fluorescent lamps through melanopsin [30]. This hypothesis can be tested by an intervention field experiment which was done [31] and introduced here.

In the case of adolescents and children, exposure to lights of 300 Lux or more during the first half of subjective night in the normal life might decrease their melatonin level and prevent the falling into sleep [32]. Japanese junior and senior students were known to study at home mainly at night and also in the private preparatory school (for upper schools). In such cases, they are exposed to bright lights in most cases from fluorescent light bulbs. Many blue or blue-green lights with 470–500 nm wave lengths which were included in the bright lights were powerful to suppress melatonin concentration [33].

In the epidemiological studies made in 2003–2013 on university students in Kochi Prefecture (33°N), 21.4% of the students used frequently (more than 4–5 days or more per week) convenience stores [34]. Twenty-two percent of convenience store users went there after sunset. Among convenience store users, 30.2 and 6.5% of junior high school students stayed there for 15–30 min and more than 30 min per one use, respectively [8]. In Japan, many junior high school students were faced to the entrance examination for the upper senior high school and went to a private preliminary school after schools. About 62.4 and 18% of the students in preparation went and studied there for 2 or 3 hours till 21:00 and 22:00, respectively [8]. Generally, in Japanese education scene, some junior and senior students use convenience stores after sunset and were exposed to bright light with high color temperature with more than 2000 Lux from the fluorescent lamp. These exposures seem to suppress the plasma melatonin level [31, 35] and also are possible to make the circadian phase delayed in junior high school and university students.

Tryptophan is one kind of amino-acid of 21 kinds and cannot be made up from another substance but only can be absorbed exclusively from meals in humans. After absorption of tryptophan, it was transported from alimentary canal through brain-vessel barrier into the pineal in the brain. There, it was metabolized first to 5-hydroxytryptamine (serotonin) in the morning time mainly, at first, by two kinds of enzymes. Serotonin was again metabolized into melatonin by another two kinds of enzymes again in the pineal at night [36, 37]. What is the function of serotonin as a precursor of melatonin? The shortage of serotonin in the human brain has been known to induce eating disorders, sleep disorders, obsessive compulsive disorder, panic disorder, and depression [38]. The lack of serotonin also seems to cause impulsive behavior and suicidal attempts, anxiety/aggression-driven depression, and aggression [39, 40]. Thus, serotonin is called the "key" substance in the psychiatry field. For example, serotonin reuptake inhibitors (SSRIs) were widely and commonly used for the treatment of affective disorders like as depression [41].

For keeping mental health, serotonin in the brain, one kind of catecholamine, would be a key substance. Medical doctors in the field of psychiatry have used serotonin reuptake inhibitors (SSRIs) widely in the past four decades for the treatment of affective disorders including depression [41]. However, mixed opinions have been expressed to whether SSRIs are effective for the treatment of depression in children and adolescents because there has been the shortage of coincident scientific evidence of SSRIs for young human beings. Synthesis of serotonin seems to be promoted by sunlight exposure after consuming protein-rich foods at breakfast [42]. This synthesis is hypothesized to occur mainly in the morning time. Another study on young Japanese children showed that the amount of tryptophan which was consumed at supper had neither related with morningness-eveningness (M-E) scores nor with sleep habits [43].

How do cow's milk proteins promote human health? Eight ways to promote human health were demonstrated by Nongonierma and FitzGerald [44]: (1) improving satiety and weight management, (2) reducing risk of heart disease, (3) having an antimicrobial role, (4) having anti-inflammatory effects, (5) showing anticancer effects, (6) exerting antioxidant effects, (7) affecting insulin secretion and serum glucose regulation, and (8) an action upon muscle protein synthesis.

Brezinova and Oswald [45] showed, using electroencephalography, that sleep was significantly improved (longer and uninterrupted night sleeps) in older people when they ate a combination of cow's milk and cereal before going to bed. Laird and Drexel [46] reported that a meal of cornflakes and milk strongly improved sleep quality (as judged from an uninterrupted night sleep), with regard to the relationship between sleep health and the intake of cow's milk. On the effects of morning-drinking cow's milk, only a few studies have been performed for any improvement in sleep health. The two results of a questionnaire study have been reported on Japanese infants aged 2–6 years old [47]. Infants who added protein-rich foods at breakfast to the usual breakfast by other infants were more morning-typed and slept with significantly better quality than the other infants. Moreover, infants who drank milk at breakfast were less frequently depressed than those who did not.

Protein intake at breakfast would mean the consumption of tryptophan from the alimentary canal to the blood. Such tryptophan could be transferred to the pineal where serotonin can be synthesized and promote mental health in the daytime as an antidepressive agent. Serotonin can be further synthesized into melatonin as a sleep-onset agent at night [27–29, 31, 48]. For Japanese children, drinking cow's milk at breakfast is an important source of tryptophan and could, on the basis of a questionnaire study [47], be supposed to promote mental and sleep health. Recently, an intervention of drinking cow's milk (200 ml) at breakfast was reported to make Japanese university soccer team athletes who were originally more evening-typed than evening-typed, and this intervention also made their soccer performances in advance [49]. Another intervention study was performed for 1 month on the Japanese university soccer team members using a leaflet entitled: "Three benefits: Go to bed early! Get up early! Eat a nutritionally rich breakfast!" [48]. As the result of this intervention, all of their soccer performance, sleep health, and mental health were improved.

An increased intake of cow's milk at breakfast, as a source of tryptophan, is hypothesized to promote the amount of serotonin in the morning and the following synthesis to melatonin at night in the Japanese university soccer team athletes. However, this hypothesis has not been tested. This study will try to test this hypothesis.

2. Effects of evening light conditions on salivary melatonin of Japanese junior high school students

2.1. Methods

2.1.1. Participants

Japanese junior high school students (four females and six males) as participants in this study were aged 14–15 years old [35]. They were Motoyama junior high school students in the third grade. This junior high school was located in the mountain area of Reihoku district (33.5°N) in Kochi Prefecture, Japan. Seven days were holidays for the participants before this study as intervention experiment. During the holidays before the experiment, they were recommended to keep usual diurnal rhythm (like as bedtime and wake-up times).

The two groups "bright light experimental group (BLEG)" and "dim light control group (DLCG)" were set up for the intervention experiment for junior high school students. For the BLEG and DLCG, participants were selected to have similar circadian typology scores as the diurnal-type scale (DTS) of the morningness-eveningness (M-E) questionnaire of Torsvall and Åkerstedt [50] (mean ± SD: 15.00 ± 4.30 by BLEG and 14.80 ± 4.09 by DLCG). Participants of BLEG showed 23.0 ± 4.2 hours (mean ± SD, bedtime), 8.4 ± 1.9 hours (wake-up time), and 9.1 ± 1.4 hours (sleep hours) just before the experiment. On the other hand, the values were 23.8 ± 1.3 hours (bedtime), 8.9 ± 1.3 hours (wake-up time), and 9.5 ± 1.5 hours (sleep hours) for the DLCG participants. Each group has two females and three males. All participants collected their own saliva using "Salivette" by collecting tubes (SARSTEDT Aktiengesellschaft & Co., Numbrecht, Germany) at 22:30–23:00 under the 200–300 Lux light from fluorescent light bulbs in their home on the day before the experimental day.

Most of the Japanese citizens are enjoying evening time under fluorescent light bulbs during the first half of the subjective night (about 19:00–24:00) based on a long-term epidemiological study [48] on 3700 small children aged 2–6 years and their mothers in 2003–2017 in Kochi.

Eighty-five percent or more of 3700 families of Japanese infants used fluorescent light bulbs as night lighting at home usually. When the illumination was measured at the level of 1 m above floor under a usual type of round-shaped fluorescent light bulb in a typical one-room apartment for university students, it was 340 Lux [31].

2.1.2. Procedure

We collected all 10 participants in front of Motoyama junior high school at 8:00 in 4 January 2003. We moved the participants by a wagon car to the experimental place which was a Japanese-style hotel located at a mountain area, Yusuhara town in Kochi Prefecture, Japan. The Yusuhara town was located 126 km west from the Motoyama town. During driving, illumination inside the car was 350–500 Lux. The car arrived at the hotel around noon on 4 January 2004. It was heavily snowing through the day around the hotel. Behavior of all participants was controlled during the experimental day in the hotel till the next morning of the experimental day. In the experimental daytime, all participants played outside and were exposed to the lights with 6000–7500 Lux at the eye level during 12:30–13:30 and 14:50.

All the participants were exposed to the sunlight with 6000–7500 Lux at the eye level during 12: 30–13:30 and 14:00–14:50 during they played in the yard of the hotel. After the playtime, they were allowed to have a rest in the living room of the hotel. The floor of the rest room was filled with 12 *tatami* mats. The illumination of the light at the eye level in the rest room was 250 Lux from fluorescent light bulbs during the resting time till 16:00. Bath was taken by the participants one by one between 16:30 and 18:00. After that, supper was together taken by all participants between 18:15 and 19:20 in the living room.

BLEG participants moved to a Japanese-style room with eight *tatami* mats at 19:25. They were exposed to the high color temperature (white-colored) light with 2000 Lux at the eye level from fluorescent light bulbs. On the other hand, the DLCG ones moved to another Japanese-style room with eight *tatami* mats at the same time. Instead, the DLCG ones were exposed to the low color temperature (orange-colored) light with 60 Lux from an electronic light bulb.

In each room for BLEG and DLCG, all the participants did homework (e.g., literatures and mathematics) or made a small wooden folk craft object which is typical in the Yusuhara district, under each light condition till 22:30. An oil heater in both rooms functioned to keep the room temperature 15 ± 2°C.

At 22:30, they moved back to the former living room (12 *tatami* mats) and stayed there under the light of 250 Lux till 23:40. After that, experimental staffs ordered female and male participants to move to separate rooms and go to bed just before 24:00. At 21:45, 22:30, and 23:40, the participants collected their own saliva using the "Salivette" as collecting tubes. Their salivary samples were preserved in a refrigerator at less than −20°C. Melatonin concentration in the samples was analyzed by a professional-analyzing company (MSL Co. Ltd.) which was a professional company for analyzing several chemicals and microbiological organisms.

All the participants of BLEG and DLCG were ordered to get up at 7:00 in the next morning by calling out. They were enforced to get up between 7:00 and 7:15. Then, they took breakfast and left the experimental place, the hotel, at 9:00 for Motoyama junior high school. Light exposure at the eye level was measured by using a digital illuminance meter through the study.

2.1.3. Ethic treatment

Detailed explanation of the objectives and methods of the experiment was provided before the experimental performance to the participants and their parents. The research project received full and complete agreement from all of them.

2.1.4. Statistical analysis

The software used for statistical analysis was SPSS 12.0 J for Windows (SPSS Inc., Chicago, IL, USA). The Wilcoxon test was used for the pair-wise test for melatonin concentration for temporal change of melatonin concentration before, through and after the intervention day.

2.2. Results

Salivary melatonin concentration in the DLCG increased from 3.00 ± 3.34 (mean ± SD) pg/ml at 21:45 to 9.18 ± 7.66 pg/ml at 23:30 in the experimental day (t-test between values at 21:45 and 23:30; $t = 3.60$, $df = 4$, $p < 0.05$) (**Figure 1**). On the other hand, it remained at less than 1.3 pg/ml till 23:30 in BLEG ($t = 2.07$, $df = 4$, $p = 0.2$). On the day before the experiment, significant difference was not shown in the melatonin concentration in saliva between BLEG and DLCG (Wilcoxon test: $z = -1.163$, $p = 0.31$). In comparison with the melatonin concentration at 22:30

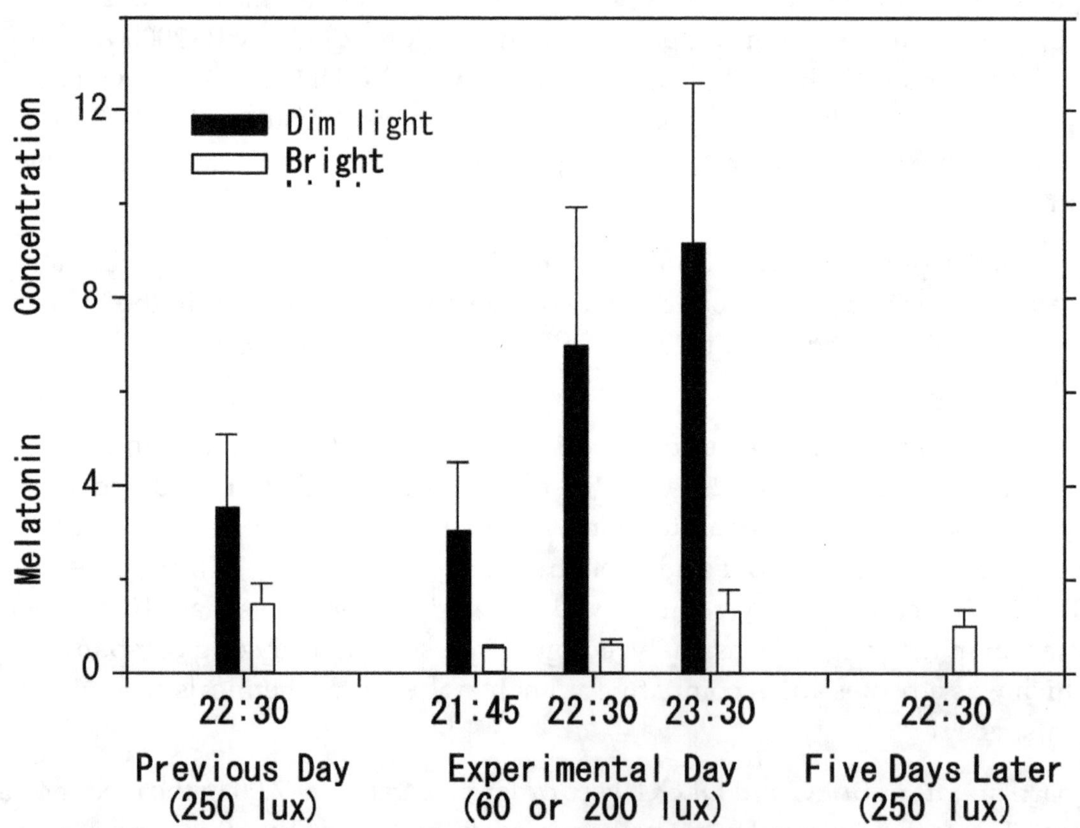

Figure 1. Effects of light condition on salivary melatonin concentration. Values shown are means (n = 5 per group) and SEM [35].

under fluorescent lamps emitting 250 Lux white lights, the value for BLEG at experimental 22:00 tended to be lower, whereas for DLEG, it was significantly higher. In the day before the experimental day, melatonin concentration under the fluorescent lamp with 200–400 Lux in each home of both BLEG and DLCG was similar and had no significant difference (Mann-Whitney U-test: $z = -1.163$, $p = 0.31$). At 22:30 of the experimental day, melatonin concentration of BLEG tended to be lower than that of BLEG on the day before the experiment (Wilcoxon test: $z = -1.604$, $p = 0.109$). On the other hand, the concentration of DLCG at 22:30 become higher than that of the previous day at home ($z = -2.023$, $p = 0.043$).

The bright light of 2000 Lux from fluorescent lamps with high color temperature seems to have suppressed the night increase of melatonin concentration of junior high school students. On the other hand, the relatively low color temperature light with 60 Lux did not. In Japan, the light condition with 2000 Lux and high color temperature can be seen usually inside all the convenience stores of Japan, which are now increasing and become common. Such bright light conditions are also common as room lightings in Japanese private schools, the so-called Juku, which are preliminary schools for preparation of going through the entrance examination, which is a very severe competition for upper schools. Therefore, exposure to bright lights in the evening "Juku" and convenience store would suppress the night increase in the plasma melatonin level as a direct effect also would make the circadian phase delayed and as a result phase of sleep wake cycle can be delayed.

2.3. Discussion

Traditional lightings by ancient Japanese citizens were mainly low color temperature lights which were emitted from a traditional Japanese hearth fire or an oil lamp or candle (20–30 Lux). Such "orange" lightings might be healthy for adolescent and children, because the ancient lightings included only a low amount of the light components with 460–480 nm wave lengths (blue or high color temperature lights), which are peaks of energy consumption by melanopsin (relative to conopsin and lodopsin). Melanopsin is included in neuro-segmental cells and key substance for melatonin suppression [30]. Such orange lights do not stimulate the melanopsin, and melatonin suppression also does not occur. Therefore, junior high school children can fall in night sleep very smoothly [51]. This part 2 was already published in [35].

3. A tryptophan-rich breakfast and exposure to light with low color temperature at night improve the sleep and salivary melatonin level in Japanese students

3.1. Methods

3.1.1. Participants

Ninety-four participants were male university students aged 19–22 years old with averaged 20.33 who were belonging to a university soccer club [31]. They participated in an intervention study; 63 of them answered to the integrated questionnaire before and after the intervention period.

Group 1 (G1) consisted of 20 soccer players without intervention, Group 2 (G2) had 22 soccer club members who were asked to have protein-rich foods such as fermented soybeans and vitamin B6-rich foods such as bananas at breakfast and sunlight exposure after breakfast, and Group 3 (G3) consisted of 21 members who were asked the same breakfast contents and sunlight exposure after that and additionally were asked to use incandescent light as night lighting. All participants were males.

For the night lighting, all the participants in the three groups have used fluorescent lamps (white light). Integrated questionnaires were administered to all participants three times to estimate the effects of the 1-month intervention. Questionnaire studies were performed just before the intervention period, soon after the end of the intervention, and 1 month after the intervention. The same questionnaire was used for study before the intervention and also 1 month after that. The contents of the questionnaire were the diurnal-type scale constructed by Torsvall and Åkerstedt [50], questions on sleep habits and meal habits [52], an Irritation Index, the General Health Questionnaire (GHQ), the Sense of Coherence (SOC) questionnaire, and FFQ (Food Frequency Questionnaire). After the intervention, the questionnaire which had been administered before it was again done. Moreover, other self-assessment questions were also administered to the members of the three groups. The self-assessment questions were on how many days during the month-long intervention period they followed the three recommendations. The first one was on protein-rich foods as breakfast contents, the second one was sunlight exposure after breakfast, and the third one was the usage of orange lightings (like light bulbs which emit orange (lower color temperature)) lights at night.

3.1.2. Procedure

Based on the two questionnaire scores of FFQ (good, mild, and bad: three groups) and the diurnal-type scale (DTS) (morning-typed, middle-typed, evening-typed), nine groups (3 × 3) were made. Members of each of nine groups were randomly divided into the three experimental groups. As the results of the treatment, no significant differences were made also in the body height, body weight, and age, among the three groups.

Through the intervention of 30 days in October–November in 2010, we asked all participants to keep a sleep diary. The sleep diary included a question and a selection list of answer: "How was the depth of your last night's sleep?" "(1) Deep, (2) Relatively deep, (3) Relatively shallow, (4) Shallow." To the members of Group 3, incandescent light bulbs (emitting orange lights) were distributed one by one before the intervention period. After that, they were asked to install the light bulbs (distributed) in their bed room. The G1 and G2 members were asked to switch fluorescent lamps on as usual, whereas the G3 ones were asked to switch incandescent light bulbs (distributed) on instead, when they were asked on the lightings when they got back to their residences after sunset. Room lights for G1 and G2 (white: fluorescent lamp) and G3 (orange: incandescent lamp) were 100–400 Lux and <100 Lux, respectively. Sixty-seven percent of the participants (63 of 94) answered the first questionnaire before intervention and 81% of participants (51 of 63) wrote their own sleep diaries during the intervention of 1 month.

On "high-protein content breakfast" and following "exposure to >30 min exposure to sunlight," the implementation scores were calculated as the sum of days when the "protein-rich breakfast and following light exposure" was implemented. On another intervention "night exposure to low color temperature light," it was defined as implementation score how many minutes per night they were exposed to the low color temperature light emitted from the incandescent bulb.

We asked the participants of G2 and G3 to mark (marking as 0–100 points as satisfaction score) the scores on "To what extent do they satisfy on their carryout of the two (G2) or three (G3) intervention contents for 30 days in the total." We measured the salivary melatonin of the 10 participants of three groups. The 10 participants in each group were selected randomly because there was financial limitation for the chemical analysis. Ninety salivary samplings were needed for the experiment, because three groups prepared one sampling at 23:00 before, in the middle, and in the end of intervention (10 × 3 × 3). We asked participants to extract their own saliva at around 23:00 with cylindrical cotton (1 cm diameter, 3 cm long). If participants put them under their tongues for 3 min, full amount of saliva (1–3 ml) for analysis can be extracted outside and absorbed into the cotton. It was kept frozen at −25°C till analysis for 1–2 weeks. Melatonin concentrations in the saliva were determined using an ELISA kit (Direct Saliva Melatonin ELISA, Bulmann, Switzerland).

3.1.3. Ethic treatment

Participants received a full explanation with the code of the guideline for a study targeting humans before the study [53]. The explanation included that the results of the study would be used only for academic purposes and that all participants completely agreed to participate in this study.

3.1.4. Statistical analysis

We used a statistical analysis software as SPSS 12.0 J for Windows (SPSS Inc., Chicago, IL, USA). As nonparametric analyses, Kruskal-Wallis test and following Bonferroni multiple comparison were used among the three groups. Wilcoxon's signed-rank sum test was used for the pair-wise test in the same group and after the intervention (**Figure 2**).

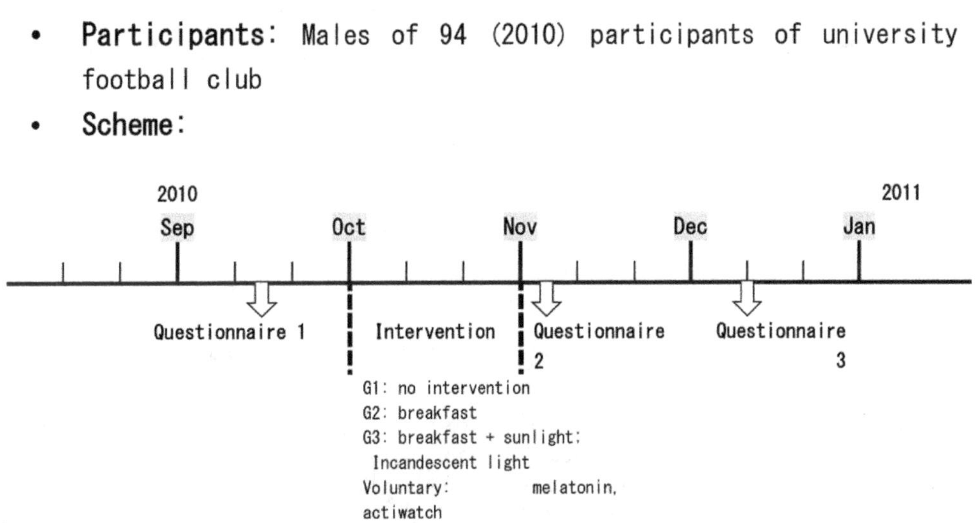

Figure 2. Graphic schema of intervention study for university soccer club athletes.

3.2. Results

We could get significant positive correlation between the feeling of sleeping well in the last week period (LWP) of the intervention period and hours spent under incandescent light at night (Pearson's correlation test $r^2 = 0.265$, $p = 0.034$). Salivary melatonin concentration by G3 participants was significantly higher than that of G1 and G2 in the midpoint and the day before the last day of intervention period (Bonferroni multiple comparison test: G1 vs. G3, $p = 0.018$; G2 vs. G3, $p = 0.011$). On the other hand, we have got no significant differences in the salivary melatonin among the three groups on the day just before the start of the intervention period (Kruskal-Wallis test: χ^2-value = 0.92, df = 2, $p = 0.63$) (**Figure 3**). In the middle period (MP) of the intervention period of G3, the "high implementation period" tended to show a higher concentration of salivary melatonin than the "low implementation group" did (Mann-Whitney U-test: $z = -2.000$, $p = -0.071$).

Group 2 participants tended to follow the morning intervention recommendations (high-protein breakfast and sunlight exposure) on less days than G3 participants did (Mann-Whitney U-test: first week period (FWP), $z = -1.952$, $p = 0.053$; MP, $z = -1.628$, $p = 0.105$;

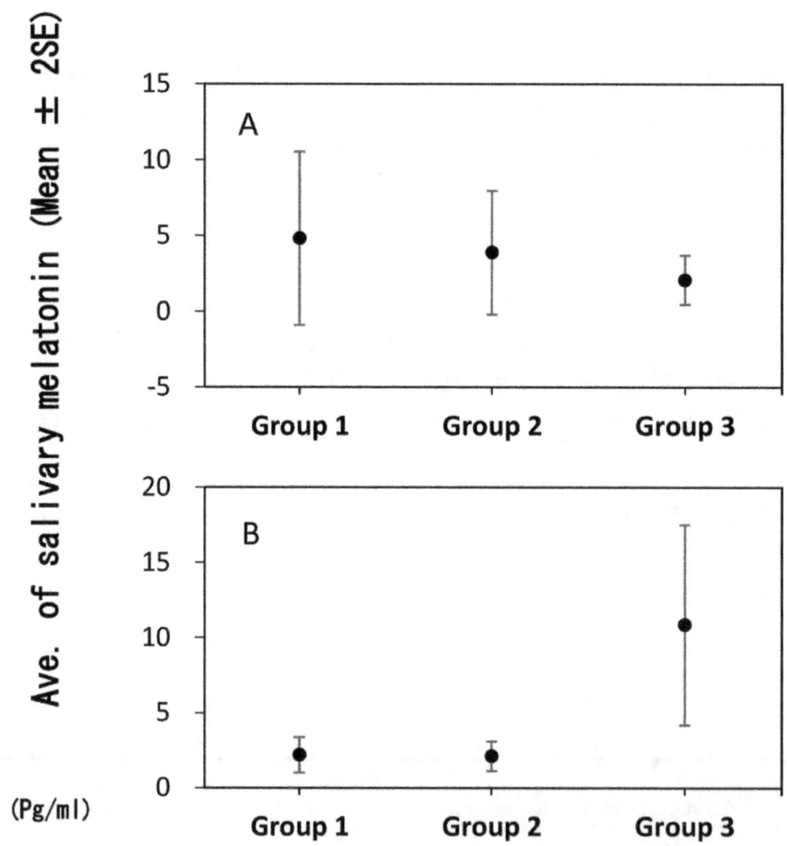

Figure 3. Salivary melatonin level just before intervention (A) (no significant difference: Kruskal-Wallis test: χ^2-value = 0.92, df = 2, $p = 0.63$). All three groups showed low salivary melatonin level of 2–5 pg/ml just before intervention. Melatonin in the saliva collected at the midpoint and on the day before the last day of the intervention (B) (Bonferroni multiple comparison test: G1 versus G3, $p = 0.018$; G2 versus G3, $p = 0.011$). Comparison of salivary melatonin concentration among the three groups. Group 1: no intervention; Group 2: recommendation of high-protein breakfast and exposure to sunlight; and Group 3: same as Group 2 plus the recommendation of exposure to orange lights from incandescent lamps.

LWP, $z = 1.253$, $p = 0.221$). The implementation rate in FWP tended to be higher than MP (Wilcoxon's signed-rank sum test: G2, $z = -1.851$, $p = 0.064$; G3, $z = -1.914$, $p = 0.056$) and LWP (G2, $z = -2.298$, $p = 0.022$, G3, $z = -2.898$, $p = 0.004$). The implementation rate in LWP in G2 and G3 tended to be lower than that in MP (G2, $z = -1.681$, $p = 0.093$; G3, $z = -2.533$, $p = 0.011$).

There was a significantly positive correlation between the regularity of time to take breakfast and supper and the implementation satisfaction index (maximum score, 100) (Kendall tau-b test: breakfast $r^2 = 0.058$, $p = 0.038$; supper $r^2 = 0.057$, $p = 0.036$). There was a significant positive correlation between the index on implementation days and the diurnal-type scale (DTS) at 1 month later after the intervention period (higher scores showing morning-typed) (Pearson's correlation test: $r^2 = 0.195$, $p = 0.006$). The index on intervention days was how many days (among intervention of 30 days) the participants satisfied the implementation on the breakfast contents as high-protein foods.

A significant positive correlation was shown between the number of nights (among 30 days) when participants were exposed to orange-colored lights emitted from incandescent lamp and the index of meal time for three meals just after the intervention (Kendall tau b-test: breakfast $r = -0.574$, $p = 0.007$; lunch $r^2 = 0.146$, $p = 0.084$; supper $r^2 = 0.215$, $p = 0.029$). In comparison with those who ate breakfast less frequently for 1 month after the intervention, participants who took breakfast more frequently took late-night snacks with less frequency (Kendall tau-b test = -142, $p = 0.003$).

In G3, participants after the intervention showed a lower anger/irritation index than those before the intervention (Wilcoxon's signed-rank sum test: $z = -3.072$, $p = 0.002$). On the other hand, G1 showed only a tendency of reduced irritation ($z = -1.786$, $p = 0.074$), and G2 had no differences in mental health index after the intervention ($z = -0.956$, $p = 0.340$). Anger/irritation indices (the frequency to be irritated and the frequency to become angry due to small trigger) were also decreased after the intervention in G3 (Wilcoxon's signed-rank sum test: irritation $z = -2.496$, $p = 0.013$; anger $z = 2.714$, $p = 0.007$).

3.3. Discussion

This study showed that a triple intervention concerning breakfast content, sunlight exposure after breakfast, and exposure to low temperature light emitted from incandescent bulbs are powerful methods for inducing secretion of high amounts of melatonin by the pineal gland inhuman adults. Underlying mechanisms can be hypothesized to consist of two components. The first component is that serotonin synthesis from tryptophan taken at breakfast may be enhanced by the exposure to sunlight just after taking breakfast. The second component is that the high potential of melatonin synthesis based on the high serotonin synthesis in the pineal during daytime might be available due to the night exposure to the "low-temperature light" emitted from incandescent bulbs. Many reports have shown that melatonin secretion is suppressed by evening or night light emitted from fluorescent lamps including shortwave length (with around 460 nm of wave length) components [10, 33, 35, 54–56]. Moreover, this study newly implies that the combined behaviors of (1) modifying breakfast content, (2) receiving sunlight exposure, and (3) receiving exposure to low color temperature lighting at night can facilitate achievement of high plasma melatonin at night in humans. Melatonin, a hormone secreted from the pineal gland, has been reported to cause the core body temperature to decrease and induces sleep [9, 12, 57]. An important role of the high plasma melatonin level at night was reported as a sleep-onset agent and sleep quality promoter [58]. There was a significant and positive correlation between the duration when participants spent under incandescent lights at night and the scores which they marked to feel deep sleep, in this study.

High sleep quality would be promoted by high plasma melatonin in human beings. The principle theory of this study is promotion of serotonin synthesis in the morning and succeeding melatonin synthesis at night. The intervention of this study is composed of three issues: (1) having sources of tryptophan and vitamin B6 at breakfast, (2) following up breakfast with exposure to sunlight, and (3) the exposure to low color temperature lights as night lighting. Serotonin works as antidepression agent, and melatonin is a natural sleep-onset pill. Moreover, these two hormones would act as a circadian clock as inner-zeitgebers. As a result, shift to morning-typed would lead to promoted mental health.

A limitation of this study of the intervention study is as follows: this intervention could not set a control group with low-tryptophan breakfast, sunlight exposure, and exposure to low-temperature light at night for finding out the importance of the intake of tryptophan at breakfast in the physiological mechanism of serotonin-melatonin synthesis. This study was not the so-called physiological experiment to set up several experimental groups and control group under controlling their usual life like as meals, lightings, and social activity in some extents. In the future, another intervention study controlling more life habits would be possible. Another limitation of this study is that this intervention study was performed only with men. In the future, women participants from sports club could add important data for making gender differences in response to breakfast modulation and the change at night lighting into orange light at night. This part 3 was already published in [31].

4. Effects of drinking cow's milk at breakfast on saliva melatonin concentration in Japanese university athletes

4.1. Methods

4.1.1. Participants

Sixty percent of 93 participants were born and grown in Shikoku island, whereas the others were from other parts of all over Japan. Participants in this study were 19–25 years old (Takeuchi et al., unpublished).

4.1.2. Procedure

Seventy-three participants of the experimental group were asked to drink 200 ml of cow's milk at breakfast each morning for a period of 21 days, from 13 November 2014 to 4 December

2014. We provided the milk for them. Twenty participants in the control group did not drink the cow's milk in the morning at breakfast. Twenty men did not like milk originally. Between the two groups, no significant differences were shown in age, diurnal-type scale [50] scores, and sleep habits (wake-up time, bedtime, and sleep hours both in the weekdays and weekends) [52]. After the questionnaires and sleep diaries had been distributed, participants were allowed to answer them at home.

4.1.3. Ethic treatment

Before administrating the intervention study, all participants were given a written explanation that detailed the concepts and purposes of the study and also stated that we would use the saliva melatonin data only for academic purpose. All participants agreed completely with the proposal and gave written consents after the explanation. The explanation stated that they could withdraw at any time and the withdrawal (canceling) had negative consequences for them. However, there were no withdrawals at fact. The intervention research was performed in accordance with the guidelines which have been established by the *Chronobiology International* journal for the conduct of research on human beings [53]. The study was also permitted by the Kochi university soccer club committee and the committee in the Laboratory of Environmental Physiology, Graduate School of Integrated Arts and Sciences, Kochi University, which carried out ethical inspections regarding the contents of the methodology in this study.

4.1.4. Statistical analysis

The software used for statistical analysis was SPSS 12.0 J for Windows (SPSS Inc., Chicago, IL, USA). ANOVA and T-test were used for the tests on spacing ratio variables between ranked variables. Friedman test was used for paired variables. We were sometimes interested in changes *during* the intervention (Friedman).

4.2. Results

In saliva collected at 22:00, melatonin concentration was increased during the intervention period in the cow's milk consumption group (ANOVA due to GLM repeating measurement analysis: df = 2, F-value = 8.038, p = 0.080; Friedman test: p = 0.044) (**Figure 4A**). Moreover, the differences in the individual levels in the saliva melatonin concentrations tended to be higher (more increased) in the cow's milk consumption group than the control group (T-test: t-value = 2.05, p = 0.061) (**Figure 4A**). On the other hand, at 23:00, there were no significant differences during the intervention in the melatonin level (ANOVA: df = 2, F-value = 1.999, p = 0.172; Friedman test: p = 0.867) in the experimental group (cow's milk consumption) (**Figure 4B**). On the other hand, there were no differences in the saliva melatonin concentrations through the intervention of 21 days both at 22:00 (**Figure 4A**) (ANOVA: df = 2, F-value = 0.794, p = 0.235; Friedman test: p = 0.867) and at 23:00 (**Figure 4B**) (ANOVA: df = 2, F-value = 0.176, p = 0.841; Friedman test: p = 0.867) in the control group (no cow's milk consumption).

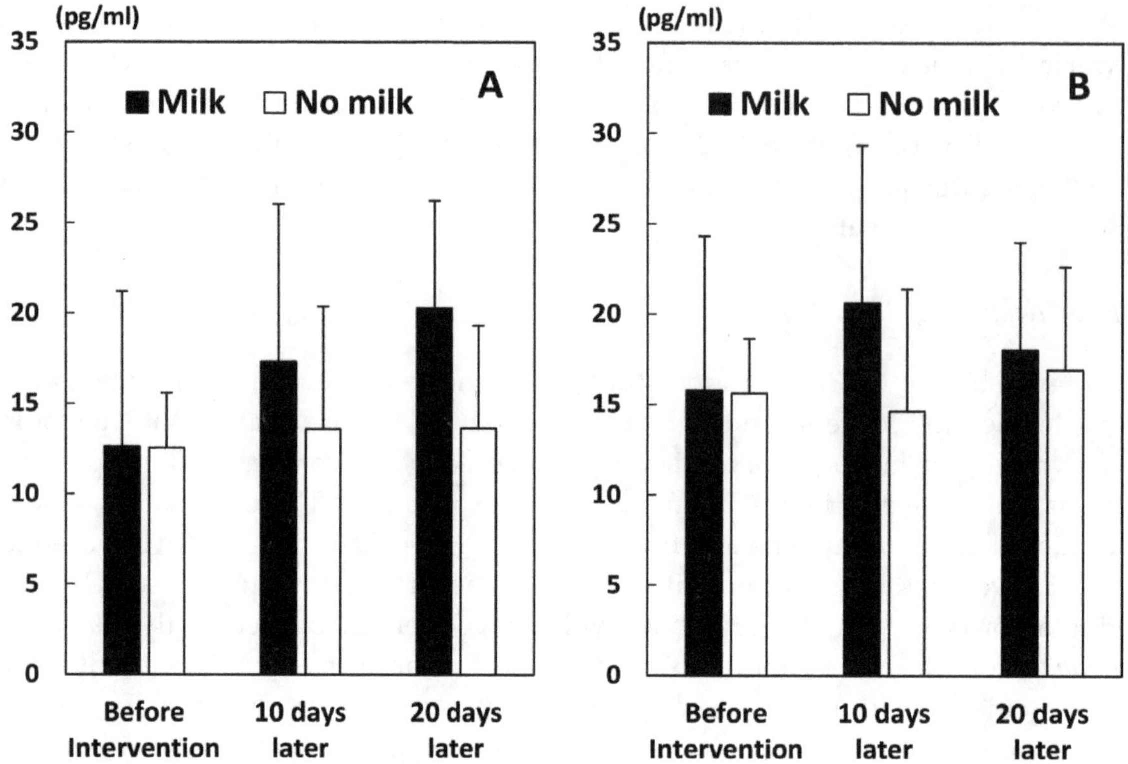

Figure 4. Comparisons of saliva melatonin concentration in saliva taken at 22:00 (A) and 23:00 (B) before intervention, 10 days later and 20 days later (just after the intervention). Black bars (cow's milk consumption group), white bars (no cow's milk group) (mean ± 95% confidence) (Takeuchi et al., unpublished).

4.3. Discussion

The intake of cow's milk at breakfast made the evening-typed members more morning-typed, whereas the diurnal type of the morning-typed members shifted to more evening-typed [49]. Tryptophan included in the cow's milk was metabolized to serotonin in the morning and serotonin again synthesized to melatonin at night [28, 29, 31, 48, 49, 59]. Therefore, the sleep latency seems to become shorter during the intervention [49] due to the melatonin synthesis which has been known as the natural sleep inducer [60] based on cow's milk intake at breakfast. This shorter sleep latency leads to the longer sleep hours for the university soccer club members.

The melatonin onset timing especially at dim light conditions can be used as a "sign" of the circadian phase [60]. For example, this melatonin-onset timing could be used for the signs of mood disorders and accompanied phase delay of the circadian phase shown by the monopolar and bipolar depression phenotypes [61]. The promotion of the melatonin concentration level at 22:00 due to morning cow's milk consumption might show the phase advance of university soccer team members. If the participants in this study would be senior high school students, the increase timing might be 1 or 2 hour(s) in advance, because the melatonin onset timing was around 21:00 to 22:00 for the senior high school students [62]. However, the number of samples was very small, and the significant differences in the saliva melatonin at 23:00 was not shown in this study. More number of samplings of saliva will be taken in the future study.

On the 10th day and 21st day of the intervention period, a questionnaire on performance/skill was administered to all participants [49]. The group who drank cow's milk showed higher frequency of improvement of soccer performance than the control group who did not drink [49]. The improved sleep quality which might be induced and enhanced at 22:00 in this study in the melatonin group could be related to such improvement of soccer performance.

5. Integrated discussion

Melatonin secretion is very important for sleep induction at bedtime and also keeping sleep quality high [62]. Moreover, night melatonin for mothers can be related to brain development of their children. Braam et al. [63] showed a hypothesis that low parental melatonin levels could be one of the contributors to autism spectrum disorder (ASD) and possibly intellectual disability (ID) etiology. If this hypothesis is correct, this could lead to policies to detect future parents who are at risk and to treatment strategies to ASD and intellectual disability risk.

Pfeffer et al. [64] reviewed that the present contribution of melatonin confirmed the synchronizing effect of endogenous melatonin and the melatoninergic system in humans and rodents. However, they discussed that these effects would be subtle. These relatively subtle effects stand in contrast with their markable, overt therapeutic successes that have been achieved using melatonin as an externally applied chronobiotic in humans [65]. Thus, melatonin does not appear as the master of internal synchronization but as one component in an integrated system of synchronizing agents. Melatonin might be one indicator of a phase point of human circadian clock. And, it can be influenced by breakfast protein consumption and also evening lighting especially modern lighting which includes "blue lights (460–480 nm)" as peak wave lengths of melanopsin [66].

Several studies including Bouwmans et al. [67] that showed the possibilities of network mapping for dynamic person-specific psychological and biological data revealed that there were not only large heterogeneity between affect and fatigue in depression and melatonin secretion which can be related to fall in sleep and sleep quality, namely, negatively and positively correlation with wide personal variety in the relationship. Meaningful generalizations can be made on the interplay of melatonin with affect and fatigue in depression.

Anyway, melanopsin is a key photoreception substance to control circadian phase shift in human beings [68, 69] and moreover to relate to sleep and mood disorders in the parents [66]. Melanopsin function might be related to melatonin synthesis via circadian phase shift indirectly. Twenty-four hours of commercialization society might be dangerous for disruption of circadian phase and normal melatonin secretion through over usage of smartphone (e.g., line and game) and watching TV program at night for children.

Acknowledgements

Thanks should be due to all the participants in this study. The following financial supports have been supplied to this study: (1) JSPS fund (Foundation No: JP 16 K01871; To H. Takeuchi:

2016–2019); (2) Fund from J-Milk "Meals and Education" (To T. Harada: 2013–2014); and (3) Fund from J-Mild "Research Study to Promote Health by Milk and Related Foods" (To T. Harada: 2016–2017). We would like to give many thanks also to Professor Emeritus Jim Waterhouse, Liverpool John Moores University, Liverpool, UK, for his valuable comments from an academic view point on this manuscript.

Author details

Hitomi Takeuchi and Tetsuo Harada*

*Address all correspondence to: haratets@kochi-u.ac.jp

Laboratory of Environmental Physiology, Graduate School of Integrated Arts and Sciences, Kochi University, Akebono-cho, Kochi, Japan

References

[1] Fukuda K, Ishihara K. Research work on life habits and tiredness in Japanese elementary, junior high and senior high school students. In: Reports of Study Supported by Ministry of Sciences and Technologies for Science Promotion Japanese Ministry of Sciences and Technologies. 2000

[2] Takahashi M, Wang G, Adachi M, Jiang F, Saito M, Nakamura K. Differences in sleep problems between Japanese and Chinese preschoolers: A cross-cultural comparison within the Asian region. Sleep Medicine. 2018;**48**:42-48. DOI: 10. 1016/j.sleep.2017.11.1145

[3] Harada T, Takeuchi H. Scientific study on "Go to bed early! Get up early! Take nutritionally rich breakfast!". Chronobiology. 2017;**23**:9-16 (Jikanseibutugaku in Japanese)

[4] Harada T, Morikuni M, Yoshii S, Yamashita Y, Takeuchi H. Usage of mobile phone in the evening or at night makes Japanese students evening-typed and night sleep uncomfortable. Sleep and Hypnosis. 2002;**4**:150-154

[5] Kawada T, Kataoka T, Tsuji F, Nakade M, Krejci M, Noji T, et al. The relationship between a night usage of mobile phone and sleep habit and the circadian typology of Japanese students aged 18-30 years. Psychology. 2017;**8**:892-902

[6] Honma K, Honma S. A human phase-response curve for brightlight pulses. The Japanese Society of Psychiatry and Neurology. 1988;**42**:167-168

[7] Harada T, Takeuchi H. Epidemiological study on diurnal rhythm and sleep habits of Japanese students aged 9-22 years. Annals of Japanese Society for Chronobiology. 2001; **3**:37-46 (in Japanese)

[8] Harada T, Takeuchi H. Do evening usages of convenience store, mobile phone and midnight programs of TV induce the sleep shortage of Japanese children? Japanese Journal of Clinical Dentistry for Children. 2003;**8**:57-67 (in Japanese)

[9] Zhdanova IV, Wurtman RJ, Lynch HJ, Ives JR, Dollina AB, Morabito C, et al. Pharmacodynamics and drug action; sleep-induced effects of low doses of melatonin ingested in the evening. Journal of Clinical Pharmacy and Therapeutics. 1995;**57**:552-558

[10] Hashimoto S, Nakamura K, Honma S, Tokura H, Honma K. Melatonin rhythm is not shifted by lights that suppress nocturnal melatonin in humans under entrainment. The American Journal of Physiology. 1996;**270**:R1073-R1077

[11] Hashimoto S, Honma K. Biological rhythms. In: Torii S, editor. Researches on Sleep Environments for Sleep. Tokyo: Asakura Shoten; 1999. pp. 23-36 (in Japanese)

[12] Cajochen C, Krauchi K, Wirz-Justice A. The acute soporific action of daytime melatonin administration: Effects on the EEG during wakefulness and subjective alertness. Journal of Biological Rhythms. 1997;**12**:636-643

[13] Peuhkuri K, Sihvola N, Korpela R. Dietary factors and fluctuating levels of melatonin. Food & Nutrition Research. 2012;**56**:17252. DOI: 10.3402/fnr.v56i0.17252

[14] Nowak R, Memillen IC, Redman J. The correlation between serum and salivary melatonin concentrations and urinary 6-hydroxymelatonin sulphate excretion rates two non-invasive techniques for monitoring human circadian rhythmicity. Clinical Endocrinology. 1987;**27**:445-452

[15] Laakso ML, Porkka-Heiskanen T, Alila A, Stenberg D, Johansson G. Correlation between salivary and serum melatonin: Dependence on serum melatonin levels. Journal of Pineal Research. 1990;**9**:39-50

[16] Nagtegaal E, Peeters T, Swart W, Smits M, Kerkhof G, Van der Meer G. Correlation between concentrations of melatonin in saliva and serum in patients with delayed sleep phase syndrome. Therapeutic Drug Monitoring. 1998;**20**:181-183

[17] Burgess HJ, Sletten T, Savic N, Gilbert SS, Dawson D. Effects of bright light and melatonin on sleep propensity, temperature, and cardiac activity at night. Journal of Applied Physiology. 2001;**91**:1214-1222

[18] Kubota T, Uchiyama M, Suzuki H, Shibui K, Kim K, Tan X, et al. Effects of nocturnal bright light on saliva melatonin, core body temperature and sleep propensity rhythms in human subjects. Neuroscience Research. 2001;**42**:115-122

[19] Aoki H, Yamada N, Ozeki Y, Yamane H, Kato N. Minimum light intensity required to suppress nocturnal melatonin concentration in human saliva. Neuroscience Letters. 1998;**252**:91-94

[20] Kohsaka M, Oyama E, Hashimoto S, Hoseki S, Honma Y, Mishima K. In: Okawa M, Honma K, editors. Lights and Health. Osaka: Matsushita Electric Co Ltd.; 1999

[21] Gooley JJ, Chamberiain K, Smith KA, Khalsa SBS, Rajaratnam SMW, Reen EV, et al. Exposure to room light before bedtime suppresses melatonin onset and shortens melatonin duration in humans. The Journal of Clinical Endocrinology and Metabolism. 2011;**96**:E463-E472

[22] Van der Meijden WP, Te Lindert BHW, Bijlenga D, Coppens JE, Gomez-Herrero G, Bruijel J, Sandra Kooij JJ, Cajochen C, Bourgin P, Van Someren EJW. Post-illumination pupil response after blue light: Reliability of optimized melanopsin-based phototransduction assessment. Experimental Eye Research. 2015;**139**:73-80

[23] Joyce DS, Feigl B, Cao B, Zele AJ. Temporal characteristics of melanopsin inputs to the human pupil light reflex. Vision Research. 2015;**107**:58-66

[24] Middleton B, Stone BM, Arendt J. Human circadian phase in 12:12 h, 200:<8 lux and 100:<8 lux light-dark cycles, without scheduled sleep or activity. Neuroscience Letters. 2002;**329**:41-44

[25] Kuller R. The influence of light on circadian rhythms in humans. Journal of Physiological Anthropology. 2002;**21**:87-91

[26] Fonken LK, Finy MS, Walton JC, Weil ZM, Workman JL, Ross J, et al. Influence of light at night on murine anxiety- and depressive-like responses. Behavioral Brain Research. 2009;**205**:349-354

[27] Harada T, Hirotani M, Maeda M, Nomura H, Takeuchi H. Correlation between breakfast tryptophan content and morningness-eveningness in Japanese infants and students aged 0-15 years. Journal of Physiological Anthropology. 2007;**26**:201-207

[28] Nakade M, Takeuchi H, Taniwaki N, Noji T, Harada T. An integrated effect of protein intake at breakfast and morning exposure to sunlight on the circadian typology in Japanese infants aged 2-6 years. Journal of Physiological Anthropology. 2009;**28**:239-245

[29] Nakade M, Akimitsu O, Wada K, Krejci M, Noji T, Taniwaki N, et al. Can breakfast tryptophan and vitamin B6 intake and morning exposure to sunlight promote morning-typology in young children aged 2-6 years? Journal of PhysiologicalAnthropology. 2012;**31**:11. DOI: 10.1186/1880-6805-31-11

[30] Alkozi HA, Wang X, De Lra MJP, Pintor LJ. Presence of melanopsin in human crystalline lens epithelial cells and its role in melatonin synthesis. Experimental Eye Research. 2017;**154**:168-176

[31] Wada K, Yata S, Akimitsu O, Krejci M, Noji T, Nakade M, et al. A tryptophan-rich breakfast and exposure to light with low color temperature at night improve sleep and salivary melatonin level in Japanese students. Journal of Circadian Rhythms. 2013;**11**:4. MS (1-7)

[32] Higuchi S, Nagafuchi Y, Lee S-I, Harada T. Influence of light at night on melatonin suppression in children. Journal of Clinical Endocrinology and Metabolism. 2014;**99**:3298-3303

[33] Wright HR, Lack LC. Effect of light wavelength on suppression and phase delay of the melatonin rhythm. Chronobiology International. 2001;**18**:801-808

[34] Harada T, Yamazaki Y, Tsuji F, Nakade M, Krejci M, Kawada T, et al. Relationship of the usages of convenience stores and personal computer at night to circadian typology and sleep habits in Japanese students aged 18-40 yrs. In: Abstract Proceedings of European Biological Rhythm Society Congress 2015 (EBRS2015); 2-6 August, 2015; Manchester, United Kingdom

[35] Harada T. Effects of evening light conditions on salivary melatonin of Japanese junior high school students. Journal of Circadian Rhythms. 2004;**2**:4. DOI: 10.1186/1740-3391-2-4

[36] Moore P, Landolt HP, Seifrizt E, Clark C, Bhatti T, Kelsoe J, et al. Clinical and physiological consequences of rapid tryptophan depletion. Neuropsychopharmacology. 2000; **23**:601-622

[37] Zheng X, Beaulieu JM, Sotnikova TD, Ganinetdiov RR, Caron MG. Tryptophan hydroxylase-2 controls brain serotonin synthesis. Science. 2004;**305**:217

[38] Suzuki E. Serotonin and Nerve Cells, the Brain and Drugs. Vol. 41-42. Tokyo: Seiwa Shoten; 2000. pp. 109-116 (in Japanese)

[39] Linnoila M, Higley D, Nielsen D, Andersen P, Suomi S, Goldman D, et al. Serotonin and impulse control: From clinic to clone. European Neuropsychoparmacology. 1993;**3**:161

[40] Van Praag HM. Anxiety/aggression-driven driven depression: A paradigm of functionalization and verticalization of psychiatric diagnosis. Progress in Neuropsychoparmacology & Biological Psychiatry. 2001;**25**:893-924

[41] Deniau E, Cohen D. Selective serotonin reuptake inhibitors in childhood and adolescent depression: Recent controversies. Psychiatry science and Human Neuroscience. 2005;**5**:109-116

[42] Rosenthal N, Schwartz P, Tumer E, Nalm S, Matthews J, Hardin T, et al. The psychobiology of SAD and the mechanism of action of light therapy. Biological Psychiatry. 1997;**42**:57S

[43] Harada T, Nakade M, Wada K, Kondo A, Maeda M, Noji T, et al. Mental health of children from a chronobiological and epidemiological point of view. In: Olisah V, editor. Essential Notes in Psychiatry. Rijeka, Croatia: Intech; 2012. pp. 439-458, 580 (Chapter 22)

[44] Nongonierma AB, FitzGerald RJ. The scientific evidence for the role of milk protein-derived bioactive peptides in humans: A review. Journal of Functional Foods. 2015; **17**:640-656

[45] Brezinova V, Oswald I. Sleep after a bedtime beverage. British Medical Journal. 1972; **2**:431-433

[46] Laird DA, Drexel H. Experimenting with food and sleep. I. Effects of varying types of foods in offsetting sleep disturbances caused by hunger pangs and gastric distress children and adults. Journal of the American Dietetic Association. 1934;**10**:89-94

[47] Takeuchi H, Wada K, Kawasaki K, Krejci M, Noji T, Kawada T, et al. Effects of cow milk intake at breakfast on the circadian typology and mental health of Japanese infants aged 1-6 years. Psychology. 2014;**5**:172-176

[48] Harada T, Wada K, Tsuji F, Krejci M, Kawada T, Noji T, et al. Intervention study using a leaflet entitled 'three benefits of "go to bed early! get up early! and intake nutritionally

rich breakfast! a message for athletes" to improve the soccer performance of university soccer team. Sleep and Biological Rhythms. 2016;**14**(Suppl. 1):S65-S74

[49] Kawada T, Takamori Y, Nakade M, Tsuji F, Krejci M, Noji T, et al. Effects of drinking cows' milk at breakfast in promoting sleep-health in Japanese university athletes. International Journal of Psychological Studies. 2016;**8**:154-163

[50] Torsvall L, Åkerstedt T. A diurnal type scale: Construction, consistency and validation in shift work. Scandinavian Journal of Work, Environment & Health. 1980;**6**:283-290

[51] Lewy AJ, Wehr TA, Goodwin FK, Newsome DA, Markey SP. Light suppresses melatonin secretion in humans. Science. 1980;**210**:1267-1269

[52] Harada T, Inoue M, Takeuchi H, Watanabe N, Hamada M, Kadota G, et al. Study on diurnal rhythms in the life of Japanese University, junior high and elementary school students including morningness-eveningness preference. Bulletin of the Faculty of Education, Kochi University Series. 1998;**1**(56):1-91 (in Japanese)

[53] Portaluppi F, Smolensky MH, Touitou Y. Effects and methods for biological rhythm research on animals and human beings. Chronobiology International. 2010;**27**:1911-1929. DOI: 10.3109/07420528.2010.516381

[54] Zeizer JM, Dijk DJ, Kronauer RE, Brown EN, Czeisler CA. Sensitivity of the human circadian pacemaker to nocturnal light: Melatonin phase resetting and suppression. The Journal of Physiology. 2000;**526**:695-702

[55] Kayumov L, Casper RF, Hawa RJ, Perelman B, Chung SA, Sokalsky S, et al. Blocking low-wavelength light prevents nocturnal melatonin suppression with no adverse effect on performance during simulated shift work. The Journal of Clinical Endocrinology and Metabolism. 2005;**90**:2755-2761

[56] Yasukouchi A, Hazama T, Kozaki T. Variations in the light-induced suppression of nocturnal melatonin with special reference to variations in the papillary light reflex in humans. Journal of Physiological Anthropology. 2007;**26**:113-121

[57] Arendt J. Melatonin: Characteristics, concerns, and prospects. Journal of Biological Rhythms. 2005;**20**:291-303

[58] Morris CJ, Aeschbach D, Sheer FAJL. Circadian system, sleep and endocrinology. Molecular and Cellular Endocrinology. 2012;**349**:91-104. DOI: 10.1186/1740-3391-11-4

[59] Harada T, Nakade M, Wada K, Akimitsu O, Noji T, Krejci M, et al. Tryptophan and sleep: Breakfast tryptophan content and sleep. In: Preedy VR, Patel VB, Le L-A, editors. Handbook of Nutrition, Diet and Sleep. Wageningen, The Netherlands: Wageningen Academic Publishers; 2013. pp. 473-487, 500 (Chapter 33)

[60] Bruni O, Alonso-Alconada D, Besag F, Biran V, Braam W, Cortese S, et al. Current role of melatonin in pediatric neurology: Clinical recommendations. European Journal of Pediatric Neurology. 2015;**19**:122-133. DOI: 10.1016/j.ejpn.2014.12.007

[61] Robillard R, Naismith SL, Rogers NL, Scott EM, Ip TKC, Hermens DF, et al. Sleep-wake cycle and melatonin rhythms in adolescents and young adults with mood disorders: Comparison of unipolar and bipolar phenotypes. European Psychiatry. 2013;**28**:412-416

[62] Crowley SJ, Shu C, Molina TA, Fogg LF, Sharkey KM, Carskadon MA. Estimating the dim light melatonin onset of adolescents within a 6-h sampling window: The impact of sampling rate and threshold method. Sleep Medicine. 2016;**20**:59-66

[63] Braam W, Ehrhart F, Maas APHM, Smits MG. Low maternal melatonin level increases autism spectrum disorder risk in children. Research in Developmental Disabilities. 2018. DOI: 10.1016/j.ridd.2018.02.017

[64] Pfeffer M, Korf H-W, Wicht H. Synchronizing effects of melatonin on diurnal and circadian rhythms. General and Comparative Endocrinology. 2018;**258**:215-221

[65] Arendt J, Skene DJ. Melatonin as a chronobiotic. Sleep Medicine Reviews. 2005;**9**:25-39

[66] Hatori M, Panda S. The emerging roles of melanopsin in behavioral adaptation to light. Trends in Molecular Medicine. 2010;**16**:435-446

[67] Bouwmans MEJ, Beltz AM, Bos EH, Oldehinkel AJ. The person-specific interplay of melatonin, affect, and fatigue in the context of sleep and depression. Personality and Individual Differences. 2018;**123**:163-170

[68] Beaulé C, Robinson B, Lamout EW, Amir S. Melanopsin in the circadian timing system. Journal of Molecular Neuroscience. 2003;**21**:73-89

[69] Van der Meijden WP, Te Lindert BHW, Bijlenga D, Coppens JE, Gómez-Herroro G, Bruijel J, et al. Post-illumination pupil response after blue light: Reliability of optimized melanopsin-based phototransduction assessment. Experimental Eye Research. 2016; **139**:73-80

9

Role of Melatonin and the Biological Clock in Regulating Lactation in Seasonal Sheep

Edyta Molik and Dorota Zięba-Przybylska

Abstract

Impact of light on animal behavior has been known for a long time—from 1925, Rowan [30] showed that lighting conditions influence gonad activity in birds and the related processes are controlled not only by means of intraorganic signals. Studies carried out in subsequent years have established that, also in mammals, the gland reacting to changes in light conditions is the pineal gland, producing a substance called melatonin. Biosynthesis of melatonin in most animals studied to date occurs at a rhythm dependent on the photocycle. The highest concentrations of this hormone—often called "the hormone of darkness"—are recorded at night. Seasonal changes in melatonin secretion conditioned by activity of the biological clock, known also as "biochemical calendar", are the key signals in the annual reproductive cycles of animals exhibiting seasonality of reproduction. Seasonality in sheep refers not only to the reproduction itself but also to lactation. One of the main hormones conditioning initiation and maintenance of lactation, synthesis of milk proteins, fat and immunoglobulins is prolactin (PRL), secreted primarily by lactotrophic cells in the adenohypophysis. Prolactin is also produced locally by the mammary gland—the hormone of this origin is identical to prolactin secreted by the pituitary gland. Until now, it was considered that the level of milk production in mammals is determined by both genetic and environmental factors. However, in recent years, many studies focused on the role of light as a modulator of prolactin levels. In livestock, changes in light-period length play a very important role as this determines their productivity and milk yield. Photoperiod is particularly important in short-day breeder animals (sheep), for which the length of light period is associated with changes in melatonin level. The modulating effect of melatonin on secretion of prolactin may take place via two different mechanisms. One is associated with the circadian rhythm, wherein—directly or through the medium of a factor popularly termed "tuberalin"—melatonin stimulates the release of prolactin. However, this effect is short-lived and is most likely applicable only to prolactin stored in lactotrophic cells of the pituitary. The second mechanism regulating the secretion of melatonin and prolactin is associated with the annual rhythms of secretion—melatonin, due to its lipophilic characteristics, has a direct effect on the secretion of prolactin. Under natural conditions, the maximum concentration of prolactin in the blood of sheep is observed over the long-day period, during which the melatonin level decreases. The lowest prolactin concentration is observed over the short-day period, where melatonin levels are at their highest. Changes in secretion of prolactin during lactation in sheep undoubtedly affect the amount of milk produced.

Keywords: seasonality sheep, melatonin, length days, biological clock lactotropic and metabolic hormone

---

1. Introduction

1.1. Genetic predispositions and impact of environmental factors on the lactation process in sheep

1.1.1. Role of melatonin and the biological clock

Sheep are short-day breeders, in which the signal for onset of estrus occurs after the summer solstice and is maintained until winter. Such a model of the reproductive cycle in which the young ones are born in the spring provides favorable conditions for rearing lambs as this period coincides with the time of abundance of food, thereby the young have time to put aside fat for the winter. Seasonality of reproductive cycle in sheep is associated with the season and the day length as a recurring reproductive cycle is an endogenous rhythm, encoded genetically. Information on changes in photoperiod reaches the animal's organism through a multineural tract. Much more studies confirm the presence of a molecular mechanism—located in the SCN (suprachiasmatic nucleus) as well as in pars tuberalis (PT)—involved in decoding the melatonin signal.

Both the SCN and PT host over a dozen genes of the circadian clock, such as *Bmal1*, *Clock*, *Per1*, *Per2*, *Cry1*, *Cry2A*, *Rev-erbα* and *CK1ε*, which are mutually coupled [1, 2]. Most likely, the summer and winter rhythm observable in sheep is conditioned by the biological clock genes. Over 24 hours, changes in the melatonin profile affect the rhythmic changes in the expression of these genes as evidenced by varying levels of clock genes mRNA in the PT and SCN. The peak gene expression of *Cry1* (Cryptochrome) gene occurs at twilight, together with the increase in melatonin level, while expression of the gene *Per1* (Period) is stimulated by approaching dawn [3, 4]. In contrast to *Cry1*, *Cry2* gene is not melatonin-induced [5]. On the other hand, expression of the *Per1* gene is melatonin-dependent as pinealectomy (surgical removal of the pineal gland) blocks the rhythm of the *Per1* gene in the PT, but does not affect the expression of this gene in the SCN.

Studies have reported that repeated multiple injections of melatonin in animals previously subjected to pinealectomy restore the cyclical transcription of *Per1* in PT [6]. The results of studies on biological clock genes in mammalian SCN showed that the BMAL1/CLOCK protein complex encoded by the genes of *Bmal1*, *Clock* induces activation of the *Per1*, *Per2*, *Cry1*, *Cry2*, *Rev-erbα* genes [2]. Studies in sheep artificially subjected to a sudden light stimulus characteristic of a long-day period have shown that the gene expression profile of *Cry1* and *Per1* mirrored that occurring in natural conditions, i.e., expression of *Cry1* increased at night, while that of *Per1* was rising during the day, indicating the presence of a rapid mechanism for regulation of *Cry1* and *Per1* gene expression in response to a melatonin impulse [1].

The neurosensory receptor of circadian rhythm in mammals is the retina of the eye, through which light stimuli are transmitted to the suprachiasmatic nucleus of the hypothalamus (SCN). The pathway the light stimulus travels from the retina to the SCN is known as the retinohypothalamic tract. Secretion of melatonin is a biochemical signal informing the body about changes occurring in the external environment. Melatonin has lipophilic properties and is secreted from the pineal gland by simple diffusion [7]. Because of a well-developed network of blood vessels in the pineal gland, this hormone is released directly into the blood and distributed throughout the entire organism. In animals sensitive to changes in day length, the melatonin profile is a biochemical signal regulating the processes of reproduction and lactation [8]. In sheep, which are short day breeders, seasonal changes in melatonin levels inform the fetus of the environmental conditions.

A large number of MT_1 melatonin receptors are present in pars tuberalis (PT) of sheep, while no similar high concentration is noted in the tuberal region of the hypothalamus and in the SCN. This suggests that melatonin may modulate the secretion of hormones secreted only in the pars tuberalis [9, 10]. Increase in melatonin secretion in sheep is stimulated already within 1 or 2 hours after sunset and lasts until the onset of dawn. According to Misztal et al. (1999) [11], the modulating effect of melatonin on prolactin (PRL) secretion could be explained by two different mechanisms. One is linked to the circadian rhythm, which may either have direct impact or act through the factor conventionally known as tuberalin. However, this effect is short-lived and most likely is only applicable to prolactin stored in the lactotropic cells of the pituitary. It is possible that tuberalin activates the expression of the prolactin gene in lactotropic cells [9]. The second mechanism modulating melatonin secretion is related to the annual rhythm of secretion—this means that melatonin, due to its lipophilic properties, has a direct effect on the lactotrophic cells of the pituitary and thus also impacts the secretion of prolactin [11, 12]

1.1.2. Role of prolactin and the growth hormone (GH)

Changes in melatonin and prolactin profiles in sheep are closely interlinked. Regulation of PRL secretion by melatonin may occur via two different mechanisms. In the case of the circadian rhythm mechanism, melatonin may directly affect PRL secretion—this option applies to the hormone stored in the lactotropic cells; the process may also be mediated by the aforementioned peptide—tuberalin, which activates PRL gene expression in lactotropic cells of the anterior pituitary [9]. In contrast, the process of annual PRL secretion rhythm is directly induced by melatonin that—due to its lipophilic nature—affects the lactotropes [13]. Synthesis of prolactin occurs in the anterior pituitary in the lactotropic cells. The main role of PRL is to initiate and control processes such as mammogenesis, lactogenesis, galactopoesis and involution. Moreover, this hormone plays an important role in biosynthesis of milk proteins (β-casein, α-lactalbumin, lactose). It has been shown that in sheep, the daily and seasonal rhythms of PRL and melatonin are characterized by volatility. Changes in prolactin levels throughout the day are strongly associated with the season. Increases in PRL concentration in the spring are observed at dawn and before dusk. In the summer, the peak level is recorded halfway through the dark cycle, while the autumn PRL profile is characterized by a spike in the first half of the photoperiod and near its end. In short-day breeders, such as sheep, the seasonal lengthening of day-light hours (spring, summer) resulting in a short melatonin signal (4–8 hours a day) does not inhibit the secretion of PRL, while in autumn and winter, a long-lasting melatonin impulse (>10 hours per day) causes a decrease in prolactin concentration [6, 14]. Melatonin modulates PRL secretion also through the intermediary of dopamine. The neurotransmitter stimulates PRL secretion acting through dopamine D1 receptors and inhibits the secretion of this hormone via its effect on dopamine D2 receptors. The presence of seasonal changes in melatonin and prolactin profiles was also confirmed by tests carried out on sheep kept for dairy purposes. It has been shown that key factors affecting milk yield in ewes are changes in the photoperiod. It has been found that milk yield in females entering lactation during the day-light lengthening season is by far (50%) higher than that in animals starting milk synthesis in short-day conditions [15]. The reaction to the shortening of the photoperiod was an increase in melatonin levels, decrease in PRL concentration and lower milk yield. Subjecting sheep to conditions of artificially prolonged day-light cycle (16L:8D) resulted in light-induced inhibition of melatonin synthesis in the pineal gland. Decrease in PRL concentration and lower milk yield were observed simultaneously. Thus, the artificial prolongation of the photoperiod during short-day season is not enough to maintain lactation in seasonal sheep [10, 14, 16, 17]. Previous observations indicate that such processes as mammogenesis, lactogenesis, galactopoesis and involution in sheep require the presence of multiple factors, strongly interdependent. Milk production is based on the impact of a number of factors and day length, as well as changes in PRL profile are only some of many [18]. An important role is also played by the somatotropic system (GH, IGF-1). The growth hormone, similar to PRL, is produced in the anterior pituitary and is involved in synthesis of proteins and fatty acids; it also lowers the concentration of glucose in the blood and is partly responsible for synthesis and secretion of prolactin [19]. Increase in concentration of the GH is stimulated by the "suckling factor"—higher growth hormone levels are observed at the beginning of lactation. Studies carried out on sheep have shown that changes in concentration of both the GH and PRL are dependent on the length of day and are linked to changes in the profile of pineal melatonin. Periodic changes in melatonin levels result in rhythmic inhibition of PRL secretion [20]. It is known that during lactation, under the impact of suckling, the GH and PRL levels in the blood are boosted [19]. Increase in GH secretion during lactation is controlled by GHRH and endogenous opioids. Recently, attention has been drawn to a compound, derivative of dopamine, known as salsolinol—it has been shown that concentration of this substance increases in the case of various dysfunctions in the dopaminergic system. Salsolinol stimulates the release of PRL in rodents and ruminants. In lactating sheep, the presence of salsolinol was confirmed in MBH and increase in its concentration in response to suckling was recorded [21]. Salsolinol administered to the third ventricle of the brain during lactation increases prolactin concentration.

Salsolinol antagonist is a compound called 1-MeDIG—this substance inhibits the release of PRL and cancels the stimulatory impact of the "suckling factor" on PRL secretion in rats. A similar effect was observed in sheep in which 1-MeDIQ acts directly on the central nervous system [22]. The compound inhibits the increase in the level of noradrenaline (NA), which acts as a mediator between salsolinol and GH. Interestingly, 1-MeDIQ does not affect the changes in GH concentration induced by stimulation of the mammary gland during suckling. In sheep, both over the period of lamb rearing and beyond, PRL levels decreased after 1-MeDIG was administered. It was proven experimentally that salsolinol has no direct influence on GH profile during lamb rearing. However, in rats subjected to simultaneous administration of both salsolinol and 1-MeDIQ, no statistically significant changes in pituitary hormone levels were observed with the exception of prolactin.

1.1.3. Role of metabolic hormones

The role of metabolic hormones in the process of lactation has garnered a lot of attention. An important role in initiating and maintaining lactation in small ruminants is played by the thyroid hormones, ghrelin and orexin. The production capacity of animals (milk yield, growth and development, coat growth) is largely dependent on proper functioning of the thyroid hormones. These hormones influence also the processes of reproduction in many species of animals, including sheep and goats [23]. In seasonal species, T4 and T3 are obligatory for the annually recurring termination of reproductive activity [24, 25]. Thyroxine in sheep with normally functioning thyroid will shorten the reproductive period and quicken the transition into anoestrus. Thyroxine level peaks in ewes in early pregnancy and decreases just before lambing and after the offspring is born. The level of thyroid hormones in sheep varies throughout lactation. At the start of the process, concentration of these substances is low [26]; however, over time, the thyroxine concentration increases. It has been shown that thyroid hormones, especially tri-iodothyronine, have a suppressive effect on expression of the prolactin gene, which can translate into milk yield as well. An important role in lactation belongs to calcitonin and the parathyroid hormone, responsible for modulation of phosphorus (P) and calcium (Ca) levels. Concentration of these elements in milk has major impact on the chemical composition of the product. The presence of the parathyroid hormone is essential for calcium absorption from the gastrointestinal tract; it also enhances synthesis of active D3 (1,25-di-hydroxycalciferol) that stimulates the process of calcium binding by proteins. It has been experimentally demonstrated that thyroid hormone secretion is correlated with day length in sheep. In vitro studies in thyroid gland explants showed higher levels of thyroxine under short-day conditions and lower in the season of elongating photoperiod (spring), while T3 reached higher levels in the summer and lower when the photoperiod was shortening. In addition, there was an increase in T3 concentration induced by exogenous melatonin [25]. Productivity of the animals depends not only on the level of nutrition, environmental factors and their genetic potential. Thyroid hormones are an important link in the key stages of life (reproduction and lactation) of all living organisms [27]. Orexin A is of particular importance in the reproductive process of animals sensitive to changes in day length. The process of initiating and maintaining lactation in sheep requires the presence of many hormones. Defining the role of orexin in regulating their secretion, especially that of prolactin, may allow to better understand the process of maintaining lactation in sheep, in particular over short-day period.

2. Influence of day length and melatonin on milking yield

Changes in day length and the related secretion of melatonin and prolactin are of particular significance in sheep as they determine reproductive processes, the last stage of which is lactation. The possibility of artificial extension of the milking period in late-lambing ewes by application of prolonged day length, 16 hours of light—8 hours of darkness (16L:8D), was introduced additionally (Group III). Measurements of plasma levels of prolactin and melatonin were used as parameters of season-dependent hormonal regulation of milk production in this seasonally breeding species [28]. Lambs remained with their mothers up to 56th day of life. Then lambs were separated from their mothers, which were allocated to the milking. During milking period, ewes were milked twice a day using Alfa-Laval machine. Individual milk yield checks were carried out every 10 days. From the 20th day of lactation to the end of this process, the blood samples were carried out from each sheep every 30 days to determine concentration of melatonin and prolactin. Blood sampling started after sunset and continued for 6 consecutive hours with a frequency of every 60 minutes. Blood after collection were centrifuged and the resulting plasma was stored at temperature −20°C until analysis. Hormones have been determined by radioimmunologically (RIA) method. During lambs' rearing period, sheep produced similar quantities of milk, since ewe Group 1 produced 48.2 ± 12.9 liters whereas Group II produced 42.4 ± 16.4 liters. Higher productivity was observed in Group III 60.5 ± 16.6 liters, which was kept in artificial light conditions. The observed differences were statistically insignificant. Distinct differences in milk yield were

Groups of sheep	Milk yield of the first 28 days of lactation (l)		Total length of lactation (days)		Days of milking (days)		Milk production during milking (l)	
	$\bar{x}$	SEM	$\bar{x}$	SEM	$\bar{x}$	SEM	$\bar{x}$	SEM
Group I Sheep lambed in January	48.2	2.3	177	8.6	102	4.8	33.0	3.6
Group II Sheep lambed in June	42.4	3.1	147	3.5	77	4.0	16.8	1.4
Group III Sheep lambed in June (16L:8D)	60.5	3.2	160	4.1	90	3.9	21.2	1.7

Table 1. Parameters characterizing lactation duration and efficiency of Polish Longwool sheep lambing in January (Group I), in June, kept under natural lighting conditions (Group II) and in June, kept under the long-artificial photoperiod (16L:8D, Group III). See text for statistical comparisons.

observed between the groups of sheep milk in the period of use. The highest milk yield of 33.0 ± 11.2 liters was found in Group I, while Group II produced only 16.8 ± 4.4 liters, the obtained differences were statistically significant ($P \leq 0.01$). Mothers who remained in artificial light conditions (Group 3) produced 21.2 ± 5.5 liters of milk (**Table 1**). The results of the total lactation length and days of milking show conclusively that the lactation period in Group I was significantly longer than that in Groups II and III ($P < 0.05$, **Table 1**). Analysis of the course of lactation with regard to the mean amount of milk obtained in particular months of milk use revealed that the milk yield of Group I in the first month of milking (0.43 ± 0.09 liters/day) was similar to the milk yield of Group III (0.42 ± 0.07 liters/day), with only 0.18 ± 0.08 liters/day in Group II ($P < 0.01$, **Figure 1, Tables 2–4**).

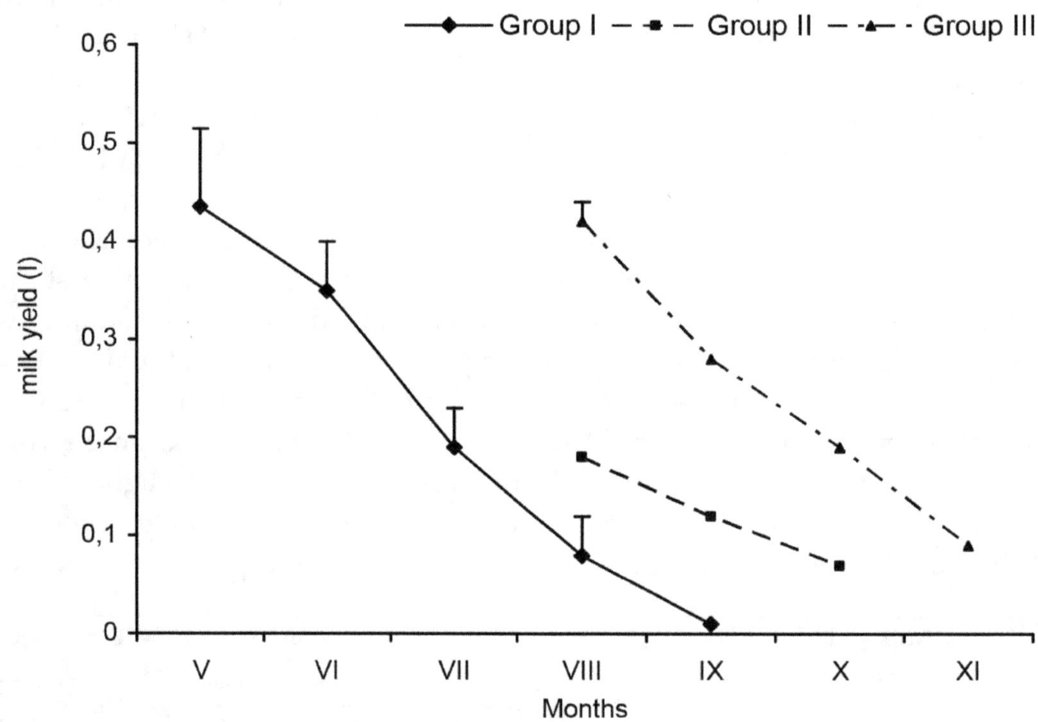

Figure 1. Mean monthly milk yield of Polish Longwool sheep lambed in January (Group I), in June, kept under natural lighting conditions (Group II) and in June, kept under the long-artificial photoperiod (16L:8D, Group III), during the milking period. See text for statistical comparisons.

Months		II	III	IV	V	VI	VII	VIII	IX
MLT (pg/ml)	$\bar{x}$	168.5	85.5	132.8	133.5	77.	73.3[c]	124.7	91.3
	SD	137.3	45.3	112.6	113.0	38.9	50.1	100.6	42.2
PRL (ng/ml)	$\bar{x}$	128.6	102.8	156.5	312.6[r]	185.7	247.0[j]	151.6	43.9
	SD	46.3	33.8	18.1	45.2	54.7	60.9	43.9	33.1
Milk (l)	$\bar{x}$	–	–	–	0.43	0.35	0.19	0.08	0.01
	SD				0.08	0.05	0.04	0.04	–

Table 2. Mean (±SEM) and SD of plasma melatonin and prolactin and milk concentrations in sheep lambed in January (Group I). See text for statistical comparisons.

Months		VII	VIII	IX	X	XI
MLT (pg/ml)	$\bar{x}$	61.1	87.8	82.3	77.5	93.2[a]
	SD	28.5	45.5	45.0	46.1	57.4
PRL (ng/ml)	$\bar{x}$	234.0	124.6	60.5	30.8	16.8
	SD	39.5	48.8	31.1	17.7	10.4
Milk (l)	$\bar{x}$	–	0.18	0.12	0.07	0.04
	SD		0.05	0.03	0.01	0.01

Table 3. Mean (±SEM) and SD of plasma melatonin and prolactin and milk concentrations in sheep lambed in June kept under natural lighting conditions (Group II). See text for statistical comparisons.

Months		VII	VIII	IX	X	XI
MLT (pg/ml)	$\bar{x}$	41.0[a]	60.4	17.6	4.4	17.0
	SD	19.7	39.8	27.6	4.1	15.5
PRL (ng/ml)	$\bar{x}$	278.8	132.7	147.9	84.3	38.3
	SD	55.3	57.4	82.4	42.5	25.2
Milk (l)	$\bar{x}$	–	0.42	0.28	0.19	0.09
	SD		0.07	0.05	0.03	0.02

Table 4. Mean (±SEM) and SD of plasma melatonin and prolactin and milk concentrations in sheep lambed in June and kept under the long-artificial photoperiod (Group III, 16L:8D, bottom). See text for statistical comparisons.

2.1. Secretion melatonin and prolactin in day length

The highest melatonin level in Group I determined in February was 168.5 ± 137.3 pg/ml, while prolactin level at this time was 128.6 ± 46.3 ng/ml. The highest prolactin concentration determined in May was 312.6 ± 45.2 ng/ml, further growth of prolactin level in July was 247.0 ± 60.9 ng/ml and the resulting differences were statistically significant ($P \leq 0.05$) compared to the level of the hormone in other administrations. With the lengthening of lactation and changes in day length light from August to September significantly decreased prolactin level from 151.6 ± 43.9 ng/ml to 43.9 ± 33.1 ng/ml and increased levels of melatonin. In August, the concentration of melatonin was the highest and amounted to 124.7 ± 100.6 pg/ml, while sheep milk production has decreased to a level of 0.08 ± 0.02 liters per day. In the last month of lactation, melatonin level was 91.3 ± 42.2 pg/ml and sheep milk production at this time was only 0.01 ± 0.02 liters/day (**Figure 4**, **Table 4**). The increase in melatonin levels from July to September of 33.4 pg/ml was accompanied by a decrease in prolactin level of 107.7 ng/ml. At that time, there was a decrease in the secretion of milk by an average of 0.11 liters/day (**Table 2**).

2.2. Secretion melatonin and prolactin in short days

In the case of Group II, the highest level (234.0 ± 39.5 ng/ml) of prolactin was also determined in July and the melatonin concentration in this period was the lowest (61.1 ± 28.5 ng/ml). With the shortening of the light day, prolactin secretion was decreasing and the level of this hormone was lower by 25.8% in September compared to the level observed in July. A clear decrease in prolactin level observed during the last 2 months of lactation, i.e, October and November was 30.8 ± 17.7 ng/ml and 16.8 ± 10.3 ng/ml, respectively. In July, as previously indicated, the lowest concentration of melatonin was 61.1 ± 28.5 pg/ml, differing significantly ($P \leq 0.05$) to the identified levels of this hormone in November (93.2 ± 57.4 ng/ml). Changes in the concentration of melatonin and prolactin during the shorter photoperiod influenced the parameters of sheep milk production, causing a drop in milk yield by 22.2% between August and November (**Table 3**). The results obtained in Group III showed that the highest level of prolactin found in July was 278.8 ± 55.3 ng/ml and much lower in September, 147.9 ± 82.4 ng/ml; however, it was higher than the level of prolactin identified in August, 132.7 ± 57.4 ng/ml. The resulting differences in the levels of prolactin in the month of July, August and September were statistically significant ($P \leq 0.05$). Despite ensuring that this group of animals underwent 16-hour lighting intensity of 200 lux, the concentration of prolactin from September to November reduced (**Table 4**).

The sheep of all groups produced similar amounts of milk during the first 28 days of lactation as estimated based on the weight gains of the lambs. The study results showed that the shift in lambing date—from winter to summer—had a negative effect on milk production parameters in ewes. Sheep that gave birth in January and were used for dairy purposes over the long-day period produced 50% more milk than ewes that gave birth in June and were then milked as the day length was gradually decreasing. Lactation in sheep milked in the summer-time was significantly longer than that in sheep milked when the photoperiod duration was shortening. Day length had no effect on milk yield in the period of rearing lambs (i.e., 28 days). Monitoring of hormone levels (prolactin and melatonin) in sheep during lactation allowed to conclude that secretion of melatonin in the fall months increased, while prolactin secretion was decreased over the same period. The increase in melatonin level during the shortening of the day in the Polish Longwool sheep reduces prolactin secretion and inhibition of the synthesis of milk. Introduction of artificial light conditions during the shortening of the photoperiod is not enough to maintain secretion of prolactin in ewes at a level that allows to maintain lactation in the autumn.

Length of illuminating day, but especially profile of melatonin has a particular meaning in sheep, because decidate of trial procreative with last stage physiology that last stage physiology reproduction is lactation. [18]. As the many physiological processes also the reproductive cycle is genetically encoded in the sheep. The course of this cycle is reflected by the seasonal changes in the secretory activity of the hypothalamopituitary gonadotropic GnRH-LH system. Sustaining of the proper duration of this cycle requires, however, constant and periodically repeated factors which enable the synchronization of the physiological processes with a suitable season of the year. Thus, the day length plays the most important role in this aspect. The information about the day length reaches the organism as the biochemical signal generated by the pineal gland via the nocturnal secretion of melatonin. The seasonal changes in the duration of melatonin secretion are of great importance in the modulation of sexual activity and lactation in the sheep with the inherent traits of seasonality. The dependence of milk yield and the duration of lactation on melatonin and prolactin secretion are also demonstrated in seasonal and aseasonal breeds of sheep lambed during the different seasons of the year. The putative mechanisms of melatonin action on luteinizing hormone and prolactin secretion are also demonstrated with reference to the melatonin-binding sites in the sheep central nervous system and pituitary gland [29].

2.3. Influence of day length and melatonin in prolactin secretion and growth hormone in suckling sheep

The effects of melatonin on the secretion of prolactin (PRL) and growth hormone (GH) were studied in ewes' nursing lambs (Polish Longwool, n = 20) under different photoperiods (March and November). The animals were divided into four groups: (a) (LDC—long-day control group, n = 5), (b) melatonin-treated (LDM—long-day group, n = 5), (c) (SDC—short-day control group, n = 5) and (d) (SDM—short-day melatonin, n = 5). Blood samples were collected from ewes 5 days after lambing. Four blood collections were performed at 10-day intervals, over a 40-day time period. Sampling started at sunset and continued for 6 hours at 20-minute intervals. Melatonin implants (exogenous melatonin) were inserted in ewes of the LDM and SDM groups after first blood collection. The plasma concentrations of PRL and GH were assayed using RIA. In ewes from the LDC group, the mean plasma PRL concentration increased gradually, reaching a significantly ($P < 0.001$) higher level, after 3 weeks. In contrast, in the LDM group, PRL concentration decreased significantly ($P < 0.001$) following 10 days, compared to that in ewes from the LDC group. The mean plasma GH concentration was significantly ($P < 0.001$) higher in the LDC group than that in the LDM group, the for the entire experimental period during the experimental period. In the SDC and SDM groups, plasma PRL concentrations did not decrease significantly ($P < 0.001$) 2 weeks after the onset of the experiment and did not differ significantly between these groups. The mean plasma GH concentration increased significantly ($P < 0.001$) in the SDM group compared with the SDC group only after the third week. The mean plasma GH concentration in the SDM group and the SDC group reached a similar level by the end of the trial. It would appear that melatonin may effectively inhibit PRL secretion in nursing ewes during long photoperiod and stimulate GH release during short photoperiod. The inhibition of PRL secretion in nursing ewes during increasing photoperiod (long days) occurs, despite the strong stimulation of suckling. At the onset of the experiment, the mean plasma PRL concentrations in the LDC and LDM groups were similar (193.2 ± 10.9 and 192.3 ± 8.7 ng/ml, respectively) (**Figure 2**). During the subsequent collection (second), the PRL concentration in the LDC group was 166.2 ± 8.0 ng/ml; however, in the LDM group a significant decrease in the plasma PRL concentration was recorded as 56.5 ± 4.2 ng/ml ($P < 0.001$). During this time, the mean concentration of PRL in LDC ewes was significantly higher ($P < 0.001$) than the LDM ewes (**Figure 2**). The mean concentration continued to increase as day length (photoperiod) increased.

During the decreasing day length period, the PRL secretion profile was similar in SDC and SDM groups (**Figure 2**). In both groups, there was a significant ($P < 0.05$) decrease in plasma of PRL concentration in during the third week of lactation (14.7 ± 1.4 and 12.6 ± 1.0 ng/ml) compared with the initial concentration (60.6 ± 7.3 and 53.4 ± 6.0 ng/ml, respectively). No differences in PRL plasma concentrations were recorded between the SDC and SDM groups.

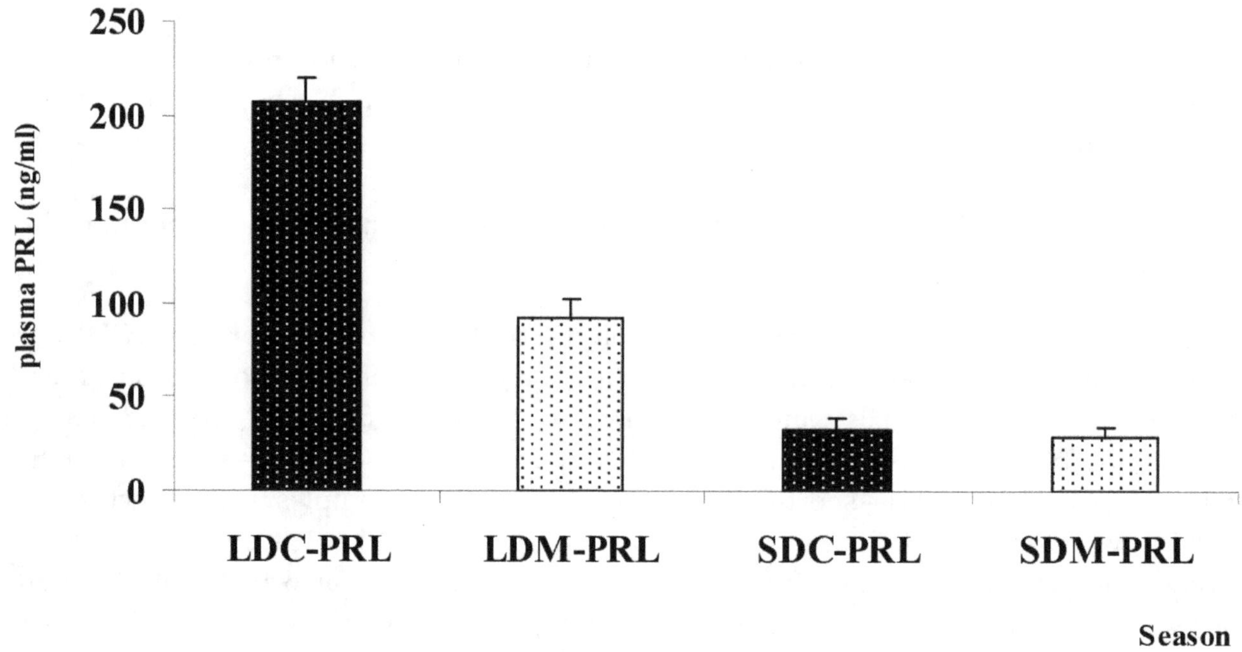

Figure 2. Mean plasma PRL concentrations in nursing-sheep lambing (LDC—a long-day control and LDM—a long-day melatonin-treated group, SDC—a short-day control and SDM—a short-day melatonin-treated group). See text for statistical comparisons.

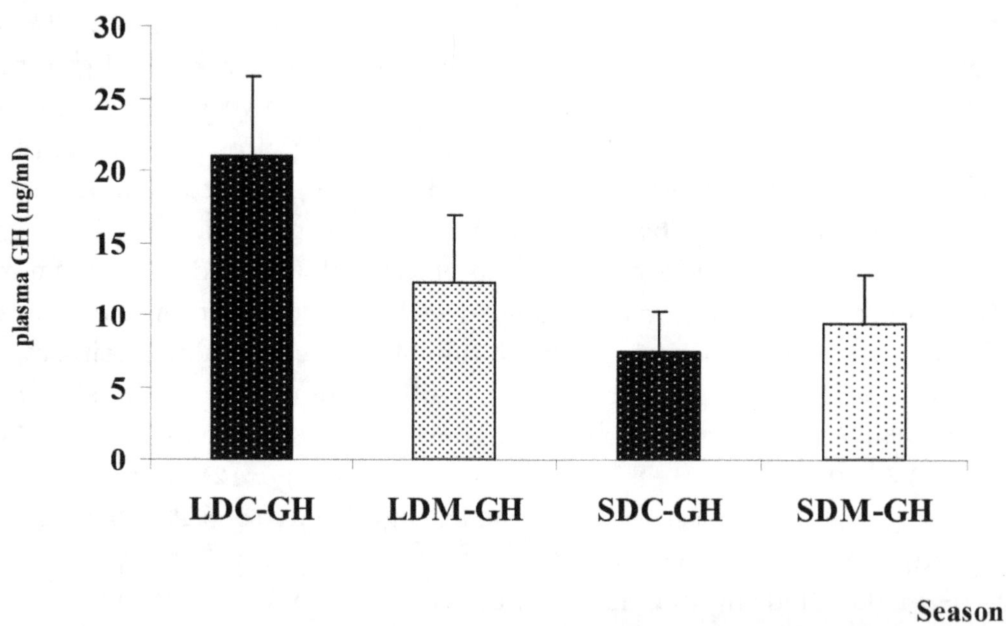

Figure 3. Mean plasma PRL concentrations in nursing-sheep lambing (LDC—a long-day control and LDM—a long-day melatonin-treated group, SDC—a short-day control and SDM—a short-day melatonin-treated group). See text for statistical comparisons.

The mean plasma GH concentration was significantly ($P < 0.001$) higher in the LDC group than the LDM group for the entire trial period. It was also observed that a gradual decrease in GH concentration took place in both groups (**Figure 3**). The mean GH concentrations in

SDC and SDM ewes were at a similar level up to the second time of blood collection day (**Figure 3**). The only significant ($P \leq 0.001$) rise in plasma GH secretion was recorded in the third week of lactation in the SDM group (12.23 ± 5.36 ng/ml) compared with the SDC group (6.58 ± 2.36 ng/ml).

In conclusion, the long-term treatment with exogenous melatonin of early-lactating sheep reduced the PRL secretion during the increasing photoperiod, despite strong stimulation by suckling. Moreover, in nursing ewes, melatonin stimulated GH secretion during the short photoperiod. It can therefore be assumed that melatonin may be indirectly affected by the level of milk production in sheep, especially following the nursing period.

3. Influence of metabolic hormones on prolactin secretion in lactation sheep

3.1. Role of orexin

Studies on the role of orexin A in the control of prolactin (PRL) and growth hormone (GH) secretion in rodents have produced inconsistent results. Orexin A may play a special role in animals' sensitivity such as sheep to the day length changes. The aim of the study was to determine the role of orexin A in the control of prolactin secretion and growth hormone in sheep during different photoperiods. In vitro studies were carried out on 10 Polish Longwool ewes on 30 days of lactation during long photoperiod (May, LD, n = 5) and short photoperiod (December, SD, n = 5). After rearing lambs to 30 days of age, ewes were decapitated and the pituitaries were dissected and then cut along the longitudinal fissure into two halves, so that each half contained the glandular and nervous parts. Pituitary glands were collected and divided along the longitudinal fissure into two halves. Glands were incubated for 3 hours at 37°C in Parker medium with addition of orexin A—experimental group or in medium alone—control group. During the following 3-hour incubation, medium was exchanged every 15 minutes and a sample of 1 ml was collected and immediately frozen at −80°C until assay. Prolactin concentrations in the medium were determined radioimmunologically (RIA).

In the long-day conditions (May), the pituitary explants of lactating sheep exhibited the strongest secretory activity during the first hour of incubation—significantly higher in orexin-treated group (O1) than the control group (K1), ($P < 0.01$). During the second hour of the incubation, PRL concentration decreased and reached the similar values in both groups. During the third hour, PRL concentration in O1 group was again significantly higher than that noted in K1 group ($P < 0.01$). In the short-day conditions (December), PRL concentration was significantly higher in orexin-treated group O2 during the first hour of incubation than the value observed in the control group—K2 ($P < 0.01$). The inverse relationship in prolactin release was observed during the second hour of incubation ($P < 0.01$), however, during the third hour, PRL concentration was again significantly higher in O2 group than the concentration noted in K2 group ($P < 0.05$). Collective analysis of the data showed that PRL concentrations were higher in experimental groups (O1 and O2) than the concentrations noted in control groups (K1 and K2) under both the long (May) and short (December) photoperiods (**Figure 4**).

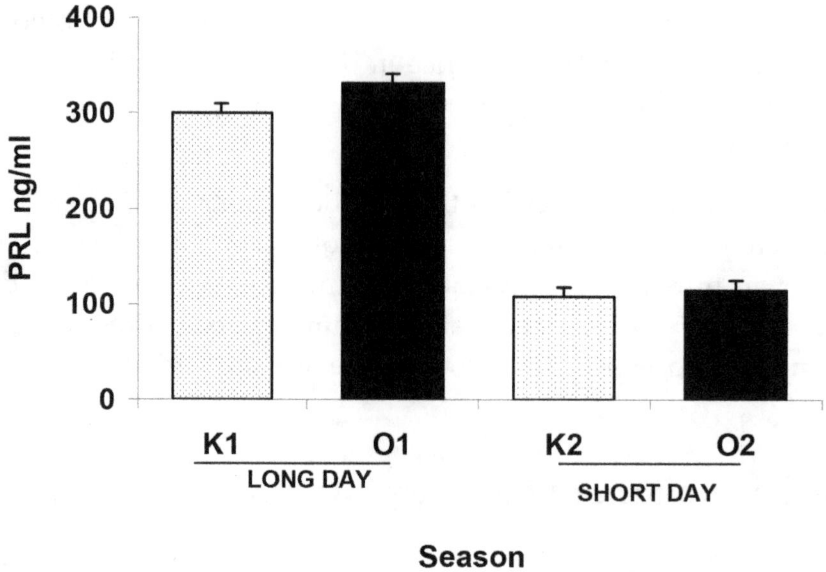

Figure 4. Mean concentrations of prolactin in control and orexin A-treated pituitary explant cultures during long-day (LD) and short-day (SD) photoperiods. See text for statistical comparisons.

GH release from the pituitary explants during the long-day conditions was maintained on significantly higher level in orexin-treated group O1 than control K1 group ($P < 0.05$), throughout the whole period of the incubation. In contrast, during the short-day period, GH release from the explants was significantly less in orexin-treated group O2 than that in the control K2 group ($P < 0.05$). The suppressive effect of orexin was observed during 2 hours. Collective analysis of the data showed that GH concentrations were higher under long-day conditions than under short-day conditions (**Figure** 5).

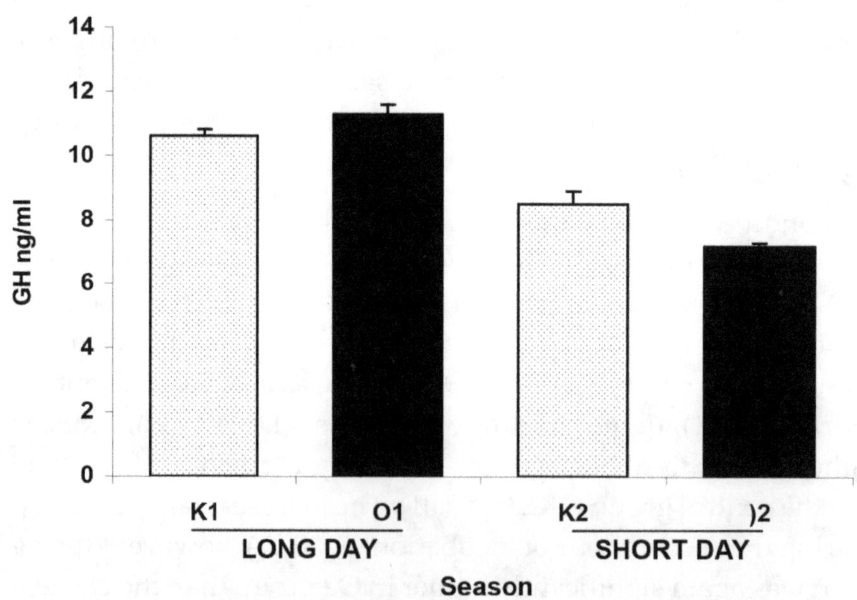

Figure 5. Mean concentrations of growth hormone in control and orexin A-treated pituitary explant cultures during long-day (LD) and short-day (SD) photoperiods. See text for statistical comparisons.

The results of experiments performed on lactating sheep, i.e., animals with strong seasonality characteristics, are difficult to compare with others, however, in ewes as in rodents, orexin A is able to stimulate PRL secretion due to its direct effect on the lactotropic cells. The slight response of ovine pituitary glands to orexin during short days is probably due to the insensitivity of lactotropic cells to the orexin signal. The initiation and maintenance of lactation in sheep require the presence of many hormones, where PRL and GH seem to be the most important. Studies on lactating sheep showed that the ewes starting lactation during the period of increasing day length produced 50% more milk compared with sheep milked during the decreasing day length [15]. When June-lambed ewes were kept under artificial conditions of the long day (16L:8D), PRL level decreased as the natural length of a day became shorter. The fact that pituitary cells become refractory to over-repeated summer signal of the darkness hormone (melatonin) makes it impossible to lengthen lactation in sheep in the autumn-winter period [15]. Determining the role of orexins, especially orexin A, in regulating prolactin secretion may help to clarify the process of lactation maintenance in sheep, especially during the decreasing photoperiod. In conclusion, our results obtained on the pituitary explants demonstrated that the pituitary tissue of lactating sheep was sensitive to photoperiod and orexin A. We conclude that the secretion of PRL and GH from the ovine pituitary gland is negatively responsive to orexin A during SD, whereas orexin may stimulate PRL and GH secretion during LD. Further studies investigating orexin—PRL and GH interactions are needed.

3.2. Role of TRH

Recently, it was observed that TRH has a role to play in the initiation and maintenance of lactation in small ruminants. The aim of the performed study was to determine the impact of the TRH factor on secretion of prolactin in lactating sheep. In vitro studies were carried out on 10 animals. The pituitary gland of each sheep was collected at day 40 of lactation. In vitro incubations were performed on 12 microwell plates in Parker medium for 1 hour at 37°C. One half of the gland was incubated in pure Parker medium (control group), while the second (test group) half was incubated in Parker medium conditioned with exogenous TRH (TRH concentration—36 ug/100 ml medium). The medium was administered every 15 minutes and collected from the wells; in each case, 1 ml of medium was administered. The first 15 minutes served as blank and both halves of the pituitary remained in the same medium; the aim was to stabilize the secretory function of lactotropic cells. Prolactin measurements were made using RIA method. The tests carried out have demonstrated a stimulating impact of the TRH factor on secretion of prolactin. In the first 15 minutes of incubation, PRL concentration in the control group was 81.83 ± 11.4 pg/ml and was significantly ($P \leq 0.05$) lower than the concentration (87.48 ± 11.6 pg/ml) observed in the test group. After 30 minutes of incubation, the control group showed significantly ($P \leq 0.05$) lower prolactin level (74.04 ± 10.03 pg/ml) than the group with TRH-enriched medium (79.9 ± 10.6 pg/ml). After 45 minutes of incubation, the concentration of PRL in the control group was 59.66 ± 9.4 mg/ml and it was significantly ($P \leq 0.01$) lower than that in the experimental group (10.2 ± 65.47 mg/ml) (**Figure 6**).

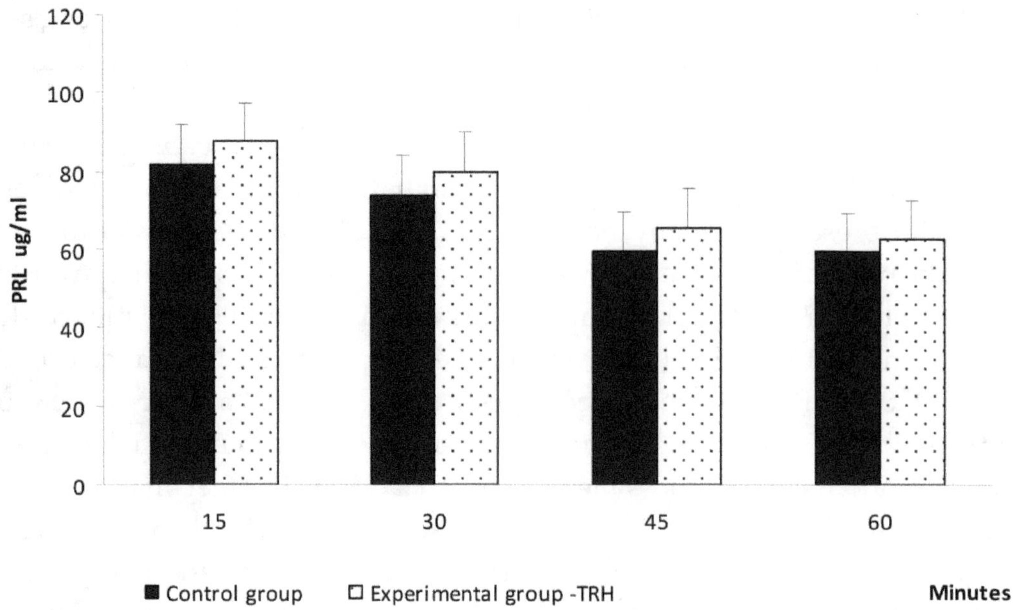

Figure 6. Mean concentrations of prolactin in control and TRH-treated pituitary explant cultures during long-day. See text for statistical comparisons.

3.3. Role of ghrelin

The process of initiation and maintenance of lactation in sheep requires the presence of a number of hormones. The aim of this study was to determine the role of ghrelin in the regulation of prolactin secretion in lactating sheep, based on the culture of in vitro pituitary. The study was conducted in May—long-day period. Pituitary was collected from 10 sheep on day 30 of lactation and divided along the longitudinal grooves so that each contains half of the glandular part and nerves. Incubations were carried out in vitro pituitary in 12 well plates for 1 hour at 37°C. The control group was incubated in a clean Parker medium and experimented in medium supplemented with exogenous ghrelin. The concentration of prolactin in the medium was determined by RIA method. The study showed stimulatory effect of ghrelin on the secretion of prolactin. The tests demonstrated a modulating effect of ghrelin on secretion of prolactin. Significant ($P \leq 0.05$) increase in prolactin secretion after 30 minutes of incubation in the test group (89.6 ± 18.1 mg/ml) compared with the control group (73.6 ± 17.4 mg/ml) was noted. After 45 minutes of incubation, the concentration (69 ± 15.2 mg/ml) of prolactin in the test group was significantly ($P \leq 0.05$) lower than the concentration (77.2 ± 17.6 mg ml) in the control group. After 60 minutes, prolactin level was significantly lower at $P \leq 0.05$ in the test group (46.3 ± 8.4 mg/ml) than that in the control group (51.8 ± 9.6 mg/ml) (**Figure 7**). The results of studies conducted have demonstrated a modulating impact of ghrelin on secretion of prolactin. While increase in prolactin secretion during the incubation period was observed, reduction in prolactin secretion has been recorded in the test group. Administration of exogenous ghrelin during the period of physiologically high prolactin concentration in lactating sheep has not given a clear answer as to whether ghrelin stimulates the secretion of prolactin. The results suggest, therefore, that ghrelin does not directly affect the secretion of prolactin from the pituitary. The hitherto obtained test results showed that the effects of ghrelin may be dependent on the species of animals. In the case of sheep, seasonal breeders, the mechanism of ghrelin activity is complicated. As revealed by the studies in lactating sheep, administration of exogenous ghrelin modulates the secretion of prolactin.

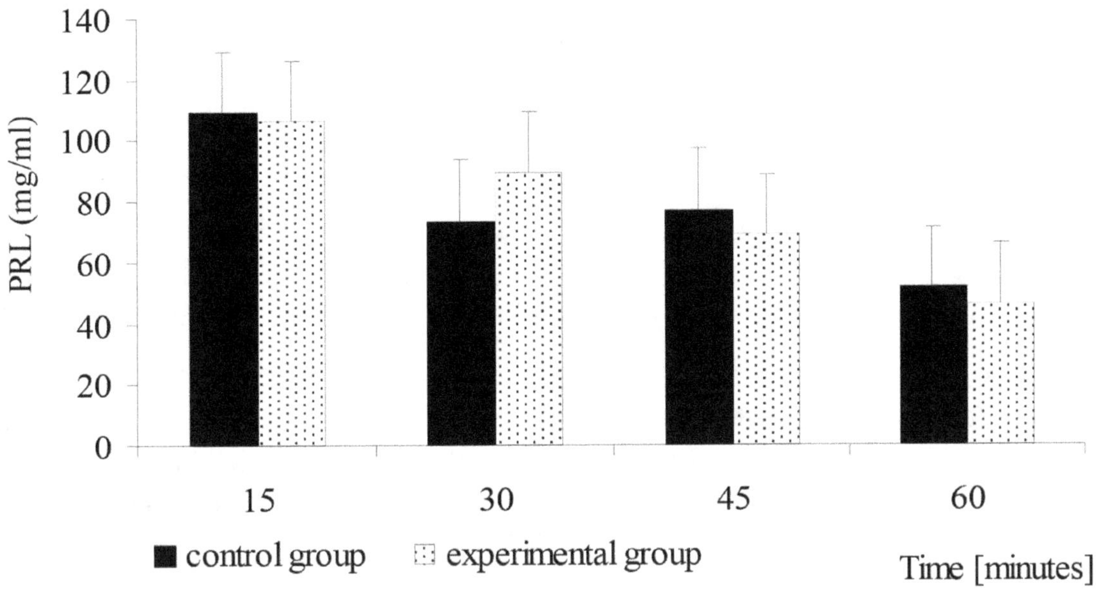

Figure 7. Mean concentrations of prolactin in control and ghrelin-treated pituitary explant cultures during long day. See text for statistical comparisons.

4. Summary

In seasonal animals, the process of triggering and maintaining lactation requires numerous hormones. The interaction of growth factors and other hormones is necessary in processes such as mammogenesis, lactogenesis and galactopoiesis. Due to the proper synchronization of pregnancy and changes in the area of the mammary gland, the gland is ready for the production of milk at the moment the offspring is born. Mammogenesis is a phenomenon that requires the participation of a number of hormones, including prolactin (PRL), growth hormone (GH), estrogens, progesterone, oxytocin, placental lactogen (PL) and insulin-like growth factor (somatomedin, e.g., IGF1). The coparticipation of IGF and GH is necessary in coordinating the differentiation and proliferation of epithelial cells. The manner in which the growth factors stimulate or inhibit the growth of cells or their influence on the cell cycle is not fully understood. The role of IGF in particular stages of functioning of the mammary gland (mammogenesis, lactogenesis, galactopoiesis and desiccation), particularly in the case of ruminants, is highly complicated. Recently, attention has been given to the metabolic hormones, particularly the role of leptin, orexin and ghrelin in mammogenesis, lactogenesis and galactopoiesis, respectively. Due to the recently increased interest in sheep's milk products, an understanding of the endocrine mechanisms facilitating the maintenance of lactation during autumn and winter may contribute to the improved profitability and usefulness of sheep's milk.

Author details

Edyta Molik* and Dorota Zięba-Przybylska

*Address all correspondence to: rzmolik@cyf-kr.edu.pl

Department of Animal Biotechnology, Agricultural University in Krakow, Kraków, Poland

References

[1] Hazlerigg DG andersson H, Johnston JD, Lincoln G: Molecular characterization of the long-day response in the Soay sheep, a seasonal mammal. Current Biology. 2004; 14, 334–339.

[2] Lincoln G, Messager S andersson H, Hazlerigg D: Proceedings of the National Academy of Sciences. Temporal expression of seven clock genes in the suprachiasmatic nucleus and the pars tuberalis of the sheep: evidence for an internal coincidence timer. 2002; 99(21), 13890–13895.

[3] Lincoln GA: Decoding the nightly melatonin signal through circadian clockwork. Molecular and Cellular Endocrinology. 2006; 252, 69–73.

[4] Lincoln GA: Melatonin entrainment of circannual rhythms. Chronobiology International. 2006; 23, 301–306.

[5] Dardente H: Does a melatonin-dependent circadian oscillator in the pars tuberalis drive prolactin seasonal rhythmicity. Journal of Neuroendocrinology. 2007; 19, 657–666.

[6] Lincoln GA, Clarke IJ: Photoperiodically-induced cycles in the secretion of prolactin in hypothalamo-pituitary disconnected rams: evidence for translation of the melatonin signal in the pituitary gland. Journal of Neuroendocrinology. 1994; 6, 251–260.

[7] Cardinali DP, Pévet P: Basic aspects of melatonin action cardinali. Sleep Medicine Reviews. 1998; 2(3), 175–190.

[8] Houghton DC, Young IR, Mcmillen IC: Photoperiodic history and hypothalamic control of prolactin secretion before birth. Endocrinology. 1997; 138, 1506–1511.

[9] Johnston JD: Photoperiodic regulation of prolactin secretion: changes in intra-pituitary signalling and lactotroph heterogeneity. Journal of Endocrinology. 2004; 180, 351–356.

[10] Molik E, Pasternak M, Błasiak M, Misztal T, Romanowicz K, Zieba D: The effect of the diversified signal of melatonin on milk yields in seasonally breeding sheep. Archive fur Tierzucht. 2013; 56(93), 924–929.

[11] Misztal T, Romanowicz K, Barcikowski B: Melatonin modulation of the daily prolactin secretion in intact and ovariectomized ewes. Neuroendocrinology. 1999; 69, 105–112.

[12] Mikolayunas CM, Thomas DL, Dahl GE, Gressley TF, Berger YM: Effect of prepartum photoperiod on milk production and prolactin concentration of dairy ewes. Journal of Dairy Science. 2008; 91(1), 85–90.

[13] Morrissey AD, Cameron AW, Tilbrook AJ: Artificial lighting during winter increases milk yield in dairy ewes. Journal of Dairy Science. 2008; 91(11), 4238–4243. doi: 10.3168/jds.2007-0918.

[14] Misztal T, Romanowicz K, Barcikowski B: Short-term modulation of prolactin secretion by melatonin in anestrous ewes following dopamine - and opiate receptor blockade. Experimental, Clinical, Endocrinology & Diabetes. 2001; 109, 174–180.

[15] Molik E, Misztal T, Romanowicz K, Wierzchoś E: Dependence of the lactation duration and efficiency on the season of lambing in relation to the prolactin and melatonin secretion in ewes. Livestock Science. 2007; 107, 220–226.

[16] Molik E, Misztal T, Romanowicz K, Wierzchoś E: The Influence of length day on melatonin secretion during lactation in aseasonal sheep. Archive fur Tierzucht. 2006; 49, 359–364.

[17] Molik E, Misztal T, Romanowicz K, Zięba D, Wierzchoś E: Changes in growth hormone and prolactin secretion in ewes used for milk under different photoperiodic conditions. Bulletin of the Veterinary Institute in Puławy. 2009; 53, 389–393.

[18] Andrade BR, Salama AA, Caja G, Castillo V, Albanell E, Such XJ: Response to lactation induction differs by season of year and breed of dairy ewes. Journal of Dairy Science. 2008; 91(6), 2299–2306. doi: 10.3168/jds.2007-0687.

[19] Misztal T, Górski K, Tomaszewska-Zaremba D, Molik E, Romanowicz K: Identification of salsolinol in the mediobasal hypothalamus of lactating ewes and its relation to suckling-induced prolactin and GH release. Journal of Endocrinology. 2008; 198, 83–89.

[20] Zieba D, Szczęsna M, Klocek-Górka B, Molik E, Misztal T, Williams GL, Romanowicz K, Stepien E, Keisler DH, Murawski M: Seasonal effects of central leptin infusion on melatonin and prolactin secretion and on SOCS-3 gene expression in ewes. Journal of Endocrinology. 2008; 198, 147–155.

[21] Górski K, Romanowicz K, Herman A, Molik E, Gajewska A, Tomaszewska-Zaremba D, Misztal T: The possible involvement of salsolinol and hypothalamic prolactin in the central regulatory processes in ewes during lactation. Reproduction in Domestic Animals. 2009;45(5), e54–e60. doi: 10.1111/j.1439-0531.2009.01521.

[22] Górski K, Romanowicz K, Molik E, Fülöp F, Misztal T: Effects of salsolinol and its antagonistic analogue, 1-MeDIQ, on growth hormone release in nursing sheep. Acta Neurobiology of Experimental. 2010; 70, 20–27.

[23] Reinert BD, Wilson FE: Hormone thyroid and the hypothalamus-pituitary-ovarian axis in American Tree Sparrows (Spizella arborea). General and Comparative Endocrinology. 1996; 103, 60–70.

[24] Karsch FJ, Dahl GE, Hachigian TM, Thrun LA: Involvement of thyroid hormones in seasonal reproduction. Journal of Reproduction and Fertility. Supplement. 1995; 49, 409–422.

[25] Klocek-Górka B, Szczęsna M, Molik E, Zieba D: The interaction of season, leptin and melatonin levels with thyroid hormone secretion, using an in vitro approach. Small Ruminant Research. 2010; 2, 231–235.

[26] Mitin V, Mikulec K, Karadjole I: Thyroid hormones and insulin concentration in sheep. Veterinarski Arhiv. 1986; 55, 73–75.

[27] Tucker HA: Hormones, mammary growth and lactation: a 41-year perspective. Journal of Dairy Science. 2000; 83, 874–884.

[28] Kokot F, Stupnicki R: Methods used radioimmunoassay and radiokompetycyjne in the clinic. PZWL, Warszawa, 1985.

[29] Morgan PJ: The pars tuberalis: the missing link in the photoperiodic regulation of prolactin secretion. Journal of Neuroendocrinology. 2000; 12, 287–295.

[30] Rowan W. Relation of light to bird migration and developmental changes. Nature. 1925; 115, 494–495.

10

Melatonin and Exercise: Their Effects on Malondialdehyde and Lipid Peroxidation

Mahsa Rastegar Moghaddam Mansouri,
Sadegh Abbasian and Mohammad Khazaie

Abstract

Melatonin as an omnipresent molecule is secreted by the pineal gland. It is a strong free radical scavenger, which reduces nitric oxide (NO) generation within mitochondria. Exercise has great impacts on many body's homeostatic systems. Most human's organisms display rhythms and have 24 hours environmental cycles, which are called circadian rhythm. Melatonin is one of the circadian rhythm generator in various physiological variables. Exercises could regulate plasma melatonin levels. Melatonin scavenges reactive oxygen spices (ROS) and reactive nitrogen spices (RNS) and acts as the antioxidant cascade. It not only decreases the exercise induced-oxidative stress in the muscles but also enhances muscle antioxidant enzymes, such as superoxide dismutase. Body lipids and unsaturated fatty acids are prone to oxidation, while the free radicals penetrate into bilayer membrane structure lipid peroxidation is going to happen. Malondialdehyde (MDA) is created by free radicals, and it is one of the most frequent marker of lipid peroxidation. Exercise, its duration, and time of the day have immediate and or delayed effects on melatonin secretion. The combination of aerobic exercise and melatonin reduces the exercise induced-free radicals agents. Melatonin supplementation, especially while it combined with aerobic training, could decrease the lipid peroxidation and malondialdehyde. Melatonin could impede exercise-induced ROS, increase body health, and exercise-related adaptation.

Keywords: exercise, health, lipid peroxidation, malondialdehyde, melatonin, reactive oxygen spices

1. Introduction

Melatonin is an omnipresent molecule that has various functional activities in plants and animals [1]. It is possibly associated with longevity in which their dysfunction is what initiates the aging process [2, 3]. Melatonin was secreted by pinecone-like gland that is deeply placed in the brain which is called the "pineal gland." This gland has sympathetic innervation as its main sources due to its special location in the brain [2]. The pineal gland is a tranquilizing organ leading to a high melatonin production in response to darkness. Serotonin (made from tryptophan) through the cascade of enzymatic reactions produces melatonin with chemical name N-acetyl-5-methoxy tryptamine. This gland is located outside the blood–brain barrier (BBB) and has large uptake of tryptophan which produces high melatonin levels [2]. This hormone is mostly secreted at night and results in sleep regulation, signaling the time of the day that acts as chronological pacemaker, and participates in various physiological functions.

2. The melatonin advantages for the body

Melatonin is a strong free radical scavenger which reduces nitric oxide (NO) generation within mitochondria. NO strongly interferes with components of the respiratory chain in the mitochondria [4, 5]. Melatonin has two direct and indirect antioxidant capacities, which directly scavenges free radicals and indirectly regulates the activity of antioxidant enzymes. When melatonin interacts with the toxic reactants, several metabolites are generated which per se act as direct free radical scavengers such as N1-acetyl-N2-formyl-5-methoxykynuramine (AFMK) [6]. Melatonin impacts toxic radicals and breaks them down, eliminates reactive oxygen species-induced H_2O_2 (one of the most important reactive oxygen species or ROS), acts on uncoupling proteins (UCPs), and decreases body heat production [7, 8]. Moreover, as melatonin decreases NO generation, melatonin leads to mitochondria function development, and due to increase in the mitochondria respiration, the ATP production and electron transportation increase as well [5, 9, 10].

To have a glance at the other importance of melatonin, we pointed to neurodegenerative diseases. Melatonin production in aged individuals declines and is known as the primary contributing factor for aged-related neurodegenerative diseases. Also, hypoxia, hypoglycemia, viruses, drug neurotoxicity, radiation, or noxious substances all could produce neural damage. Through antioxidant effects of melatonin, it has been proposed as a neuroprotective agent. Over the melatonin therapeutic value, it is used as treatment of Alzheimer disease (AD), Parkinson disease (PD), amyotrophic lateral sclerosis (ALS), stroke, and brain trauma. Neurodegenerative disorders mostly happen due to free radical-mediated damage and mitochondria dysfunction as common pathophysiological mechanism [11].

3. What is exercise, and how does it affect the melatonin?

According to the Center for Disease Control and Prevention (CDC), exercise is a subcategory of physical activity that is planned, structured, repetitive, and purposive that improves or maintains one or more components of physical fitness. Physical activity also refers to any bodily movement which is produced by the skeletal muscle contraction that increases energy expenditure more than basal level and enhances health. Furthermore, health is a human condition with three dimensions as physical, social, and psychological. To clarify the benefit of exercise and physical activity, we have to define the physical inactivity which refers to those physical activities less than what is required for optimal health and prevention of premature death [12, 13].

There are huge differences between physical activity and physical fitness which should not be interchangeably used. According to CDC physical fitness is the ability to carry out daily tasks without fatigue and of course with plenty of energy to enjoy leisure time and respond to emergencies. Physical fitness has a number of components consisting of cardiorespiratory endurance, skeletal muscle endurance, skeletal muscle strength, skeletal muscle power, flexibility, balance, speed of movement, reaction time, and body composition. Physical activity according to above definition refers to any bodily movement produced by skeletal muscle contraction [12, 13].

Muscular strength is an essential factor for health and functional ability and consequently increases life quality. The importance of progressive resistance exercise had been clarified seen in World War II which was recommended for veteran rehabilitation. The important point of all resistance training is that the training must be "progressive" and progression is the act of advancing toward a specific goal which leads to continued improvement in muscle ability. Muscle development is under the effects of program variables such as exercise selection and order, number of sets and repetitions, and rest period length [14].

Physical activity and exercises are so important strategies to face chronic conditions, lower cancer risk, and synchronize the circadian system. Increasing physical activity and taking part in aerobic endurance activities, resistance training, and flexibility exercises have been shown to decrease the risk of several chronic diseases such as coronary heart disease, obesity, diabetes, low back pain, osteoporosis, and sarcopenia [12, 14–16]. Physical activities and exercises are nonphotic signals that entrain human circadian clock [16]. Physical activity could increase the melatonin levels, decrease estrogen production, and improve fat metabolism [15].

Cardiorespiratory fitness also is the capacity of the cardiovascular (both heart and vessels) and respiratory (lungs) systems to supply oxygen to the blood and consequently to the working skeletal muscles and the capacity of the muscles to use oxygen to produce energy for movement. The best test to determine the cardiorespiratory fitness is the maximum aerobic fitness; moreover in the human studies, length of time running or cycling in standardized test could examine the physiological/biochemical/psychological exhaustion [12].

Strength fitness is also another health component that is defined as the capacity of the skeletal muscle to move an external load. Balance is defined as the ability to control the body during the body movement, and flexibility is also defined as range of joint motion or range of motion (ROM) [12, 14].

To continue the importance of the combination of the exercise and melatonin on the body system, we have to deliberate some fundamental concepts of training. Overload as the first concept is the "gradual increase of stress placed upon the body during exercise training." Specificity of training is that training should be specific to the body needs or both movement patterns and force-velocity characteristics. Also, the good training program should have variation to support the training needs to remain optimal. In this case training periodization is defined as utilizes variation in training program design [14]. Exercise and physical activity can also act as preventer of chronic disease and regulate body systems. Regular activity and structured exercises are related to vast health benefits and body hormone regulation [12, 17, 18].

Exercise has great impacts on many body's homeostatic systems. Most human organisms display rhythms in their physiology and have 24 hour environmental cycle which is called circadian rhythm. Melatonin is one of the circadian rhythm generators in various physiological variables. Also, there are some voluntary rhythm modifiers such as activity or physical exercise; meal time can also act as circadian rhythm modifier signal [16]. Physical activity and exercise are nonphotic signals that regulate the human circadian clock and synchronize circadian system. Melatonin is one of the main signals of body clock that is commonly measured to report the effects of exercise on the circadian clock. Noteworthy almost different kinds of exercises and physical activities both acute and chronic could modify plasma melatonin levels. Meanwhile, endogenous profile of melatonin has different responses such as increase, decrease [19], or even unaffected to exercises that time of the day, and lighting condition is the most effective item on the melatonin secretion cycle even in response to exercises. As an overall consensus, those exercises which have been done at night or in the dark whether of moderate or high intensity result in delay in melatonin secretion. Indeed, the age does not influence the exercise-induced circadian rhythm of melatonin as nocturnal hormone. Besides the effects of exercises on the different phases of melatonin secretion, the exercises also transiently affect the melatonin levels. The mechanism of this transient changes in melatonin levels could be due to the circadian phase at that time exercise was undertaken. A bout of exercise increases the plasma melatonin levels, while regular training and exercises attenuate the melatonin [16]. There are several potent physiological factors that describe the melatonin changes. Melatonin acts as an antioxidant, and exercise especially strenuous exercise increases oxidative stress, hence melatonin which is secreted by the human body or even ingested capable of protecting against potential molecular damage [6]. It was reported that proximately after exercise melatonin levels increase and following 1 hour after physical activity, it returns to pre-exercise level [20]. Melatonin levels of trained individuals is higher in the morning compared to the evening, but in the following 3 weeks of hard training, the evening melatonin levels were higher than morning levels. Interestingly both morning and evening levels of melatonin decreased compared to pre-3 weeks of hard training. Well-trained individuals show an adaptive response to each training that they take part as their oxidative stress regulates and diurnal melatonin levels temporarily increase [16, 21]. Total mechanisms of the melatonin alteration following exercises remained unknown, but exercise-induced absolute rise in melatonin levels is more pronounced in the morning compared to the evening [22].

4. Exercises on the melatonin

4.1. Acute and strenuous exercises

Acute sport trainings and resistance exercises lead to change in the energy demands and are strong stimulation of muscle tissue. Intense exercises produce free radicals, inflammatory responses, hormonal and biochemical disturbances, and metabolic and defensive changes [6]. Acute exercise increases oxygen consumption much more than rest time which makes muscles prone to oxidative stress. Oxygen molecule is a radical species per se and also results in generation of various free radicals, and those free radical species that are forming due to oxygen and nitrogen are the most important in the living organisms [23]. While subjects have routine life pattern, their energy demands and blood vessel contribution are balanced. During the acute or resistance exercise training, oxygen consumption of both striated and smooth muscles increases dramatically which leads to increase in reactive oxygen/nitrogen species that is called RONS. While exercise-derived RONS are generated, the body antioxidant defense system starts to work and protects cells and tissues against free radicals. The imbalance between body antioxidant defense system and RONS is called oxidative stress [24]. Low levels of ROS regulate muscle force through calcium release mechanism, and influencing myofilament structure creates adaptive response to training. However, high levels of ROS reduce force production and result in muscular fatigue [25].

Melatonin due to its scavenging ability could directly interact with a variety of oxygen- and nitrogen-based radicals. It is an antioxidant that regulates the activities of other antioxidant enzymes [6, 25]. Strenuous sport activities lead to acute muscle injuries that are indicated by muscle soreness, prolong loss of muscle function, and leakage of muscle proteins. Acute exercise-induced muscle injuries consist of 30–67% of athletic injuries, while exercise-induced severe muscle injuries could impede the athletic progression. Muscle damages result in multidimensional changes in muscle tissue such as inflammation that per se encourage the free radical production and muscle atrophy [26, 27]. This condition could be reduced with optimal nutrition mostly by increasing dietary content of nutritional antioxidant. Melatonin as one of the body-secreted natural antioxidants could cross all barriers and reduce the oxidative damage in almost every environment in the body. Intensive exercises cause abundant changes in immunity and also change the carbohydrate and lipid metabolism that make athletes vulnerable to infection. In this case melatonin protects heart muscle cells and other body parts from exercise-induced inflammation [6, 27]. As previously mentioned, strenuous exercise muscle injuries lead to protein degradation that encourages muscle injury. Whenever exercise-induced protein degradation and consequent muscle atrophy are limited, the extent of muscle injuries could be blunted. Melatonin is one of the most effective factors that could limit muscle injuries. It was shown that melatonin inhibited the nuclear factor kappa-B (NFKB) activation that prevents the cytokine-induced atrophy and thus muscle injury. Melatonin also decreases proinflammatory cytokines, tumor necrosis factor-alpha (TNF-alpha), and interleukin-6 (IL-6) expression within the muscle. Also, muscle atrophy F-box (MAF_{BX}) and muscle RING finger 1 (MURF-1) are inhibited by melatonin. MAFBX is a muscle-specific ubiquitin ligase that mediates the degradation of muscle-specific transcription factor MyoD. MURF-1 also is a member of ubiquitin ligase family which interacts with the giant protein titin in the muscle and is called titin-associated protein that expert antihypertrophic activity [28, 29]. In this case melatonin through the elevation of the expression of the muscle Akt could reduce the ratio of the MAFBX/MURF-1 and inhibits the breakdown of the structural muscle protein such as myosin heavy chain (**Figure 1**). The functional role of the melatonin and strenuous muscle injury prevention is not fully understood, but the melatonin effects on the muscle cytokines, NFKB activation, muscle Akt elevation, and consequent decline in the MAFBX/MURF-1 could open new points of view to the melatonin protection mechanism [26].

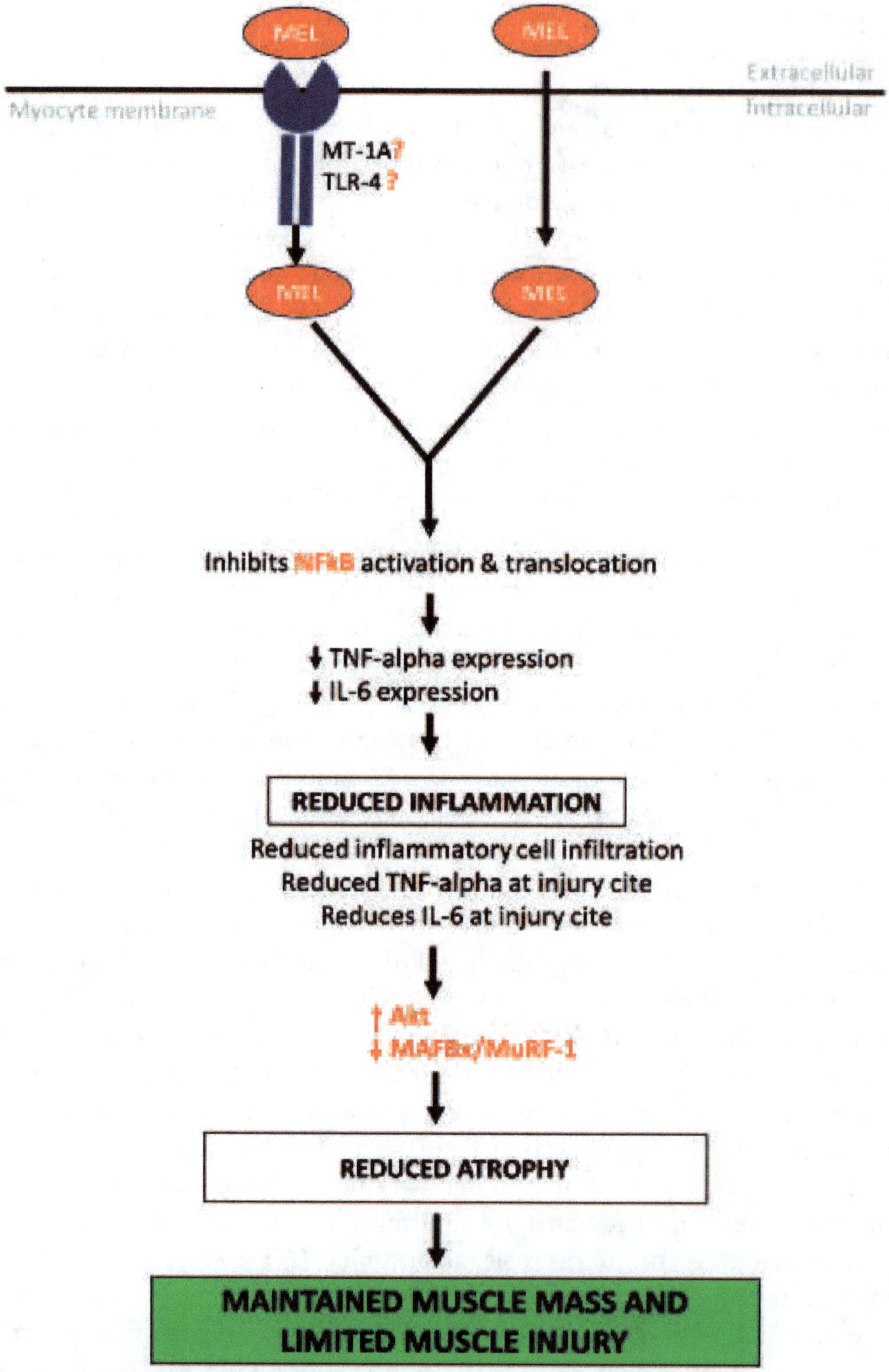

Figure 1. Advantages of melatonin on the muscle injury that contribute to the strenuous exercise. Melatonin inhibits the activation of the nuclear factor kappa-light-chain-enhancer of activated B cells (NFKB) and translocates it that reduces the expression of tumor necrosis factor-alpha or TNF-alpha and interleukin-6 or IL-6 in exercise-induced injured muscle. Consequently melatonin could limit inflammation and increase the activation of the protein kinase B also known as Akt to control protein deprivation and downregulate the atrophy via NFKB/MAFBX/MURF-1/Akt pathway during injury. NF-κB, nuclear factor kappa-B; TNF-alpha, tumor necrosis factor-alpha; IL-6, interleukin-6; Akt, serine/threonine kinase; MAFBX, muscle atrophy F-box; and MuRF-1, muscle RING finger 1 [26].

Melatonin and all its metabolites could scavenge ROS and reactive nitrogen species (RNS) and act as the antioxidant cascade. Melatonin not only decreases the exercise-induced oxidative stress in the muscles but also enhances muscle antioxidant enzymes such as superoxide dismutase. Moreover, melatonin reduces muscle inflammatory factors such as IL-6 and TNF-alpha [25–27]. Melatonin could successfully manage the strenuous exercise-induced muscle damage through several ways. It increases the strength of injured muscle, reduces severity of the injury, increases number of satellite cells, inhibits NF-κB activation/translocation, causes TNF-alpha and IL-6 to decline, and increases muscle Akt and thus decreases MAFBX/MuRF-1 ratio. Due to its broad-spectrum antioxidant, it could protect DNA, proteins, and biological membrane lipids from the effects of ROS and other oxidative stress [6, 24, 26].

4.2. Aerobic training

Physical exercise is performing some activities to keep healthy weight, building and conserving healthy bone, muscle, and joints to develop physiological health. Exercise also promotes the immune system. Immune system responses to exercise are directly dependent on the intensity, duration, and body adaptive responses. It has been suggested that moderate exercise through endocrine hormone elevation could reverse immunosenescence. Moderate exercise training modulates exercise-induced ROS and DNA damage and regulates cytokine levels [30].

Aerobic training and regular physical activity are highly associated with vast beneficial health issues including limiting cardiovascular disease (CVD), diabetes type 2, and age-related mortality. Aerobic training also induces vast acute and chronic adaptation in various physiological systems. Furthermore, physical inactivity is one of the four main causes of premature mortality. Although the aerobic physical activity increases in the current society, the level of the physical inactivity is still high [17, 31]. It was shown that physical activity could elevate melatonin levels, decrease estrogen production, improve fat metabolism, and reduce cancer risk as well. It has been reported that short- or even long-term physical activity has no substantial effects on the melatonin levels [15]. Moderate exercise, in another study, could modulate ROS, cytokines, and hormone levels that all affect apoptosis. Melatonin as one of this regulating hormones has diverse physiological aspects that it can counteract the immune depression following acute stress or aging and also upregulate TNF [30]. Exercise has immediate and/or delayed effects on melatonin secretion, in which duration, type of exercise, time of the day, fitness status, and age have also been identified as intervening factors in exercise-induced changes in the melatonin levels (**Figure 2**).

Melatonin also plays an important role in the exercise-induced metabolic adaptation. Pinealectomized animals do not show adaptive metabolic changes due to aerobic training. Melatonin acts as a mediator between environment situation and physiological regulatory manner. Besides melatonin effects on the blood pressure and endocrine regulation, it also acts on the GLUT 4 (glucose transporter) gene expression (31). In this case aerobic training is coworker of melatonin in which both of them stimulate glucose uptake through

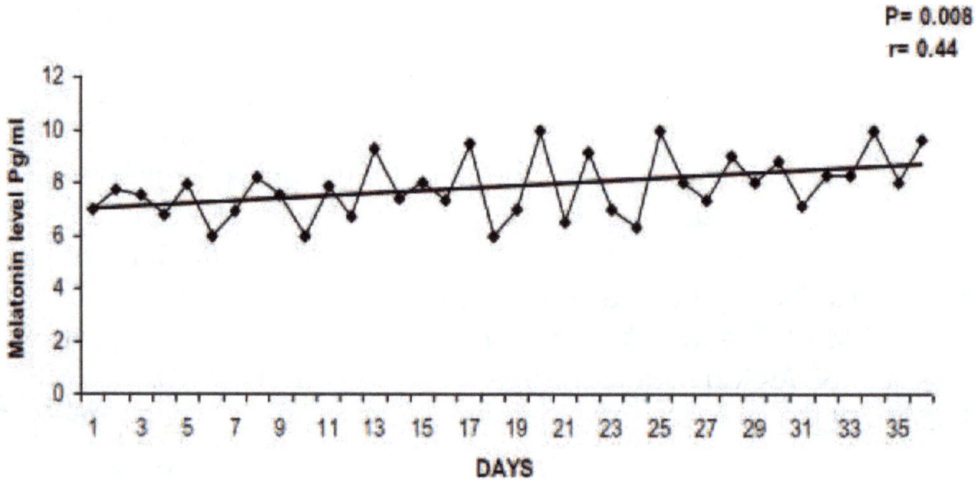

Figure 2. The effects of exercise time duration on the melatonin levels [30].

insulin-independent process and increase GLUT 4 protein expression. It was reported that those pinealectomized rats that undergo aerobic training did not show any metabolic development. So melatonin plays key role in metabolic adaptation in both adipose and muscle tissues. As it was mentioned, melatonin has circadian rhythm and regulates body clock; it also regulates energy metabolism circadian timing in which period of activity and adaptation to activity affect this timing [16, 31]. In one study the effects of melatonin supplementation on the aerobic exercise-induced adaptation were examined. For this purpose male wistar rats are divided into four groups: sedentary control, trained control, sedentary treated with melatonin, and trained treated with melatonin. Glucose tolerance, physical capacity, citrate synthesis, phosphatidylinositol 3-kinase (PI3K), mitogen-activated protein kinas (MAPK), and GLUT4 were examined. Following the 8-week aerobic exercise training on treadmill, those trained animals that treated with melatonin showed better results in their measured parameters that are mentioned above. Briefly, melatonin supplementation plus aerobic training creates great metabolic adaptation and improves metabolism efficiency [31]. The combination of aerobic exercise and melatonin, also, reduces the exercise-induced free radical agents. Low to moderate levels of free radicals have regulatory roles, but their high levels create cellular damages and induce oxidative stress [24]. Melatonin elevation or melatonin supplementation especially while it is combined with aerobic training could decrease the lipid peroxidation and malondialdehyde—lipid peroxidation most frequent marker—in sedentary individuals [18]. Long-term aerobic training could manage the lipid profile of sedentary individuals. Meanwhile when combined with melatonin, the protective effects of aerobic training against free radicals advance, and the body antioxidant defense system improves [18].

Two central and direct ways guide the melatonin effects on the brown adipose tissue to increase exercise-energy expenditure. The nervous system is the central way that controls the melatonin through the sympathetic system. Sympathetic nerve-secreted norepinephrine controls the daily variation in melatonin synthesis [16]. Also, exercise leads to high increase in the activity of the sympathetic nervous system and catecholamine secretion which could modulate melatonin secretion [16]. Melatonin acts as antioxidant [6]. Its secretion is affected by daytime and especially the nervous system. Exercise training stimulates sympathetic

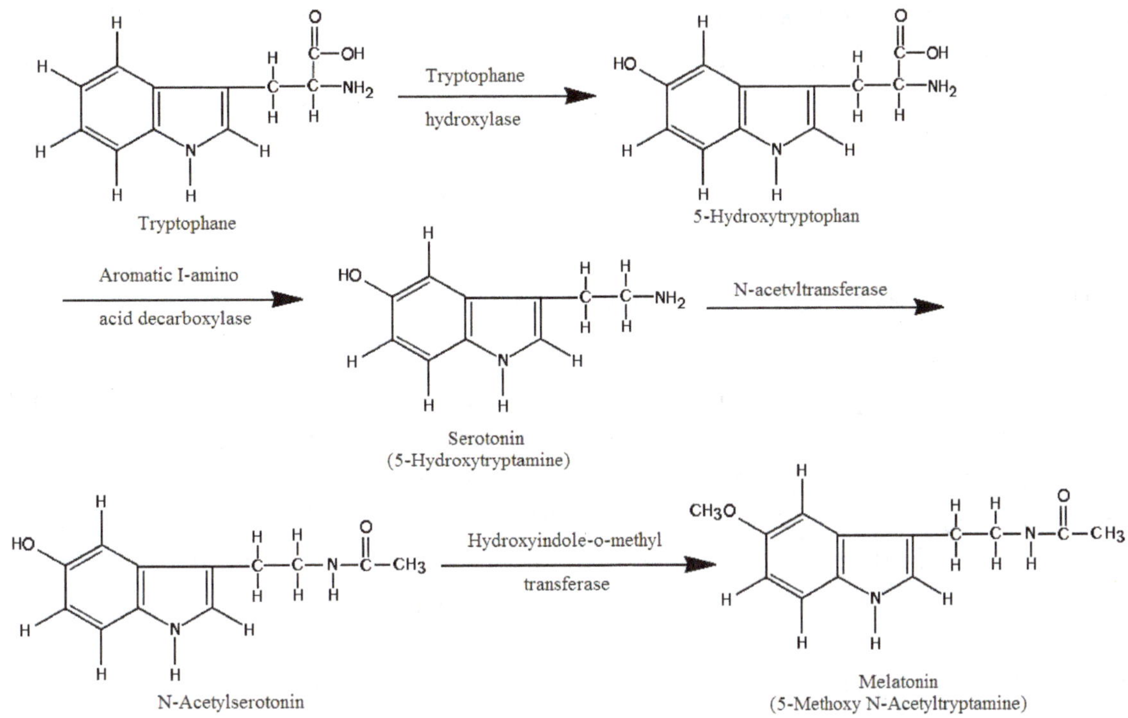

Figure 3. Tryptophan to melatonin cascade process. Tryptophan is the precursor of serotonin and melatonin [32].

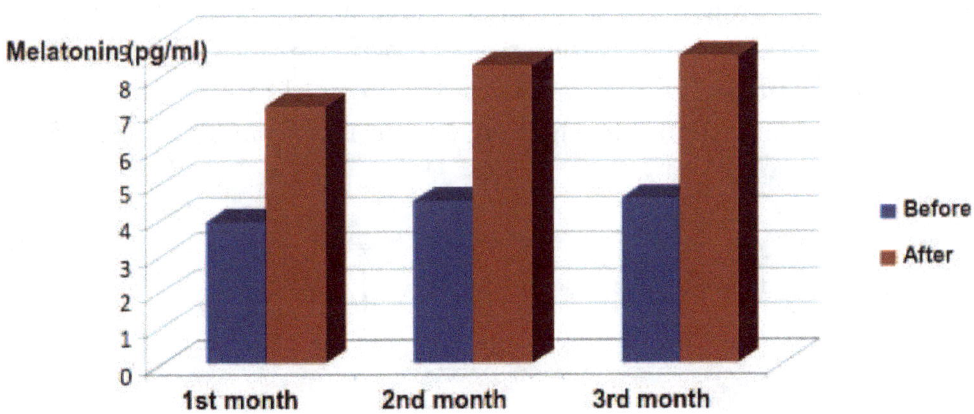

Figure 4. Direct positive correlation between melatonin levels and exercise duration. As the training days progress, the melatonin levels increase [30].

nervous system and releases noradrenaline. Noradrenaline increases the tryptophan levels [30]. Tryptophan is uptaken by the pineal gland and decarboxylated to form serotonin (or 5-hydroxytryptamine). Serotonin during the daylight is stored in the pineal gland. Darkness causes noradrenaline to activate the enzymes (serotonin-N-acetyltransferase) and finally convert serotonin into melatonin (**Figure 3**) [32].

Also, in the direct way, protein kinase C (PKC) pathway leads to increase growth factor and mitochondria biogenesis [33]. Melatonin also could increase LDL receptor and inhibit cholesterol synthesis which is even useful for control obesity [33].

Regarding long-term endurance training, the melatonin hormone reaches steady state. Furthermore, there is direct positive correlation between melatonin levels and exercise duration (**Figure 4**) [30]. Following exercise melatonin gradually increases, and due to endurance training which should last for about 3 months, the melatonin reaches to steady state [30]. It was reported that the low-intensity aerobic training has better adaptation and lipid peroxidation prevention in sedentary individuals. Melatonin supplementation for about 2 months improves dyslipidemia, decreases LDL, and improves lipid metabolism [25].

5. What is lipid peroxidation, and what is malondialdehyde?

Free radicals are those species that are created as a result of cellular oxygen consumption and are mediator of lipid peroxidation. Different elements and situations affect the lipid peroxidation such as heat, oxygen, and enzymes. Free radicals have one or even more than one free electron(s). All of these ingredients could damage the molecules' organisms and create oxidative stress. Body natural defense system impedes the oxidative stress; whenever an imbalance occurs between the free radical production and antioxidant defense system effectiveness, the oxidative stress happens [18, 34]. Lipids are one of the important agents either in food or body's biological system. Body lipids are prone to oxidation, and it would happen during several stages as food storage process or even in physiological/pathological conditions. Unsaturated fatty acids are prone to oxidation; while the free radicals penetrate into bilayer membrane structure, lipid peroxidation is going to happen [18, 35]. Oxygen and free radicals damage the unsaturated fatty acids under lipoperoxide formation. This compound is unstable and could break down into wide range of reactive species which bind to free amino groups and decrease the proteolytic degradation [34]. Free radical-induced lipid peroxidation happens in three stages: initiation, propagation, and termination [35]. In the first stage, free

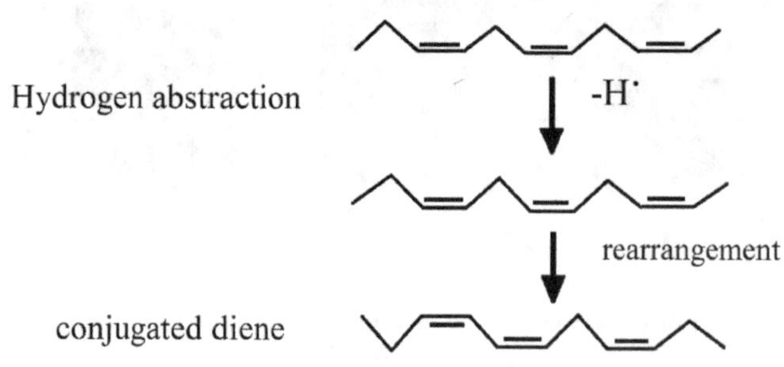

Figure 5. The first stage (initiation stage) of lipid peroxidation process [36].

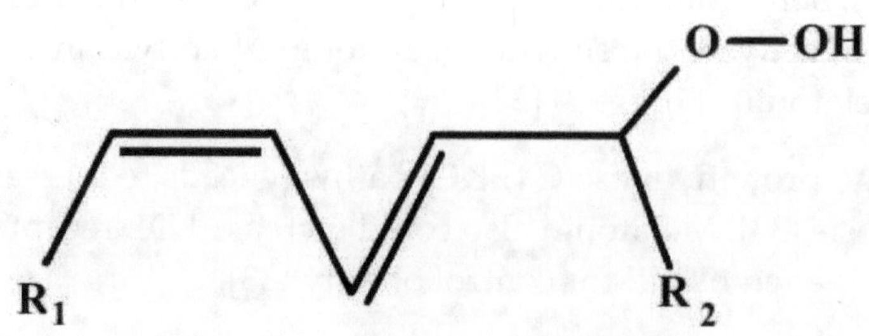

Figure 6. Structural formula of conjugated diene during lipid peroxidation [34].

radicals attack fatty acid molecule which detach hydrogen ion and create fatty acid radical. Due to reordering of double bond, two double bonds between carbon atoms contain and create conjugated diene. The diene structure reacts with oxygen molecule and creates lipoperoxyl radical (**Figures 5** and **6**).

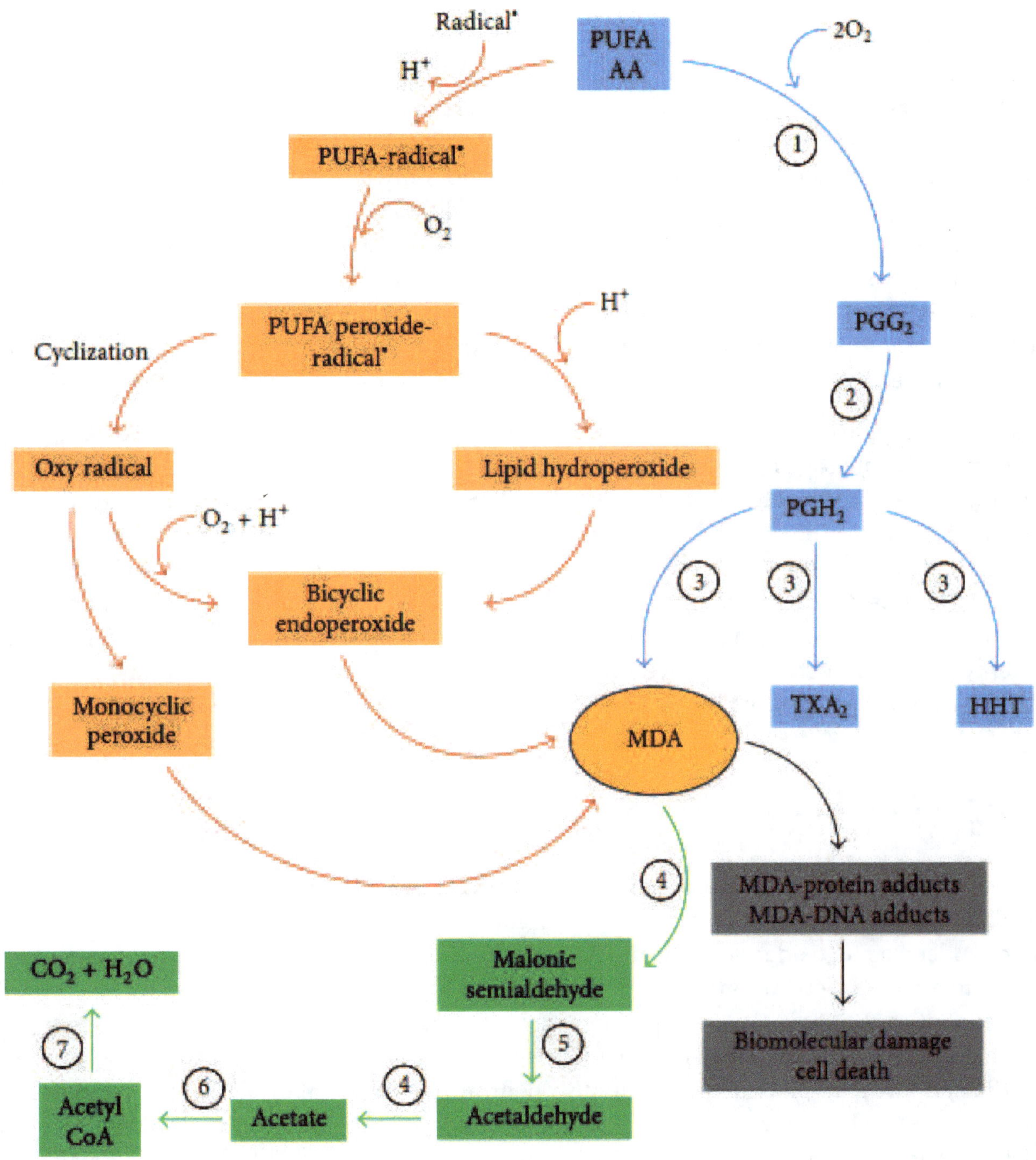

Figure 7. Malondialdehyde formation and metabolism process. Decomposition of arachidonic acid (AA) and PUFAs as side products of enzymatic process during the biosynthesis of thromboxane A_2 (TXA_2) and 12-l-hydroxy-5,8,10-hepadecatrienoic acid (HHT) (blue pathway) or nonenzymatic process by lipid peroxidation-induced bicyclic endoperoxides (red pathway) generates malondialdehyde. Malondialdehyde could enzymatically be metabolized (green pathway); those key enzymes in both malondialdehyde formation and metabolism are cyclooxygenase [1], prostacyclin hydroperoxidase [2], thromboxane synthase [3], aldehyde dehydrogenase [4], decarboxylase [5], acetyl CoA synthase [6], and tricarboxylic acid cycle [7] [38].

In the second phase named propagation, the lipoperoxyl radical, the first phase product, reacts with other fatty acid molecules. Further this reaction a hydrogen atom detaches due to lipid hydroperoxide formation. Following propagation the last stage which is called termination occurs. In this phase enzymatic lipid peroxidation which catalyzes cyclooxygenase and lipoxygenase enzymes happens [34, 36].

Lipid peroxidation leads to two results as structural damage into membrane and creates secondary products. Broken fatty acyl chains and lipid-lipid or even lipid-protein cross-links could damage membrane and affect biological systems and impair membrane function and enzymatic inactivation [36]. Malondialdehyde, which is known as MDA, is a three-carbon molecule that is created by free radicals, and it is not only a secondary product but also the most frequent marker of lipid peroxidation [18, 37]. MDA is generated by decomposition of arachidonic acid and polyunsaturated fatty acids (PUFAs) (**Figure 7**). MDA is stable and membrane permeable which may act as signaling messenger [38]. MDA is one the most popular oxidative stress markers, and due to its toxicity, it becomes very relevant to biomedical condition, and several technologies are used to determine MDA such as liquid chromatography-mass spectrometry (LC–MS) and several derivatization-based strategies [38].

There are multiple methods to prevent lipid peroxidation and MDA harmful effects that among them antioxidant usage is the most effective and suitable approach [39]. Antioxidants scavenge free radicals and inactivate peroxides and other ROS consequently could prevent or even delay oxidation process. The chemical structure, concentration, temperature, and type of oxidation substrate determine the efficiency of antioxidants. It means that to select the best antioxidant, we have to consider many points of view and take many factors into account [39]. Antioxidant defense system helps organism to battle with oxidative stress. This system has three lines of defense. In the first stage, ROS overproduction impedes. The second defense line is mainly created by enzymes, and in the third line of defense, molecules should scavenge ROS [24].

6. Conclusion

Melatonin as pineal gland hormone is secreted according to circadian rhythm. Melatonin is also a strong antioxidant that could cross physiological barrier due to its amphiphilic feature, thereby decreasing oxidative damage. Melatonin has direct (direct scavenging of free radical and activate DNA reparation enzymes) and indirect (support superoxide dismutase or SOD) antioxidant capacities [24]. Amphiphilic feature of melatonin makes it strong scavenging factor that increases the efficiency of melatonin's radical scavenging which could pass between lipidic and aqueous phases. Melatonin also neutralizes singlet oxygen, peroxynitrite anion, and nitric oxide [24]. A wide range of biological systems such as linoleate model system or LDL contributes in melatonin antioxidant properties [39, 40]. Melatonin supplementation decreases the MDA and also lipid peroxidation [18]. In an experimental study, it was shown that melatonin supplementation during long-term aerobic exercise could diminish the exercise-induced lipid peroxidation and also malondialdehyde [18]. Exercise training generates almost twofold elevation in oxygen species, lipid peroxidation, and MDA levels [41]. Another report represented that melatonin administration 30 min before the exercise impressively decreases triglyceride and MDA [6]. Four-week melatonin supplementation followed by single exercise that lasts about 30 min decreases oxidative stress and MDA as well [42].

Acknowledgements

We would like to express our gratitude to many people who saw us through this book. The authors would like to acknowledge the help of all the people involved in this project. We would also like to show our gratitude to all those researchers and their pearls of wisdom and knowledge that help us in writing this chapter.

Author details

Mahsa Rastegar Moghaddam Mansouri[1,2]*, Sadegh Abbasian[1,2] and Mohammad Khazaie[2,3]

*Address all correspondence to: rastegar.moghadam.mansouri@gmail.com

1 2020 Olympic Sport School, Tehran, Iran

2 Center of Sport Talent Identification and Development, Department of Education, Malard, Tehran, Iran

3 Faculty of Physical Education and Sport Sciences, University of Tehran, Tehran, Iran

References

[1] Pandi-Perumal SR, Srinivasan V, Maestroni GJ, Cardinali DP, Poeggeler B, Hardeland R. Melatonin: Nature's most versatile biological signal? The FEBS Journal. 2006;**273**(13): 2813-2838

[2] Masters A, Pandi-Perumal SR, Seixas A, Girardin JL, McFarlane SI. Melatonin, the hormone of darkness: From sleep promotion to Ebola. Brain Disorders & Therapy. 2014;**4**(1): 151-157

[3] Oaknin-Bendahan S, Anis Y, Nir I, Zisapel N. Effects of long-term administration of melatonin and a putative antagonist on the ageing rat. Neuroreport. 1995;**6**:785-788

[4] Maldonado MD, Mora-Santos M, Naji L, Carrascosa-Salmoral MP, Naranjo MC, Calvo JR. Evidence of melatonin synthesis and release by mast cells. Possible modulatory role on inflammation. Pharmacological Research. 2010;**62**(3):282-287

[5] Cardinali DP, Pagano ES, Scacchi Bernasconi PA, Reynoso R, Scacchi P. Melatonin and mitochondrial dysfunction in the central nervous system. Hormones and Behavior. 2013;**63**(2):322-330

[6] Maldonado MD, Manfredi M, Ribas-Serna J, Garcia-Moreno H, Calvo JR. Melatonin administrated immediately before an intense exercise reverses oxidative stress, improves immunological defenses and lipid metabolism in football players. Physiology & Behavior. 2012;**105**(5):1099-1103

[7] Acuna-Castroviejo D, Escames G, Rodriguez MI, Lopez LC. Melatonin role in the mitochondrial function. Frontiers in Bioscience. 2007;**12**:947-963

[8] Nishida S. Metabolic effects of melatonin on oxidative stress and diabetes mellitus. Endocrine. 2005;**27**(2):131-136

[9] Acuna-Castroviejo D, Martin M, Macias M, Escames G, Leon J, Khaldy H, et al. Melatonin, mitochondria, and cellular bioenergetics. Journal of Pineal Research. 2001;**30**(2):65-74

[10] Brown GC. Control of respiration and ATP synthesis in mammalian mitochondria and cells. The Biochemical Journal. 1992;**284**(Pt 1):1-13

[11] Pandi-Perumal SR, BaHammam AS, Brown GM, Spence DW, Bharti VK, Kaur C, et al. Melatonin antioxidative defense: therapeutical implications for aging and neurodegenerative processes. Neurotoxicity Research. 2013;**23**(3):267-300

[12] Booth FW, Roberts CK, Laye MJ. Lack of exercise is a major cause of chronic diseases. Comprehensive Physiology. 2012;**2**(2):1143-1211

[13] Centers for Disease Control and Prevention. Physical activity for everyone. 2011. http://wwwcdcgov/physicalactivity/everyone/glossary/indexhtml

[14] ACSM. American College of Sports Medicine position stand. Progression models in resistance training for healthy adults. Medicine and Science in Sports and Exercise. 2009;**41**(3):687-708

[15] Thrift AP, Xiao L, Patel SR, Tworoger SS, McTiernan A, Duggan C. Effects of physical activity on melatonin levels in previously sedentary men and women. Cancer Epidemiology, Biomarkers & Prevention. 2014;**23**(8):1696-1699

[16] Escames G, Ozturk G, Bano-Otalora B, Pozo MJ, Madrid JA, Reiter RJ, et al. Exercise and melatonin in humans: Reciprocal benefits. Journal of Pineal Research. 2012;**52**(1):1-11

[17] Riebe D, Franklin BA, Thompson PD, Garber CE, Whitfield GP, Magal M, et al. Updating ACSM's recommendations for exercise preparticipation health screening. Medicine and Science in Sports and Exercise. 2015;**47**(11):2473-2479

[18] Ziaadini F, Aminae M, Rastegar MM, Abbasian S, Memari AH. Melatonin supplementation decreases aerobic exercise training induced-lipid peroxidation and malondialdehyde in sedentary young women. Polish Journal of Food and Nutrition Sciences. 2017;**67**(3):225-232

[19] Davis GR, Etheredge CE, Marcus L, Bellar D. Prolonged sleep deprivation and continuous exercise: effects on melatonin, tympanic temperature, and cognitive function. BioMed Research International. 2014;**2014**:781863

[20] Theron JJ, Oosthuizen JM, Rautenbach MM. Effect of physical exercise on plasma melatonin levels in normal volunteers. South African Medical Journal;**1984**(66):838-841

[21] Lucia A, Diaz B, Hoyos J, Fernandez C, Villa G, Bandres F, et al. Hormone levels of world class cyclists during the Tour of Spain stage race. British Journal of Sports Medicine. 2001;**35**(6):424-430

[22] Marrin K, Drust B, Gregson W, Morris CJ, Chester N, Atkinson G. Diurnal variation in the salivary melatonin responses to exercise: Relation to exercise-mediated tachycardia. European Journal of Applied Physiology. 2011;**111**(11):2707-2714

[23] Fisher-Wellman K, Bloomer RJ. Acute exercise and oxidative stress: A 30 year history. Dynamic Medicine. 2009;**8**:1-25

[24] Bonnefont-Rousselot D, Collin F. Melatonin: Action as antioxidant and potential applications in human disease and aging. Toxicology. 2010;**278**(1):55-67

[25] Leonardo-Mendonca RC, Ocana-Wilhelmi J, de Haro T, de Teresa-Galvan C, Guerra-Hernandez E, Rusanova I, et al. The benefit of a supplement with the antioxidant melatonin on redox status and muscle damage in resistance-trained athletes. Applied Physiology, Nutrition, and Metabolism. 2017;**42**(7):700-707

[26] Maarman GJ, Reiter RJ. Melatonin therapy for blunt trauma and strenuous exercise: A mechanism involving cytokines, NFkappaB, Akt, MAFBX and MURF-1. Journal of Sports Sciences. 2018:1-5

[27] Ochoa JJ, Diaz-Castro J, Kajarabille N, Garcia C, Guisado IM, De Teresa C, et al. Melatonin supplementation ameliorates oxidative stress and inflammatory signaling induced by strenuous exercise in adult human males. Journal of Pineal Research. 2011;**51**(4):373-380

[28] Okada A, Ono Y, Nagatomi R, Kishimoto KN, Itoi E. Decreased muscle atrophy F-box (MAFbx) expression in regenerating muscle after muscle-damaging exercise. Muscle & Nerve. 2008;**38**(4):1246-1253

[29] Willis MS, Ike C, Li L, Wang DZ, Glass DJ, Patterson C. Muscle ring finger 1, but not muscle ring finger 2, regulates cardiac hypertrophy in vivo. Circulation Research. 2007;**100**(4):456-459

[30] Ja'afar IF, Jassim HA, Hussein AG. Effect of moderate exercise on the level of melatonin hormone and lymphocyte apoptosis in healthy subjects. The Iraqi Postgraduate Medical Journal. 2010;**9**(1):88-94

[31] Mendes C, Lopes AM, do Amaral FG, Peliciari-Garcia RA, Turati Ade O, Hirabara SM, et al. Adaptations of the aging animal to exercise: role of daily supplementation with melatonin. Journal of Pineal Research. 2013;**55**(3):229-239

[32] Wurtman R, Cooper D. Physiology and available preparations of melatonin. Dostupno: 2015. www.uptodate.com (datum zadnjeg pristupa: 275, 2015)

[33] Agil A, Navarro-Alarcón M, Ruiz R, Abuhamadah S, El-Mir MY, Vazquez GF. Beneficial effects of melatonin on obesity and lipid profile in young Zucker diabetic fatty rats. Journal of Pineal Research. 2011;**50**:207-212

[34] Sochor J, Ruttkay-Nedecky B, Babula P, Adam V, Hubalek J, Kizek R. Automation of Methods for Determination of Lipid Peroxidation. In: Catala A, editor. Lipid Peroxidation. UK: InTech; 2012. p. 131-154

[35] Gutteridge JM. Lipid-peroxidation and antioxidants as biomarkers of tissue damage. Clinical Chemistry. 1995;(41):1819-1828

[36] Repetto M, Semprine J, Boveris A. Lipid Peroxidation: Chemical Mechanism, Biological Implications and Analytical Determination, Lipid Peroxidation Angel Catala. UK: IntechOpen; August 29th 2012. DOI: 10.5772/45943. Available from: https://www.intechopen.com/books/lipid-peroxidation/lipid-peroxidation-chemical-mechanism-biological-implications-and-analytical-determination

[37] Spirlandeli AL, Deminice R, Jordao AA. Plasma malondialdehyde as biomarker of lipid peroxidation: Effects of acute exercise. International Journal of Sports Medicine. 2014;**35**: 14-18

[38] Ayala A, Munoz MF, Arguelles S. Lipid peroxidation: Production, metabolism, and signaling mechanisms of malondialdehyde and 4-hydroxy-2-nonenal. Oxidative Medicine and Cellular Longevity. 2014;**2014**:360438

[39] Natalia Fagali AC. The antioxidant behaviour of melatonin and structural analogues during lipid peroxidation depends not only on their functional groups but also on the assay system. Biochemical and Biophysical Research Communications. 2012;**423**:873-877

[40] Mekhloufi J, Bonnefont-Rousselot D, Yous S, Lesieur D, Couturier M, Therond P, et al. Antioxidant activity of melatonin and a pinoline derivative on linoleate model system. Journal of Pineal Research. 2005;**39**(1):27-33

[41] Dillard CJ, Litov RE, Savin WM, Dumelin EE, Tappel AL. Effects of exercise, vitamin E, and ozone on pulmonary function and lipid peroxidation. Journal of Applied Physiology: Respiratory, Environmental and Exercise Physiology. 1978;**45**(6):927-932

[42] Tutkun E. Melatonin administration in rats with acute swimming exercise prevents lipid peroxidation in muscle tissue. International Journal of Academic Research. 2013;**5**(3):1-5

11

How Can Molecular Pharmacology Help Understand the Multiple Actions of Melatonin: 20 Years of Research and Trends

Jean A. Boutin

Abstract

Melatonin actions are so numerous that a naive reader might become suspicious at such wonders. In a systematic way, we would like to summarize the various approaches that led to what is scientifically sounded in terms of molecular pharmacology: where and how melatonin is acting as a molecule, what can be its action as an antioxidant per se, and its side effects at a molecular level not as a drug or in vivo. Finally, the nature of the relationship between melatonin and mitochondria should be decrypted as well. The road we took from 1987 up to now, and particularly after 1995, will be mentioned with special considerations to the receptors from various species and our goals beyond that; the synthesis and catabolism of melatonin and their link to other enzymes; the discovery of the MT_3 binding sites, and what's left to understand on this particularly interesting target; and the search for agonists that occulted part of the potential discovery of true and potent antagonists, a situation quite unique among the G-protein-coupled receptors.

Keywords: melatonin, molecular pharmacology, MT_1, MT_2, catabolism

1. Introduction

Melatonin is a neurohormone synthesized by the pineal gland at night. The longer the night, the higher the concentration of melatonin in the blood. Even if new information is modulating this basic principle, this rhythmicity has been the basis of many published observations linking melatonin to many physiological features of animals, including human. This comprises the daily changes in light and the way the body understands the successions of dark and clear periods but also the circannual rhythmicity, during which animals prepare for the harsher winter period during which access to food is more difficult. By "measuring" the length of melatonin synthesis periods (directly proportional to the length of the nights), animals start to modify their physiology in order to prepare the time to come: accumulation of fat (fat storing) for some, food storing for others, and preparing the bodies to reproduction for all animals at the best period to avoid the exposure of the newborns to cold and difficult conditions. Apparently, humans have lost this advanced capacity in our ever lit-up society.

New evidences recently caught our attention and challenge our ways of understanding the melatonin actions and pathways, whether because it seems that light can be "seen" by the body without the relay of melatonin or because one finds that melatonin is synthesized in mitochondria in all parts of the brain, as opposed to the pivotal and ancient statement: melatonin is synthesized by the pineal gland only. Nowadays, one can also see many publications claiming that melatonin helps cure cancer as well as so many other diseases (see a non-exhaustive selection of such actions since 2015 in **Table 1**). All these information should be treated with respect, integrated inside our decade-old knowledge and carefully evaluated as a contribution to a bigger picture. The basics on melatonin can be found in some recent reviews [1–5]. The present chapter concentrates on the molecular pharmacology of melatonin. This small molecule, derived from tryptophan, has a limited number of recognized targets. It is synthesized and catabolized by a limited and well-known number of enzymes that have been described in the past (see **Figure 1** for a simplistic summary). The core of the discussion seems always to be the same: how this molecule can be active on so many pathological events?

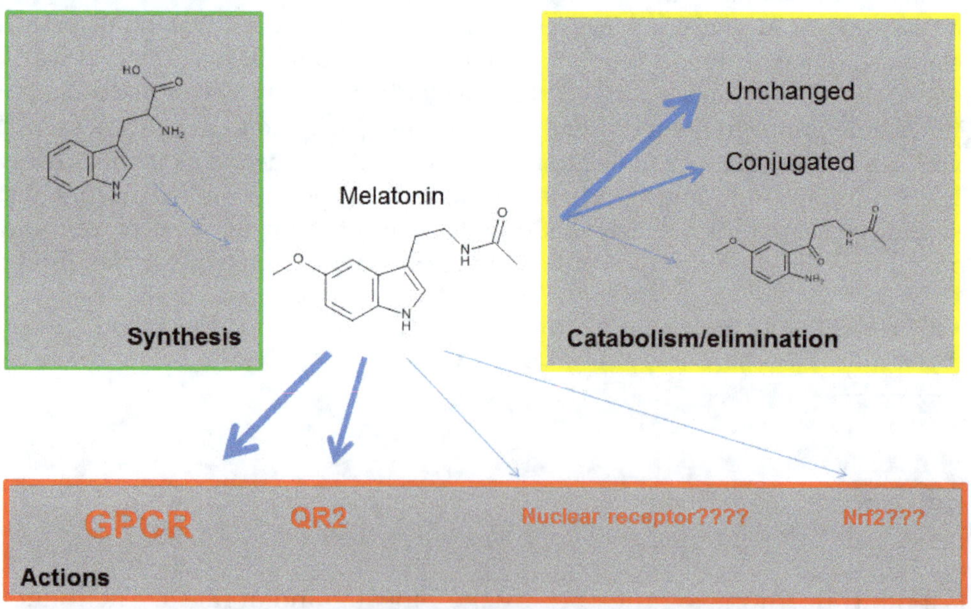

Figure 1. A simplistic summary of melatonin-related proteins. Melatonin is synthesized from tryptophan by a series of enzyme the the limiting step of which is catalyzed by Arylalkylamine N-acetyl transferase (green box); melatonin is excreted mainly unchanged from mammalian bodies or conjugated either by UDP-glucuronosyltranserases or by sulfotranferases, but it is also catabolized by indoleamine-2,3-dioxygenase, myeloperoxidase or cytochrome c (yellow box). At the molecular level, the targets of melatonin are mainly: Its two melatonin receptors, MT_1 and MT_2, QR2 (formerly known as MT_3). Furthermore, putative targets might exist such as nuclear receptors and particularly Nrf2 that might explain some of the anti-oxidant capacities of melatonin (red box).

How antioxidant this molecule is and why? What makes it so special? Some of these points are reviewed in the present chapter based on two decades of research in this area.

Beyond these biochemical features, melatonin has two unique features: it is very soluble but seems to travel freely through biological membranes, and its possible toxicity is extremely low (although some human cases of undesirable effects were reported), permitting scientists to give on many models very large amounts of the compound in cellulo and in vivo without apparent associated major toxicity. It was thus obvious that in many cases, the activity at those "pharmacological" dosages led to surprisingly numerous therapeutic properties of this molecule. Furthermore, the discovery that melatonin had, in cellulo and in vivo, antioxidant properties added to the multiple possibilities of use of melatonin, leading to this apparent paramount of therapeutic properties.

2. Melatonin synthesis

Melatonin is mostly synthesized starting from tryptophan in the pineal gland by a series of enzymes, the limiting one being arylalkylamine *N*-acetyltransferase (AANAT) also known as the timezyme [6]. Many studies have been performed on this enzyme and its requirements in terms of substrate specificity and inhibitor research, in particular in human [7, 8]. Over the years, several groups hypothesized and reported the possibility that melatonin was also synthesized in mitochondria (see also below, Section 6.4), suggesting that the antioxidant properties of the molecule would confer a strong resistance of mitochondria to the generation of ROS, a common feature of those subcellular organelles. Indeed, if the dogma was, in the 1950s and later on, that melatonin was mainly synthesized in the pineal gland, a fact that was clearly confirmed by surgical removing of the gland would lead to a major reduction of circulating melatonin and to the loss of some of the circadian and circannual rhythms; several papers co-indicated that such local synthesis that does exist should be taken into consideration (see, for instance, Stehle et al. [9]). What is more troubling is the recent precise description of melatonin synthesis in mitochondria, at least in brain-derived organelles [10] as well as the presence of a functional GPCR (MT_1). Intuitively, many previous strong knowledge would go against the finding that melatonin is synthesized in mitochondria, even if that was recently restricted to brain-derived mitochondria [11]. But melatonin is also known to "travel" freely inside membranes. Thus in order to stay inside mitochondria, it should be sequestered inside them in order to prevent the damages of ROS production—a common and key feature of the respiratory chain—thanks to the antioxidant properties of melatonin (see below, Section 6.1.2, for further discussion).

No revolution, nevertheless, occurred in the way melatonin is synthesized. It comes from several steps. All those enzymes have been cloned and studied, including from human origin. The particular case of AANAT catalyzing the limiting step of the synthesis has been at the source of the seminal work of David Klein's laboratory (see, for instance [6, 7]). This enzyme is destroyed during the day and active only at night. The way it is regulated is different according to species, but it seems a formidable waste of energy to handle it that way (synthesis and immediate destruction for "nothing") [12, 13], strongly suggesting by the way this pathway is regulated that it is of major importance for physiology. The enzyme was cloned in our laboratory, and a thorough study of its substrate and co-substrate specificities was reported [8]. It was attempting, at one stage, to try to find specific inhibitors of the enzyme, in order to better understand in in situ situations the roles of melatonin at various locations. Several publications including ours reported those efforts [14–18]. If one particular point should be stressed, it is the elegant ways analogues of an intermediary state of the substrate/co-substrate complex permitted to turn molecules into powerful inhibitors, although overall fragile ones [19], as well as the way that the incorporation of an exotic amino acid in place of a serine permitted to stabilize the enzyme, rendered insensitive to proteolysis [20–22].

3. Melatonin receptor molecular pharmacology

3.1. Melatonin receptors

To somewhat summarize the situation, there were two GPCRs (MT_1 and MT_2) found throughout the animal kingdom, an elusive binding site (MT_3) that turned out to be an enzyme—quinone reductase 2 (QR2) [23] (see below, Section 6.3), another receptor (Mel1c) that was present in fishes, birds, and reptilians and that evolved to a GPR50 in mammals [24], with the curious property to have lost the recognition of melatonin, with a single exception (in platypus [25]), and finally the elusive nuclear receptovr, first described by Becker-André et al. [26] and then retracted [27]. Several other research papers [28] pointed at nuclear receptor(s) to explain the circadian rhythm of some key metabolism enzymes that could logically be dependent on the circadian rhythm of melatonin (see discussion in Jan et al. [29]).

What are the most characterized in the melatonin field, besides the multiple functions of the molecule itself (see below), are the binding characteristics at its receptors. The receptors were first discovered and cloned/characterized by Reppert's group [30] from both hamster and human. This première was followed by a series of cloning, including the discovery that hamster had only one functional melatonin receptor [31], to the contrary of most of the mammals that possess two (MT_1 and MT_2): human, rat, mice, sheep (although it was long believed to possess also a single receptor form [32]), etc. Cloning was also reported for other species, including birds and fishes [33, 34] and probably insects [35]. This led to the possibility to establish the binding pharmacology of those receptors in several laboratory species—mouse [36], rat [37], and sheep [32]—as well as in human [38]. For years, then, our goal has been to synthesize analogues of melatonin and use them to better understand the MT_1 and MT_2 roles, as well as to be able to somehow modulate them. It is not the place, here, to review the chemistry that has been explored around melatonin, but recent reviews could be looked at: Mor et al. [39], Garrat and Tsotinis [40], Rivara et al. [41], and Zlotos et al. [42]. The field would have benefit from a quest of specific and stable in vivo binders, particularly antagonists, permitting to explore and understand the limit of the melatonin actions, at least through these particular targets.

Incidentally, one must point out that there are still no antibodies against the receptors. We and many others tried over the last decades to produce such tools with a general negative endpoint. This, of course, has been an obstacle to a better understanding of those receptors.

Nevertheless, the repartition of the receptors in various organs, and particularly throughout the brain, has been nicely reviewed by Ng et al. [43] with some precisions of their respective functions: these seem to be as follows—improvement of neurogenesis (hippocampus with a memory maintenance via the inhibition of long-term potentiation by MT_2 receptor); MT_1 would regulate the REM sleep; MT_1 would also confer a protection against Huntington disease. In terms of melatonin receptor actions, those are the strongest information available. It seems clear, for example, that most of the protection offered by melatonin in multiple pathological situations (as summarized in **Table 1**) are not mediated by its receptors.

It would be very complicated to be exhaustive in terms of characterization of those binding sites, as the data is scattered throughout the literature. What is "easy" is that we and others using the binding assay developed around Vakkuri et al.'s 2-[^{125}I] iodomelatonin [44] for establishing the basic molecular pharmacology of the MT_1 and MT_2 receptors from several key laboratory species and from humans, but basic data can be found in Jockers et al. [45].

In the next sections, three aspects must be covered: the binding, heterodimerization, and structure of the melatonin receptors.

3.2. Binding, functionality, and heterodimerization

Initially, several reports were done using [^{3}H]melatonin, but the specific activity of the tracer was not sufficient to gain robust information on the receptors. It is only recently that heavily labeled [^{3}H]melatonin became available. This radiotracer permitted to better understand the various states of the receptors and their behavior in that context [46]. Historically the binding studies were largely facilitated by the use of the super-agonist, 2-[^{125}I]-iodomelatonin [44]. Not only this compound is easy to synthesize, but its sensitivity counteracted the very high affinity of melatonin for its receptors, as well as the paucity of the expression of these receptors in relevant tissues. Almost all the laboratories involved in melatonin research have been using this radiotracer. It must be pointed out, though, that attempts to use alternative ligands have been reported, mainly in the spirit of using specific ligands of one or the other of melatonin receptors [47]. Unfortunately, only ligands specific of MT_2 have been reported, so far. MT_1-specific binders have been elusive, despite the wide variety of melatonin analogues that have been synthesized. As stated elsewhere in the present essay, the main focus of chemistry research in this melatonin domain over the last decades was to find alternative ligand agonists at the receptors with strong stability in vivo.

Functionality of seven-transmembrane domain receptors is a complex science, providing daily new data. The number of coupling pathways at receptors in general is important, and more are discovered often. An excellent review has been published very recently [48], and the contribution of the same authors to the IUPHAR compendium on melatonin receptor functionality [45] should be considered as reference documents to understand the various pathways, at least as of today.

Nevertheless relatively few publications address the functionality of ligands in a global way. Indeed, if some functional data has been produced around a series of chemical analogues completing the classical binding displacement approach, rather few address the global and "standardized" characterizations of a series of ligands on MT_1 and/or MT_2. There are cases where given compounds were characterized as partial agonists that turned out to be inverse agonists instead [49], leading to a yet another level of complexity of melatonin receptor pharmacology. We recently embarked in such a task, by screening the agonist/antagonist behavior of a series of compounds (Legros & Boutin, in preparation) after assessing the various methods [50]. We also extended these coupling measurements to a small series of potential antagonists specific of MT_2 [51], to conclude that the compounds were not antagonists but rather partial agonists. As stated and described by Kenakin [52], one should further dig the concept of biased ligands. Indeed, it seems clear, now, that some at least of the downstream pathways of melatonin receptors are elicited by some agonist ligands while not by other ones. This concept has been a bias of the approach to melatonin research. Indeed, while seeking for tools to understand these pathways and their implications in various pathological models, we never had access to real, stable, and potent antagonists, despite past claims for such compounds [53, 54]. Even when large-scale screening campaigns were attempted [55], the poor affinity (compared to the already existing compounds: low μM affinity in the best cases *versus* low nM already available ones) of those newly discovered compounds was not in favor of trying to develop series of chemicals around those hits. A similar situation occurred when we attempted to find peptide ligands at melatonin receptors [56].

After the first evidences that crystallogenesis of membrane proteins would be a challenge, we thought we would continue to search for ligands with a trial-and-error approach as we did for years, without the help of the visualization of the compounds in the protein as it became "mundane" these last years concerning co-crystallizations of compounds in their soluble protein targets. By multiplying the number of ligands in attempts to better describe the topography of the melatonin-binding site, even using mutagenesis [57–60], we also multiplied the assays on the functionality of the receptors, because we more and more discovered the ways the receptors were transferring their message to the cell. The simplistic view that a handful of such pathways between the receptors and the inner cell existed became obsolete. The by-product of such variety was that we found biased ligands that activated one but not the other(s) signaling pathways downstream melatonin receptor, as it is briefly discussed elsewhere.

Then, another new aspect came up: receptors can dimerize, a feature that was known for quite some time (see Rodbell [61], and see seminal review by Bockaert and Pin, [62]). Even though it was often believed to be an artifact of the purification attempts, the reality of such structures in situ was evidenced when one realized and demonstrated heterodimerisation between various types of such receptors: heterodimers between isoforms of a receptor, GABA [63], heterodimers between two unrelated GPCRs or even between GPCR, and another type of protein [64]. A paramount of examples were published, and their studies were made possible using the BRET technology [65]. In brief, engineering two receptors to make each of them fused with a carefully chosen fluorescent protein leads to a system in which the excitation of one of them results in the emission of fluorescent in the region exciting the other one. This cannot occur if the proteins are not physically in a very close vicinity of one another. Melatonin receptors have been also shown to be able to dimerize with serotonin 5HT2c receptor [66], as well as between MT_1 and MT_2 [67] or between MT_1 and GPR50 [68], the melatonin-related receptor (evolved from Mel1c [24] and that has lost its property to bind melatonin [69]). More recently, the heterodimerisation of GPR50 and the transforming growth factor-β receptor [70] potentially open interesting routes toward the role of this orphan receptor as well as its implication in cancer development. Obviously many control experiments should be run in these explorations, as it would be attempting to conclude that any receptor can dimerize—and thus regulate the signaling pathway of—any other receptor (see Damian et al. [71] for a counter example, among some others).

3.3. Purification/structure

Attempts to crystallize GPCRs have been done for years with various successes. Beside several reports of models of the receptors [72–74], that turned to be more or less disappointing because they poorly brought new information—somewhat as expected. Thus, several lines of strategies were further explored. One of them led to a pure, functional MT_1 receptor, after several years of technical challenges: expression, stabilization, purification, and functionality measurement [75, 76]. We embarked several years ago in an approach that attempted to be original: as a first step in this purification/crystallization of melatonin receptor(s) project, we cloned melatonin receptors from as many and as various species as possible. Many such melatonin receptors have been reported in the literature, such as various sheep strains, buffalo, fishes, and even coral, many of which has been deposited in GenBank but not described in a publication. The rationale behind this Noah-ark type of research was to systematically use melatonin receptors from those variously evolved species (birds, reptilians, mammals from various environments, some harsh insects, etc.) that have in common their capacity to recognize melatonin—by definition. We aimed at comparing their thermal stability once they were stably expressed in CHO cells. We would choose the most resistant one and use that as a model in the process of purification/reconstitution established previously by Logez et al. in our laboratory [75, 76]. Despite a few success [25], we terminated the program for resource limitation reasons.

4. Melatonin catabolism

Melatonin catabolism has been described and discussed in-depth by Hardeland throughout the living kingdom [77]. In short, the main route of melatonin elimination (from the body) is not catabolism but rather conjugation and excretion via the urine. Thus there are three ways to consider: (i) the unchanged melatonin that one can find in urine; (ii) the conjugates, mostly glucuronides and sulfates; and (iii) the catabolism itself. Catabolism means that the molecule is transformed into something quite different from the original molecule. For example, in melatonin case, several reports demonstrated the opening of the indol ring. This opening possibly occurred through cytochrome c [78] or through 1,2-dioxygenase [79]. This was of importance because not too many compounds bear a formyl moiety such as the one produced during the cleavage of the indol cycle by either of these enzymes. This catabolism process would generate several products including N1-acetyl-N2-formyl-5-methoxykynuramine (AFMK) and N1-acetyl-5-methoxykynuramine (AMK) [80]. The same paper, though, pointed out the absence of such metabolite(s) in human urine, strongly suggesting that the main catabolic route of melatonin would rather be through conjugation, even after oxidative stress.

5. The melatonin paradox

The field suffered from two paradoxes: safety and high affinity to natively poorly expressed receptors. First, melatonin is a very safe molecule, as far as we know; there is no report of human toxicity for overdose, and in mice the lethal dose is superior to 800 mg/kg [81]. Nevertheless, the French Agency for Food, Environmental and Occupational Health & Safety (www.anses.fr) emitted a report—in French—pointing at several cases of toxicity linked to melatonin consumption. Although they were ~100 cases in France reported during a 30-year period survey (i.e., a relatively modest number of cases, some of which have not been univocally linked to melatonin intake), the literature on clinical trials of melatonin is large enough to consider melatonin as reasonably safe [82], with the usual cases of deliberate overdose. In any case, it is not unusual to find reports in the literature where the dosage of melatonin in vivo or in cellulo is important. It was reported at several occasions—even if it probably depends on the cell type—cells treated with 1 mM of melatonin without apparent cell toxicity and even, in some cases, with beneficial effects [83–87]. Why is it a flaw? Because one can treat almost anything with this compound, at almost whatever dosage, and observe something, including relevant benefits for the situation (see **Table 1** and further examples in Boutin [88]). Furthermore, melatonin has a friendly behavior in terms of pharmacokinetics. When compared to another multi-card compound, resveratrol, it seems that unlike it, melatonin circulates in the blood after oral consumption at a fairly high concentration, while only 1 to 2% of resveratrol was found at the peak after ingestion of 25 mg/kg of resveratrol [89].

Finally, as stated elsewhere in the present essay, the affinity of melatonin for its receptors is in the low nanomolar range [45]. Many strict analogues have been synthesized with similar high affinities for the receptors. Thus, it has been complicated and sometimes impossible to start new chemical programs ad initio, or at least starting from molecules issued from high-throughput screening campaigns, for example, from which hits are rather in the high micromolar range. Therefore, new compounds with unexpected structures have been slowly emerged in the field. As a representative example, D600 (hydroxyl-verapamil) is one of the few compounds showing strong specificity for MT_1 [90]. No chemical program to date has been published to explore this observation and to deliver a specific ligand at MT_1 receptor with some pharmacological properties (and specificity) rendering it amenable to in cellulo or in vivo experiments.

6. Melatonin actions

6.1. Overall

Melatonin is the core master of rhythms. This part of the story is beyond any doubt. It translates the succession of days (light) and night (darkness) to the body. In the absence of light, the pineal gland (and more particularly the AANAT, the limiting step of melatonin biosynthesis) synthesizes melatonin. Nevertheless, a report [91] shows that, at least in the European hamster, the circannual rhythm could be maintained even after pinealectomy, thanks to light action in an accelerated photoperiodic regime, demonstrating the hypothalamic integration of the photoperiodic signal even in pinealectomized animals and, thus, in the absence of pineal gland synthesis of melatonin.

Melatonin circadian rhythm can be measured in the blood from healthy volunteers and is clearly linked to the successions of days and nights. The timezyme (AANAT) is the master key of this process: active during dark periods and inactive during day (as the enzyme is destroyed by the light-induced proteasome).

6.1.1. *Foreword*

Melatonin exerts protective actions far beyond mammals, as several reports showed the role of melatonin in protecting yeast [92], bacteria [93], zebrafish [94], and plants [95] from various types of insult. For a discussion of melatonin throughout evolution, see also Tan et al. [96]. For decades, melatonin has been described as a compound able to fight almost any pathological situations. Tekbas et al. [97] even seriously considered melatonin as an antibiotic and Anderson et al. as an anti-Ebola virus agent [98]. A sample of those numerous actions can be found in Boutin [88], up to 2015. **Table 1** of the present essay is the follow-up of that particular list of beneficial properties. Many of those properties of melatonin seem to be linked to the capacity of the compound to limit reactive oxygen species (ROS) actions. ROS have been first documented as an "infamous" group of highly reactive molecules responsible for oxidative stress. In an enlightening review, Roy and coworkers [99] defined the field of reactive oxygen species, by starting to recall that ROS are also regulating signaling pathways in physiological situations. They also emphasized the fact that treatments with so-called antioxidants failed to show efficacy or/and positive effects in the prevention of diseases or health complications coming from oxidative stress. Nevertheless, it seems that according to a common belief, melatonin falls outside that particular category and is the ultimate scavenger/antioxidant molecule that has multiple capacities to prevent almost any diseases.

It is sometimes complicated to find common sense in such a plethora of actions. **Table 1** lists some of these many actions, as published between 2015 and today. There is no way to be able to understand why melatonin has been reported for so many years in so many pathological situations. And the purpose of the present essay is not to do so. It is rather to make a compendium of those actions and to let the community know that such papers exist and that the reason why melatonin is so ubiquitously active remains a mystery.

It is attempting, though, to make a rapid survey of those publications and to conclude that the common factor is the production of ROS. Then, we can hypothesize that most of these beneficial actions were due to a capacity of melatonin to induce antioxidant enzymatic defenses. To conclude on this working hypothesis, one will have to identify the nuclear receptor mediating this property. Nuclear factor erythroid 2-related factor 2 (Nrf2) might be a good candidate, but a wishful thinking is certainly not a proof of fact.

Authors	Date	Protection against	Targets	Amount	Species	Ref
Abdel-Moneim et al.	2015	*Naja naja* venom toxicity	—	10 mg/kg	Rat	[100]
Allagui et al.	2015	Aluminum-induced toxicity	/	10 mg/kg	Rat	[101]
Al-Olayan et al.	2015	Aluminum-induced injury	Neurons	10 mg/kg	Rat	[102]
Al-Rasheed et al.	2016	CCl4-induced toxicity	Liver	20 mg/kg	Rat	[103]
Amin et al.	2015	Diabetes-induced apoptosis	Heart	10 mg/kg	Rat	[104]
Asghari et al.	2017	Aluminum phosphide toxicity	Heart	20–50 mg/kg	Rat	[105]
Banaei et al.	2016	Ischemia–reperfusion injury	Kidney	10 mg/kg	Rat	[106]
Barberino et al.	2017	Cisplatin-induceddamage	Ovaries	5–20 mg/kg	Mouse	[107]
Berkiks et al.	2017	Ccognitive disorders	Brain	5 mg/kg	Rat	[108]
Cao et al.	2017	Subarachnoid hemorrhage	Brain	150 mg/kg	Rat	[109]
Cebi et al.	2018	Radioiodine treatment	Testicles	12 mg/kg/day	Rat	[110]
Chang et al.	2016	Ischemia–reperfusion injury	Kidney	90 mg	Rat	[111]
Chang et al.	2015	Ischemia/reperfusion injury	Adipose stem cells	120 mg/kg	Rat	[112]
Chen et al.	2016	Endoplasmic reticulum stress	Pancreas	0.5–2 mM	Rat	[113]
Chen et al.	2017	Neuropathic pain	/	???	Rat	[114]
Czechowska et al.	2015	Thioacetamide-induced fibrosis	Liver	10 mg/kg	Rat	[115]
Das et al.	2017	Mitochondrial dysfunction	Hepatocytes	10–20 mg/kg/day	Mouse	[116]
Ding et al.	2018	Post-traumtic cardiac function	Heart	100 μM	Rat	[117]
Ding et al.	2015	Traumatic injury-induced apoptosis	Brain	10 mg/kg	Mouse	[118]
Dos Santos et al.	2018	Lupus nephritis injury	Kidney	10 mg/kg/day	Mouse	[119]
Drag-Kozak et al.	2018	Cadmium-induced toxicity	Reproductive organ	4 mg/L	Carp	[120]
Ewida et al.	2016	Metabolic syndroma	Kidney	5 mg/kg	Rat	[121]
Favero et al.	2017	Fibromyalgia-related alterations	Muscle	2.5–5 mg/kg	Rat	[122]
Fernandez-Gil et al.	2017	Radiotherapy-iondued toxicity	Intestine	45 mg/day	Rat	[123]
Galley et al.	2017	Paclitaxel-induced dysfunction	Mitochondria	5–50 mg/kg	Rat	[124]

Authors	Date	Protection against	Targets	Amount	Species	Ref
Ghaznavi et al.	2016	Gentamicin-induced toxicity	Kidney	15 mg/kg/day	Rat	[125]
Ghosh et al.	2017	Copper ascorbate-induced damage	Heart mitochondria	1 μM	Goat	[126]
Goc et al.	2017	Sodium nitroprusside toxicity	Organs	10 mg/kg	Mouse	[127]
Goudarzi et al.	2017	Cyclophophamide-induced stress	Kidneys	5–20 mg/kg	Mouse	[128]
Hermoso et al.	2016	Steatosis	Liver	10 mg/kg	Rat	[129]
Hsu et al.	2017	Trauma-induced hemorrhage	Liver	2 mg/kg	Rat	[130]
Hu et al.	2017	BBB damage	BBB	15 mg/kg	Rat	[131]
Ji et al.	2017	Sepsis-associated encephalopathy	Brain	10 mg/kg	Mouse	[132]
Jiang et al.	2016	Diabetic-induced inflammation	Retina	10 mg/kg/day	Rat	[133]
Jin et al.	2016	Non-alcoholic fatty liver disease	Liver	/	Mouse	[134]
Karaer et al.	2015	Radiation damage	Inner ear	5 mg/kg	Rat	[135]
Karimfar et al.	2015	Cryopreservation stress	Sperm	0.001–1 mM	Human	[136]
Khaksar et al.	2017	Fluoxetine-induced tissue injury	Organs	1 mg/kg	Rat	[137]
Khalil et al.	2015	Zonisamide-induced toxicity	/	10 mg/kg	Rat	[138]
Koc et al.	2016	Apoptosis	Olfactive neurons	10 mg/kg/day	Rat	[139]
Lebda et al.	2018	Thioacetamide-induced fibrosis	Liver	5 mg/kg/day	Rat	[140]
Lee et al.	2016	H_2O_2-mediated cell death	Keratinocytes	2.5–10 μM	Human	[141]
Li et al.	2016	Cadmium-induced toxicity	Testicles	1 mg	Mouse	[142]
Li et al.	2015	Maturation defect	Oocyte	0.001–1 μM	Pig	[143]
Lopez et al.	2017	MPTP-toxicity	Brain	10 mg/kg	Mouse	[144]
Lv et al.	2018	Cr(VI) toxicity	Testicles	25 mg/kg	Mouse	[145]
Ma et al.	2018	Oxidative injury	Heart	100 μM	Rat	[146]
Ma et al.	2017	Tripterygium glycosides toxicity	Ovaries	20 mg/kg/day	Mouse	[147]
Ma et al.	2015	Adriamicyn-toxicity	Breast cancer cells	10 mg/kg/day	Rat	[148]
Mehrzadi et al.	2016	Gentamicin-induced toxicity	Kidney	20 mg/kg/day	Rat	[149]

Authors	Date	Protection against	Targets	Amount	Species	Ref
Mirhoseini et al.	2017	Torsion/detorsion model	Testicles	25 μg/kg	Rat	[150]
Montasser et al.	2017	Methotrexate-induced toxicity	Liver	10 mg/kg	Rat	[151]
Mukherjee et al.	2015	Isoproterenol-induced damage	Heart mitochondria	0.125–4 μM	Goat	[152]
Munoz et al.	2017	Cumene peroxide-induced stress	Pineal gland	10 mg/kg/day	Rat	[153]
Naseri et al.	2017	Irradiation-induced toxicity	Brain	100 mg/kg	Rat	[154]
Naskar et al.	2015	MPTP-induced Parkinsonism	Brain	10–30 mg/kg	Mouse	[155]
O'Neal-Moffitt et al.	2015	Alzheimer neiuropathology	/	Ad libitum???	Mouse	[156]
Ortiz et al.	2015	Radiation-induced mucositis	Mouth	45 mg/kg/day	Rat	[157]
Othman et al.	2016	Bisphenopl A-induced toxicity	Testicles	10 mg/kg	Rat	[158]
Ozsoy et al.	2016	Mitochondrial dysfunction	Liver	10 mg/kg	Rat	[159]
Ozsoy et al.	2015	6-hydroxydopamine stress	Neurons	10 mg/kg	Rat	[160]
Pal et al.	2016	Stress-induced behavior changes	/	10–100 mg/kg	Rat	[161]
Pang et al.	2016	Frozen–thawed cycles	Sperm	0.01–1 mM	Bovine	[162]
Patino et al.	2016	o2 & Glucose deprivation	Brain slices	10–30 μM	Rat	[163]
Paul et al.	2018	Oxidative stress	Substancia nigra	10–30 mg/kg	Rat	[164]
Rajput et al.	2017	Alcohol-induced stress	Brain	20 mg/kg	Mouse	[165]
Sadek and Khattab	2017	Arginine-induced pancreatis	Pancreas	50 mg/kg	Rat	[166]
Sarihan et al.	2015	TCDD-induced injury	Heart	5 mg/kg/day	Rat	[167]
Scheuer et al.	2016	UVR-induced erythrema	Skin	0.5–12.5%	Human	[168]
Shahrokhi et al.	2016	Ischmia/reperfusion-oxidative stress	Estomac	10 mg/kg	Rat	[169]
Shang et al.	2016	Colitis-induced neuron damage	Colon	2.5 mg/kg/day	Rat	[170]
Shao et al.	2015	LPS-induced mastitis	Breast	5–20 mg/kg	Mouse	[171]
Shokri et al.	2015	Pilocarpine-induced epilesy	Brain	5–20 mg/kg	Rat	[172]
Shokrzadeh et al.	2015	Cyclophosphamide toxicity	Lung	2.5–20 mg/kg	Mouse	[173]
Sinha et al.	2018	Hypoxy/Ischemy	Brain	10 mg/kg	Mouse	[174]
Tanabe et al.	2015	Oxidative stress	???	100 μg/kg	Mouse	[175]
Tang et al.	2017	Abdominal aortic aneurysm	Aorta	10 mg/kg/day	Rat	[176]
Tas et al.	2015	Ischemia/reperfusion injury	Intestine	50 mg/kg	Rat	[177]

Authors	Date	Protection against	Targets	Amount	Species	Ref
Torabi et al.	2017	Cyclophosphamide-induced toxicity	Testicles	10 mg/kg/day	Rat	[178]
Uygur et al.	2016	As-induced apoptosis	Testicles	25 mg/kg/day	Rat	[179]
Vazan et al.	2015	Epinephrine-induced injury	Heart	50 μM	Rat	[180]
Vinod et al.	2016	Aging-induced NO rhythm loss	Brain	30 μg/kg/day	Rat	[181]
Wang et al.	2018	Intracerebral Hemorrahge	Brain	???	Rat	[182]
Wang et al.	2016	Smoke-induiced vascular injury	Blood samples	10 mg/kg	Rat	[183]
Wang et al.	2016	Smoke-induiced vascular injury	Blood samples	3 mg/day	Human	[183]
Xue et al.	2017	Kainic-induced cell death	Brain	20 mg/kg	Mouse	[184]
Yang et al.	2018	Subarachnoid hemorrhage	Brain	0.1–10 μM	Mouse	[185]
Yi et al.	2017	Stress-induced inflammation	Macrophages	50–100 mg/kg	Mouse	[186]
Yildirim et al.	2016	Ureteral obstruction-induced injury	Kidney	10 mg/kg	Rat	[187]
Yu et al.	2018	Ischemia–reperfusion injury	Heart	10 mg/kg	Rat	[188]
Yu et al.	2018	MEHP-induced meiosis defect	Oocytes	???	Pig	[189]
Yu et al.	2015	Ischemia/reperfusion injury	Heart	10 mg/kg/day	Rat	[190]
Yu et al.	2015	Ischemia/reperfusion injury	Heart	20 mg/kg/day	Rat	[191]
Zasada et al.	2015	Nitrobenzene-induced peroxidation	Thyroids	0.001–10 mM	Pig	[192]
Zhai et al.	2017	Pathological cardiac hypertrophy	Heart	20 mg/kg/day	Mouse	[193]
Zhang et al.	2017	Bisphenol A-induced toxicity	Oocytes	30 mg/kg	Mouse	[194]
Zhang et al.	2017	Diabetic cardiomyopathy	Heart	20 mg/kg/day	Mouse	[195]
Zhang et al.	2017	Arsenic-induced injury	Liver	5–20 mg/kg	Rat	[196]
Zhang et al.	2016	β-amyloid-induced damages	Brain	50 μM	Rat	[197]
Zhao et al.	2017	NaF-induced injury	Embryos	50–100 μM?	Mouse	[198]
Zhou et al.	2017	Ischemia/reperfusion injry	Heart	20 mg/kg	Mouse	[199]
Zhu et al.	2018	Oxidative stress	Heart endothelium	10 μM	Rat	[200]
Plants						
Kobylinska et al.	2017	Lead-induced cell death	Tobacco cells	200 nM	Plant	[201]
Wang et al.	2017	Drought stress	Arabidopsis	???	Plant	[202]

Authors	Date	Protection against	Targets	Amount	Species	Ref
Xu et al.	2016	Thermotolerance	Tomato plants	10 μM	Plant	[203]
Zheng et al.	2017	Salt-stress	Plant cells	—	Plant	[204]
Cells						
Baburina et al.	2017	Aging	Mitochondria	7 mg/kg/day	Rat	[205]
Bardak et al.	2017	2-ethylpyridine-induced stress	ARPE-19 cells	200 μM	Human	[206]
Charao et al.	2015	Paraquat-induced toxicity	A549 cells	10 μg/mL	Human	[207]
Chen et al.	2015	Bile acid-induced oxidative stress	L02 cells	1 μM	Human	[208]
Fu et al.	2017	Chloranil-induced toxicity	PC12 cells	25–200 μM	Mouse	[209]
Gurer-Orhan et al.	2016	b-amyloid-induced damage	Cells	10–100 μM	Hamster	[210]
Han et al.	2017	Obesity-associated stress	Oocytes	30 mg/kg/day	Mouse	[211]
Janjetovic et al.	2017	UVB-induced damage	Melanocytes	50 μM	Human	[212]
Ji et al.	2016	Angiotensin-II-indued injury	Podocytes	0.1–1 mM	Mouse	[83]
Jumnongprakhon et al.	2015	Methamphetamine-toxicity	C6 cells	1–100 nM	Rat	[213]
Liu et al.	2015	Hypoxia-induced	N2a cells	5 μg/mL	Mouse	[214]
Lu et al.	2015	LPS-induced hypertrophy	Myocardial cells	1.5–6 mg/mL	Rat	[215]
Maarman et al.	2017	Uric acid-induced toxicity	C2C12 myotubes	10 nM	Mouse	[216]
Miao et al.	2018	benzo(a)pyrene meiotic failure	Oocytes	1 nM–1 mM	Pig	[84]
Mehrzadi et al.	2017	H2O2-induced toxicity	MSC	10 nM–1 mM	Human	[85]
Ozerkan et al.	2015	CCl4-induced cytotoxicity	HepG2 & Hep3B	10 nM	Human	[217]
Pang et al.	2017	Early apoptosis	Oocytes	1 nM	Bovine	[218]
Sagrillo-Fagundes et al.	2016	Hypoxia-reoxygenation toxicity	Trophoblasts	1 mM	Human	[86]
Sanchez-Bretano et al.	2017	H_2O_2-induced cell death	661 W cells	0.1–1 μM		[219]
Song et al.	2015	LPS-induced inflammation	Stem cells	100 nM	Mouse	[220]
Tan et al.	2016	Oxidative stress-induced cell death	Adipocytes	100 μM	Human	[221]
Waseem et al.	2017	Oxaliplatin-induced toxicity	SHSY-5Y cells	10 μM	Human	[222]
Wongprayoon et al.	2017	Methamphetamine-induced stress	SH-SY5Y cells	0.01–1 μM	Human	[223]
Xie et al.	2015	Hypoxia-induced hypertrophy	Cardiomycyte cell line	1 mM	Rat	[87]

Authors	Date	Protection against	Targets	Amount	Species	Ref
Xue et al.	2017	Kainic-induced cell death	N2a cells	50–100 μM	Mouse	[184]
Yang et al.	2017	Iron overload senescence	MSCstem cells	10 nM–100 μM	Mouse	[224]
Yang et al.	2017	Glucocorticoid-induced impairment	Isolated knee joints	1 μM	Mouse	[225]
Yu et al.	2017	Ischemia–reperfusion injury	H9c2	10 μM	Rat	[226]
Zhao et al.	2018	Ab-induced neurotoxicity	Primary neurons	0.1–100 μM	Mouse	[227]
Zhou et al.	2018	rotenone-induced cell death	SH-SY5Y cells	50–500 μM	Human	[228]
Zhu et al.	2015	Myocardial infarction	Adipose stem cells	5 μM	Rat	[229]

Table 1. Some of the actions of melatonin observed in various pathophysiological situations.

6.1.2. Melatonin as an antioxidant molecule

Forman et al. in two seminal papers explained that the notion of hydroxyl radical scavengers is an extreme case of wishful thinking [230, 231]. Later on, he and his coworkers clearly showed that a unique molecule could not be a scavenger of superoxides, hydrogen peroxides, or other hydroperoxides or hydroxyl radicals. Indeed, all chemicals inside a cell react chemically with radical species, that is, proteins, lipids, nucleic acids, etc. Thus, because all organic compounds react with radicals with rate constants approaching the diffusion limitation, no compound can be better than the sum of the others to scavenge those ROS [231]. This can apply to melatonin. Like many other chemicals, whether indol-based or not, this compound, even at large concentrations, cannot be, per se, a scavenger. Therefore claims that melatonin is a super scavenger, with many advantages over other similar naturally occurring compounds, must be taken with extreme caution, despite several in-depth reviews, such as the one by Galano et al. [232]. Even the use of "direct" detection methods of radicals (to prove this hypothesis) should be handled with much caution [233]. Nevertheless, melatonin sustains antioxidant properties (see Rodriguez et al. [234] for review). Indeed, it can increase the expression of antioxidant enzymes (see, e.g., Mahrzadi et al. [149] and references therein). Melatonin can also act as a potent antiapoptotic agent in many cells [235], maybe through an antioxidant type of activity, as a relationship between ROS and apoptosis and autophagy has been well documented. How can melatonin induce those antioxidant defenses?

6.1.3. Melatonin as a ligand of Nrf2?

At the time (2003) Rodriguez et al. wrote their review [234] on antioxidant capacities of melatonin, Nrf2 was not really an identified and recognized partner in this process. The relationship between melatonin actions and the role of nuclear factor erythroid 2-related factor 2 (Nrf2) has been reported more than 50 times in the literature these last years, starting around 2009 [236].

Nrf2 is a key factor in the induction of antioxidant protein defenses of the cell. It binds to a region called EpRE—also known as ARE [230]. This transcription factor (belonging to the huge family of Cap'n'collar transcription factors) is neutralized in cellulo by another factor, Kelch-like ECH-associated protein 1 (Keap1). The heterodimer is directed to the proteasome where the proteins are destroyed. Upon some conditions, including pharmacological ones (for instance, sprout-derived chemicals [237]), the dimer is open, and the free Nrf2 migrates to the nucleus of the cell where it associates with the EpRE region. This translates by the induction of several key proteins of the antioxidant cellular armada, such as heme oxygenase 1, quinone reductase 1, glutathione S-transferase π1, etc., but also enzymes from the phase 2 drug metabolism, such as UDP glucuronosyltransferases. There is a large literature indicating that melatonin induces Nrf2 expression and/or its separation with its corepressor, Keap1 (about 50 publications reported at least the induction of Nrf2 by melatonin). Furthermore, it has been shown several times that upon melatonin treatment, the cytosolic Nrf2 migrates to the nucleus where it can exert its inductive function. One question remains unanswered, though; it is the possibility that Nrf2 was the elusive nuclear factor described at several occasions [26]? Unfortunately, the tridimensional structure of Nrf2 and/or of its complex with Keap1 has not been reported. It seems that Nrf2 has no a priori structure and is only adopting define 3D shape either once linked to Keap1 (a complex that is then directed to the proteasome) or when in complex with a ligand. Much more need to be done to understand this relationship that might enlighten part of the observation of **Table 1**.

6.2. Through MT_1/MT_2

The specificity of actions linked to the binding of melatonin to one of its receptors, MT_1 and MT_2, is still a matter of debate. Indeed, a thorough survey of its action is not possible in vivo in wildtype animals, because we are still lacking reliable and isoform-specific antagonists (see discussion in Jockers et al. [45]). It is possible, though, to study the role of one or the other of the receptors using either natural KO animals [such as the Siberian hamster, but not the European hamster (Gautier & Boutin [281])] or, alternatively, MT_1 or MT_2 (or both) KO animals, which have been engineered [238–240], but results are slow to be issued [241–243] (see also discussion in Jockers et al. [45]). Nevertheless, general conclusions can be drawn from accumulated data, as reviewed by the same authors [45]. It is difficult, as of today, without drowning in the 3970 available reviews on melatonin, to clearly segregate between the subtype roles. Among the clearest facts, mice lacking MT_1 receptors exhibit higher mean blood glucose levels than wildtype mice [244]. Those KO animals tend to be more glucose intolerant and insulin resistant than their wildtype counterparts. Through many different parameters, both MT_1 and MT_2 receptors seem to have a role in the phase shift of circadian rhythms, as demonstrated by several lines of indications, including knockout animals, the use of specific MT_2 antagonists (luzindole, 4P-PDOT), as well as ex vivo experiments. Melatonin can activate an immune response. Remarkably, that was proposed as early as 1926 by Berman. This activity seems to depend on the MT_1 receptor [245], but opposite claims have also been published [246]. Liu et al. showed that it was MT_2 that was the receptor implicated in axogenesis and the formation of functional synapses [247].

Nevertheless, it seems to me improbable that even only some of the actions in **Table 1** were through the binding of melatonin onto its receptors.

6.3. Through QR2

As stated previously, it was rapidly discovered that two melatonin-binding sites were GPCR in mammals and an extra one, Mel1c, in reptilians and birds. The group of Dubocovich also pointed at a binding site, ML2 [248, 249], with rather unconventional properties (particularly with very fast exchange) baptized MT_3. In 1999 we embarked in an attempt to clone this particular receptor, after having obtained similar results for the pharmacological description of this particular "receptor" [250]. We had the chance to identify it by using a series of inverse pharmacology techniques, comprising an analogue of a specific MT_3 ligand, MCA-NAT, on which affinity chromatography succeeded. The binding site was an enzyme with a peculiar story, quinone reductase 2 (QR2 a.k.a. NQO2) [23]. The activity of this enzyme was first described in the early 1960s as a reductase using unconventional donors as co-substrates, such as *N*-benzyl, *N*-methyl, or *N*-ribosyl dihydronicotinamides, and Talalay's group established that the enzyme was the enzyme once described by Liao et al. [251]. Interestingly, they clearly established the nature of the enzyme and particularly its incapacity to recognize NADH or NAD(P)H as co-substrates, as well as its sensitivity to some chemical, in an orthogonal way to QR1. For instance, QR2 is insensitive to the reference QR1 inhibitor, dicoumarol. When we discovered that QR2 was indeed MT_3, we had to reinforce this observation by generating KO cell lines [252], KO mouse strain [253] and various tools that would help to understand the potential role of this enzyme (see Vella et al. [254] and references there in). Although the enzyme was identified during a pure melatonin-related program, it turned out to have nothing in common, a priori, with the melatoninergic systems. Indeed, while able to bind melatonin with a rather strong affinity—in the nM range—QR2 is only poorly inhibited by melatonin, in the 50 μM range, suggesting that melatonin regulation was not a player in the QR2 game. Indeed, as often in the drug metabolism area, enzymes from both phases I and II, such as cytochrome P450, UGTs, or glutathione S-transferases, are often enzymes with enough plasticity in their catalytic sites in order to accommodate xenobiotics that are, by definition, molecules of various chemical structures issued from the environment at large.

Nevertheless, I suggested that QR2 inhibition at high dose of melatonin could be an explanation for melatonin exerting its antioxidant capacities [88].

6.4. Through mitochondria

Incidentally, a couple of papers reported not only the synthesis of melatonin in mitochondria but also the presence in these organelles—at least those isolated from the brain—of a measurable binding, signing the presence of MT_1 receptors. Again, as long as the mitochondrial DNA is not reported for genes encoding for these GPCRs, it seems possible to hypothesize that those binding sites were a leftover from the brain preparation of mitochondria, a possibility reinforced by the difficulty of preparing "pure" mitochondria from these lipid- and membrane-rich organs. Beyond these hypothetical technical considerations lays also the fact that our laboratory had experienced "very" often cells with no binding activity, suggesting that mitochondria would express melatonin receptors only in melatonin receptor-rich organs—such as the brain—an indirect suggestion that the presence of those receptors in these organelles might be a "simple" signature of a difficult separation between all the kinds of membranes present in a neuronal cell. There were several reports over the last decade showing a protective effect of melatonin onto mitochondria functions (see **Table 2**). Then several reviews suggested that melatonin was synthesized by mitochondria (see, for instance, Manchester et al., 2015 [255], Reiter et al., 2017 [256] and 2018 [257]). Particularly interesting is the fact that Cellular and Molecular Life Science published a special issue in 2017 (volume 74, issue 21) dealing with melatonin and mitochondria, emphasizing the interest of the community for these observations and their consequences. A reason for this hypothesis was given: mitochondria, like chloroplasts in plants, evolved from bacteria. Because originally cyanobacteria were subjected to heavy exposition to toxic free radicals, they evolved in keeping melatonin as an antioxidant, scavenging these radicals and thus preserving their integrity. Because this happened about 3 billion years ago, melatonin has been selected to protect and defend those microorganisms.

Of course, when bacteria colonized eukaryotic cells, the trait was maintained throughout evolution, including in mammals. Thus, no matter how high or low the blood melatonin concentration is, this particular intra-mitochondria concentration remains constant (not depending on the circadian rhythm), protecting mitochondria from the never ending production of free radicals that is the signature of sane mitochondria. An impressive series of publications were issued in these last few years (see **Table 2**) dealing with situations where toxicity was prevented by melatonin. This can be further extended to the protection afforded by mitochondria-synthesized melatonin to oocytes [278]. Finally, one can also add the observation that mitochondria melatonin protects plants from drought episodes [202]. Particularly interesting was the last one in which Suofu et al. [10] demonstrated the presence of the main melatonin synthesis enzymes, arylalkylamine *N*-acetyltransferase (AANAT) and acetylserotonin *O*-methyltransferase (HIOMT), in mitochondria matrix, as well as the high concentration of melatonin inside those mitochondria matrix. Furthermore, they showed the presence of MT_1 receptor and the actual coupling of this receptor, turning this observation into a major progress in the domain, as rare are the receptors signaling in the mitochondria. This observation was challenged by Ahluwalia et al. [279] (replied by Suofu et al. [11]) that was able to show the presence of the melatonin receptors in muscle fibers, but not in mitochondria thereof. It is clear that this breakthrough information will be better understood after the observation will be confirmed independently. Of course, questions remain in the skeptical reader mind: if the melatonin system evolved from bacteria over several billion years, then the genetic material should have evolved together with it, meaning that the mitochondrial DNA should encode for MT_1, AANAT, and ASMT, which does not seem to be the case. This observation would also lead to an extra complexity involving the protein importation system (TOM, Tim, etc.) and the *ad hoc* addressing sequence(s) onto those proteins, all of which have not been seen so far. Furthermore, the discovery and description of an inward transport of melatonin in mitochondria [280] are not fitting an in situ synthesis. For those of us who have been working with subcellular organelles, it is very hard to assess the purity of those organelles because of the continuum that exists between all the membranes from cells. One should also add to this the particular complexity of the brain tissue that is by essence very lipid-rich, leading to an extra difficulty in preparing pure membranes or pure subcellular organelles. Nevertheless, the several evidences on the melatonin actions at the level of mitochondria cannot be doubted and change our view of its role and of the role of MT_1, as MT_2 seems to be absent from the organelle.

Protection against	Authors	Year	Reference
Doxorubicin	Xu and Ashraf	2002	[258]
Oxidative stress	Jou et al.	2004	[259]
NO synthase induced dysfunction	Escames et al.	2006	[260]
Apoptosis	Han et al.	2006	[261]
Ischemia-Reperfusion	Petrosillo et al.	2006	[262]
Apoptosis	Luchetti et al.	2007	[263]
Oxidative stress	Jou et al.	2007	[264]
UV exposition	Fischer et al.	2008	[265]
Aging	Petrosillo et al.	2008	[266]
Oxidative stress	Hibaoui et al.	2009	[267]
Permeability transition	Jou et al.	2010	[268]
Permeability transition	Jou et al.	2011	[269]
Bisphenol A	Anjum et al.	2011	[270]
CCl_4	Chechshevik et al.	2012	[271]
Isoproterenol	Mukherjee et al.	2012	[272]
Ischemia-Reperfusion	Yang et al.	2013	[273]
UV exposition	Canonico et al.	2013	[274]
Demyelination induced stress	Kashani et al.	2014	[275]
Cd	Guo et al.	2014	[276]
Isoproterenol	Mukherjee et al.	2015	[272]
Ischemic-Stroke	Yang et al.	2015	[277]
Lipid toxicity	Ozsoy et al.	2016	[159]
Aging	Baburina et al.	2017	[205]
Lipid toxicity	Das et al.	2017	[116]
Paclitaxel	Galley et al.	2017	[124]
Copper	Ghosh et al.	2017	[126]

Table 2. Melatonin protects mitochondria against various stresses.

7. Future paths?

Trying to summarize the literature on subjects like melatonin is obviously impossible. One will give his/her view on some of the points that are the most attractive to him/her. It was thus vain to attempt to solve issues with such an essay on this neurohormone. The future will tell if melatonin is an exceptional molecule with many capacities. What is clear, as of today, is that melatonin has been described on a plethora of situations with beneficial endpoints. If melatonin is an antioxidant—but the concept behind this word is different from one author to another—it is not as a scavenger of radical oxygen species, but most probably through its capacity to induce cellular defenses against oxidative stress. Melatonin has different known targets; two, MT_1 and MT_2, are well described, but these receptors bring more unexpected novelties over the years, an enzyme—QR2—the study of which could be part of an explanation for the antioxidant properties of melatonin, and, finally, a pathway, linked to Nrf2 that seems to be another part of the explanation for these properties. There are many routes still to explore to understand what is behind this molecule, and the spectacular associated with it should be concealed and mastered until beyond (and despite) our hopes; facts will be revealed.

Author details

Jean A. Boutin

Address all correspondence to: jean.boutin@servier.com

Institut de Recherches Internationales SERVIER, Suresnes, France

References

[1] Majidinia M, Reiter RJ, Shakouri S-K, Mohebbi I, Rasteghar M, Kaviani M, Darband SG, Jahanban-Esfahlan R, Nabavi SM, Yousefik B. The multiple functions of melatonin in regenerative medicine. Ageing Research Reviews. 2018;**45**:33-52. DOI: 10.1016/j.arr.2018.04.003

[2] Zisapel N. New perspectives on the role of melatonin in human sleep, circadian rhythms and their regulation. British Journal of Pharmacology. 2018; in press. DOI: 10.1111/bph.14116

[3] Pevet P, Klosen P, Felder-Schmittbuhl MP. The hormone melatonin: Animal studies. Best practice & research. Clinical Endocrinology & Metabolism. 2017;**31**:547-559. DOI: 10.1016/j.beem.2017.10.010

[4] Tordjman S, Chokron S, Delorme R, Charrier A, Bellissant E, Jaafari N, Fougerou C. Melatonin: Pharmacology, functions and therapeutic benefits. Current Neuropharmacology. 2017; **15**:434-443. DOI: 10.2174/1570159X14666161228122115

[5] Liu J, Clough SJ, Hutchinson AJ, Adamah-Biassi EB, Popovska-Gorevski M, Dubocovich ML. MT 1 and MT 2 melatonin receptors: A therapeutic perspective. Annual Review of Pharmacology and Toxicology. 2016;**56**:361-383. DOI: 10.1146/annurev-pharmtox-010814-124742

[6] Klein DC. Arylalkylamine N-acetyltransferase: "the Timezyme". The Journal of Biological Chemistry. 2007;**282**:4233-4237. DOI: 10.1074/jbc.R600036200

[7] Ganguly S, Gastel JA, Weller JL, Schwartz C, Jaffe H, Namboodiri MA, Coon SL, Hickman AB, Rollag M, Obsil T, Beauverger P, Ferry G, Boutin JA, Klein DC. Role of a pineal cAMP-operated arylalkylamine N-acetyltransferase/14-3-3-binding switch in melatonin

synthesis. Proceedings of the National Academy of Sciences. 2001;**98**:8083-8088. DOI: 10.1073/pnas.141118798

[8] Ferry G, Loynel A, Kucharczyk N, Bertin S, Rodriguez M, Delagrange P, Galizzi JP, Jacoby E, Volland JP, Lesieur D, Renard P, Canet E, Fauchère JL, Boutin JA. Substrate specificity and inhibition studies of human serotonin N-acetyltransferase. The Journal of Biological Chemistry. 2000;**275**:8794-8805

[9] Stehle JH, Saade A, Rawashdeh O, Ackermann K, Jilg A, Sebestény T, Maronde E. A survey of molecular details in the human pineal gland in the light of phylogeny, structure, function and chronobiological diseases. Journal of Pineal Research. 2011;**51**:17-43. DOI: 10.1111/j.1600-079X.2011.00856.x

[10] Suofu Y, Li W, Jean-Alphonse FG, Jia J, Khattar NK, Li J, Baranov SV, Leronni D, Mihalik AC, He Y, Cecon E, Wehbi VL, Kim J, Heath BE, Baranova OV, Wang X, Gable MJ, Kretz ES, Di Benedetto G, Lezon TR, Ferrando LM, Larkin TM, Sullivan M, Yablonska S, Wang J, Minnigh MB, Guillaumet G, Suzenet F, Richardson RM, Poloyac SM, Stolz DB, Jockers R, Witt-Enderby PA, Carlisle DL, Vilardaga J-P, Friedlander RM. Dual role of mitochondria in producing melatonin and driving GPCR signaling to block cytochrome c release. Proceedings of the National Academy of Sciences. 2017;**114**:E7997-E8006. DOI: 10.1073/pnas.1705768114

[11] Suofu Y, Carlisle DL, Vilardaga J-P, Friedlander RM. Reply to Ahluwalia et al.: Contributions of melatonin receptors are tissue-dependent. Proceedings of the National Academy of Sciences of the United States of America. 2018;**115**:E1944. DOI: 10.1073/pnas.1800449115

[12] Foulkes NS, Whitmore D, Sassone-Corsi P. Rhythmic transcription: The molecular basis of circadian melatonin synthesis. Biology of the Cell. 1997;**89**:487-494

[13] Schomerus C, Korf HW, Laedtke E, Weller JL, Klein DC. Selective adrenergic/cyclic AMP-dependent switch-off of proteasomal proteolysis alone switches on neural signal transduction: An example from the pineal gland. Journal of Neurochemistry. 2000; **75**:2123-2132

[14] Ferry G, Boutin JA. High-capacity screening of arylalkylamine n-acetyltransferase inhibitors using a high-performance liquid chromatography system. Journal of Biomolecular Screening. 2000;**5**:361-368. DOI: 10.1177/108705710000500508

[15] Beaurain N, Mésangeau C, Chavatte P, Ferry G, Audinot V, Boutin JA, Delagrange P, Bennejean C, Yous S. Design, synthesis and in vitro evaluation of novel derivatives as serotonin N-acetyltransferase inhibitors. Journal of Enzyme Inhibition and Medicinal Chemistry. 2002;**17**:409-414. DOI: 10.1080/1475636021000005721

[16] Mesangeau C, Yous S, Chavatte P, Ferry G, Audinot V, Boutin JA, Delagrange P, Bennejean C, Renard P, Lesieur D. Design, synthesis and in vitro evaluation of novel benzothiophene derivatives as serotonin N-acetyltransferase (AANAT) inhibitors. Journal of Enzyme Inhibition and Medicinal Chemistry. 2003;**18**:119-125. DOI: 10.1080/1475636031000093552

[17] Lepailleur A, Lemaître S, Feng X, Sopkova-de Oliveira Santos J, Delagrange P, Boutin J, Renard P, Bureau R, Rault S. Receptor- and ligand-based study on novel 2,2′-Bithienyl derivatives as non-Peptidic AANAT inhibitors. Journal of Chemical Information and Modeling. 2010;**50**:446-460. DOI: 10.1021/ci9004805

[18] Zheng W, Cole PA. Novel bisubstrate analog inhibitors of serotonin N-acetyltransferase: The importance of being neutral. Bioorganic Chemistry. 2003;**31**:398-411

[19] Szewczuk LM, Saldanha SA, Ganguly S, Bowers EM, Javoroncov M, Karanam B, Culhane JC, Holbert MA, Klein DC, Abagyan R, Cole PA. De novo discovery of serotonin N-acetyltransferase inhibitors. Journal of Medicinal Chemistry. 2007;**50**:5330-5338. DOI: 10.1021/jm0706463

[20] Zheng W, Zhang Z, Ganguly S, Weller JL, Klein DC, Cole PA. Cellular stabilization of the melatonin rhythm enzyme induced by nonhydrolyzable phosphonate incorporation. Nature Structural Biology. 2003;**10**:1054-1057. DOI: 10.1038/nsb1005

[21] Zheng W, Schwarzer D, Lebeau A, Weller JL, Klein DC, Cole PA. Cellular stability of serotonin N-acetyltransferase conferred by phosphonodifluoromethylene alanine (Pfa) substitution for Ser-205. The Journal of Biological Chemistry. 2005;**280**:10462-10467. DOI: 10.1074/jbc.M412283200

[22] Scheibner KA, de Angelis J, Burley SK, Cole PA. Investigation of the roles of catalytic residues in serotonin N-acetyltransferase. The Journal of Biological Chemistry. 2002;**277**:18118-18126. DOI: 10.1074/jbc.M200595200

[23] Nosjean O, Ferro M, Cogé F, Beauverger P, Henlin J-M, Lefoulon F, Fauchère J-L, Delagrange P, Canet E, Boutin JA. Identification of the melatonin-binding site MT3 as the Quinone Reductase 2. The Journal of Biological Chemistry. 2000;**275**:31311-31317. DOI: 10.1074/jbc.M005141200

[24] Dufourny L, Levasseur A, Migaud M, Callebaut I, Pontarotti P, Malpaux B, Monget P. GPR50 is the mammalian ortholog of Mel1c: Evidence of rapid evolution in mammals. BMC Evolutionary Biology. 2008;**8**:105. DOI: 10.1186/1471-2148-8-105

[25] Gautier C, Guenin S-P, Riest-Fery I, Perry TJ, Legros C, Nosjean O, Simonneaux V, Grützner F, Boutin JA. Characterization of the Mel1c melatoninergic receptor in platypus (*Ornithorhynchus anatinus*). PLoS One. 2018;**13**:e0191904. DOI: 10.1371/journal.pone.0191904

[26] Becker-André M, Wiesenberg I, Schaeren-Wiemers N, André E, Missbach M, Saurat JH, Carlberg C. Pineal gland hormone melatonin binds and activates an orphan of the nuclear receptor superfamily. The Journal of Biological Chemistry. 1994;**269**:28531-28534

[27] Becker-André M, Wiesenberg I, Schaeren-Wiemers N, André E, Missbach M, Saurat JH, Carlberg C. Pineal gland hormone melatonin binds and activates an orphan of the nuclear receptor superfamily. The Journal of Biological Chemistry. 1997;**272**:16707

[28] Lardone PJ, Guerrero JM, Fernández-Santos JM, Rubio A, Martín-Lacave I, Carrillo-Vico A. Melatonin synthesized by T lymphocytes as a ligand of the retinoic acid-related orphan receptor. Journal of Pineal Research. 2011;**51**:454-462. DOI: 10.1111/j.1600-079X.2011.00909.x

[29] Jan JE, Reiter RJ, Wong PKH, Bax MCO, Ribary U, Wasdell MB. Melatonin has membrane receptor-independent hypnotic action on neurons: An hypothesis. Journal of Pineal Research. 2011;**50**:233-240. DOI: 10.1111/j.1600-079X.2010.00844.x

[30] Reppert SM, Weaver DR, Ebisawa T. Cloning and characterization of a mammalian melatonin receptor that mediates reproductive and circadian responses. Neuron. 1994; **13**:1177-1185

[31] Weaver DR, Liu C, Reppert SM. Nature's knockout: The Mel1b receptor is not necessary for reproductive and circadian responses to melatonin in Siberian hamsters. Molecular Endocrinology (Baltimore, Md.). 1996;**10**:1478-1487. DOI: 10.1210/mend.10.11.8923472

[32] Cogé F, Guenin SP, Fery I, Migaud M, Devavry S, Slugocki C, Legros C, Ouvry C, Cohen W, Renault N, Nosjean O, Malpaux B, Delagrange P, Boutin JA. The end of a myth: Cloning and characterization of the ovine melatonin MT(2) receptor. British Journal of Pharmacology. 2009;**158**:1248-1262. DOI: 10.1111/j.1476-5381.2009.00453.x

[33] Gaildrat P, Becq F, Falcón J. First cloning and functional characterization of a melatonin receptor in fish brain: A novel one? Journal of Pineal Research. 2002;**32**:74-84

[34] Park Y-J, Park J-G, Kim S-J, Lee Y-D, Saydur Rahman M, Takemura A. Melatonin receptor of a reef fish with lunar-related rhythmicity: Cloning and daily variations. Journal of Pineal Research. 2006;**41**:166-174. DOI: 10.1111/j.1600-079X.2006.00350.x

[35] Van Kirk T, Powers E, Dowse HB. Melatonin increases the regularity of cardiac rhythmicity in the Drosophila heart in both wild-type and strains bearing pathogenic mutations. Journal of Comparative Physiology. B, Biochemical, Systemic, and Environmental Physiology. 2017;**187**:63-78. DOI: 10.1007/s00360-016-1019-8

[36] Devavry S, Legros C, Brasseur C, Cohen W, Guenin S-P, Delagrange P, Malpaux B, Ouvry C, Cogé F, Nosjean O, Boutin JA. Molecular pharmacology of the mouse melatonin receptors MT1 and MT2. European Journal of Pharmacology. 2012;**677**:15-21. DOI: 10.1016/j.ejphar.2011.12.009

[37] Audinot V, Bonnaud A, Grandcolas L, Rodriguez M, Nagel N, Galizzi J-P, Balik A, Messager S, Hazlerigg DG, Barrett P, Delagrange P, Boutin JA. Molecular cloning and pharmacological characterization of rat melatonin MT1 and MT2 receptors. Biochemical Pharmacology. 2008;**75**:2007-2019. DOI: 10.1016/j.bcp.2008.02.022

[38] Audinot V, Mailliet F, Lahaye-Brasseur C, Bonnaud A, Le Gall A, Amossé C, Dromaint S, Rodriguez M, Nagel N, Galizzi J-P, Malpaux B, Guillaumet G, Lesieur D, Lefoulon F, Renard P, Delagrange P, Boutin JA. New selective ligands of human cloned melatonin MT1 and MT2 receptors. Naunyn-Schmiedeberg's Archives of Pharmacology. 2003;**367**:553-561. DOI: 10.1007/s00210-003-0751-2

[39] Mor M, Plazzi PV, Spadoni G, Tarzia G. Melatonin. Current Medicinal Chemistry. 1999; **6**:501-518

[40] Garratt PJ, Tsotinis A. Synthesis of compounds as melatonin agonists and antagonists. Mini Reviews in Medicinal Chemistry. 2007;**7**:1075-1088

[41] Rivara S, Pala D, Bedini A, Spadoni G. Therapeutic uses of melatonin and melatonin derivatives: A patent review (2012-2014). Expert Opinion on Therapeutic Patents. 2015;**25**:425-441. DOI: 10.1517/13543776.2014.1001739

[42] Zlotos DP, Jockers R, Cecon E, Rivara S, Witt-Enderby PA. MT 1 and MT 2 melatonin receptors: Ligands, models, oligomers, and therapeutic potential. Journal of Medicinal Chemistry. 2014;**57**:3161-3185. DOI: 10.1021/jm401343c

[43] Ng KY, Leong MK, Liang H, Paxinos G. Melatonin receptors: Distribution in mammalian brain and their respective putative functions. Brain Structure & Function. 2017;**222**: 2921-2939. DOI: 10.1007/s00429-017-1439-6

[44] Vakkuri O, Lämsä E, Rahkamaa E, Ruotsalainen H, Leppäluoto J. Iodinated melatonin: Preparation and characterization of the molecular structure by mass and 1H NMR spectroscopy. Analytical Biochemistry. 1984;**142**:284-289

[45] Jockers R, Delagrange P, Dubocovich ML, Markus RP, Renault N, Tosini G, Cecon E, Zlotos DP. Update on melatonin receptors: IUPHAR review 20. British Journal of Pharmacology. 2016;**173**:2702-2725. DOI: 10.1111/bph.13536

[46] Legros C, Devavry S, Caignard S, Tessier C, Delagrange P, Ouvry C, Boutin JA, Nosjean O. Melatonin MT1 and MT2 receptors display different molecular pharmacologies only in the G-protein coupled state. British Journal of Pharmacology. 2014;**171**:186-201. DOI: 10.1111/bph.12457

[47] Legros C, Matthey U, Grelak T, Pedragona-Moreau S, Hassler W, Yous S, Thomas E, Suzenet F, Folleas B, Lefoulon F, Berthelot P, Caignard D-H, Guillaumet G, Delagrange P, Brayer J-L, Nosjean O, Boutin JA. New radioligands for describing the molecular pharmacology of MT1 and MT2 melatonin receptors. International Journal of Molecular Sciences. 2013;**14**:8948-8962. DOI: 10.3390/ijms14058948

[48] Cecon E, Oishi A, Jockers R. Melatonin receptors: Molecular pharmacology and signalling in the context of system bias. British Journal of Pharmacology. DOI: 10.1111/bph.13950

[49] Devavry S, Legros C, Brasseur C, Delagrange P, Spadoni G, Cohen W, Malpaux B, Boutin JA, Nosjean O. Description of the constitutive activity of cloned human melatonin receptors hMT(1) and hMT(2) and discovery of inverse agonists. Journal of Pineal Research. 2012;**53**:29-37. DOI: 10.1111/j.1600-079X.2011.00968.x

[50] Dupré C, Bruno O, Bonnaud A, Giganti A, Nosjean O, Legros C, Boutin JA. Assessments of cellular melatonin receptor signaling pathways: B-arrestin recruitment, receptor internalization, and impedance variations. European Journal of Pharmacology. 2018;**818**:534-544. DOI: 10.1016/j.ejphar.2017.11.022

[51] Boutin JA, Bonnaud A, Brasseur C, Bruno O, Lepretre N, Oosting P, Coumailleau S, Delagrange P, Nosjean O, Legros C. New MT2 melatonin receptor-selective ligands: Agonists and partial agonists. International Journal of Molecular Sciences. 2017;**18**:e1347. DOI: 10.3390/ijms18071347

[52] Kenakin T. Is the quest for signaling bias worth the effort? Molecular Pharmacology. 2018;**93**:266-269. DOI: 10.1124/mol.117.111187

[53] Dubocovich ML. Luzindole (N-0774): A novel melatonin receptor antagonist. The Journal of Pharmacology and Experimental Therapeutics. 1988;**246**:902-910

[54] Dubocovich ML, Masana MI, Iacob S, Sauri DM. Melatonin receptor antagonists that differentiate between the human Mel1a and Mel1b recombinant subtypes are used to assess the pharmacological profile of the rabbit retina ML1 presynaptic heteroreceptor. Naunyn-Schmiedeberg's Archives of Pharmacology. 1997;**355**:365-375

[55] Yan J-h, Su H-r, Boutin JA, Renard MP, Wang M-w. High-throughput screening assay for new ligands at human melatonin receptors. Acta Pharmacologica Sinica. 2008;**29**: 1515-1521. DOI: 10.1111/j.1745-7254.2008.00903.x

[56] Boutin JA, Lahaye C, Pegurier C, Nicolas JP, Fauchere JL, Langlois M, Renard P, Delagrange P, Canet E. Screening of ligand binding on melatonin receptor using non-peptide combinatorial libraries. Journal of Receptor and Signal Transduction Research. 2000;**20**:105-118. DOI: 10.3109/10799890009150040

[57] Clement N, Renault N, Guillaume J-L, Cecon E, Journé A-S, Laurent X, Tadagaki K, Cogé F, Gohier A, Delagrange P, Chavatte P, Jockers R. Importance of the second extracellular loop for melatonin MT1 receptor function and absence of melatonin binding in GPR50. British Journal of Pharmacology. 2018; in press. DOI: 10.1111/bph.14029

[58] Gubitz AK, Reppert SM. Chimeric and point-mutated receptors reveal that a single glycine residue in transmembrane domain 6 is critical for high affinity melatonin binding. Endocrinology. 2000;**141**:1236-1244. DOI: 10.1210/endo.141.3.7356

[59] Kokkola T, Watson MA, White J, Dowell S, Foord SM, Laitinen JT. Mutagenesis of human Mel1a melatonin receptor expressed in yeast reveals domains important for receptor function. Biochemical and Biophysical Research Communications. 1998;**249**:531-536. DOI: 10.1006/bbrc.1998.9182

[60] Conway S, Mowat ES, Drew JE, Barrett P, Delagrange P, Morgan PJ. Serine residues 110 and 114 are required for agonist binding but not antagonist binding to the melatonin MT(1) receptor. Biochemical and Biophysical Research Communications. 2001;**282**:1229-1236. DOI: 10.1006/bbrc.2001.4722

[61] Rodbell M. The role of GTP-binding proteins in signal transduction: From the sublimely simple to the conceptually complex. Current Topics in Cellular Regulation. 1992;**32**:1-47

[62] Bockaert J, Pin JP. Molecular tinkering of G protein-coupled receptors: An evolutionary success. The EMBO Journal. 1999;**18**:1723-1729. DOI: 10.1093/emboj/18.7.1723

[63] Jones KA, Borowsky B, Tamm JA, Craig DA, Durkin MM, Dai M, Yao WJ, Johnson M, Gunwaldsen C, Huang LY, Tang C, Shen Q, Salon JA, Morse K, Laz T, Smith KE, Nagarathnam D, Noble SA, Branchek TA, Gerald C. GABA(B) receptors function as a heteromeric assembly of the subunits GABA(B)R1 and GABA(B)R2. Nature. 1998;**396**: 674-679. DOI: 10.1038/25348

[64] Hall RA, Premont RT, Chow CW, Blitzer JT, Pitcher JA, Claing A, Stoffel RH, Barak LS, Shenolikar S, Weinman EJ, Grinstein S, Lefkowitz RJ. The beta2-adrenergic receptor interacts with the Na+/H+–exchanger regulatory factor to control Na+/H+ exchange. Nature. 1998;**392**:626-630. DOI: 10.1038/33458

[65] Boute N, Pernet K, Issad T. Monitoring the activation state of the insulin receptor using bioluminescence resonance energy transfer. Molecular Pharmacology. 2001;**60**:640-645

[66] Kamal M, Gbahou F, Guillaume J-L, Daulat AM, Benleulmi-Chaachoua A, Luka M, Chen P, Kalbasi Anaraki D, Baroncini M, La Mannoury CC, Millan MJ, Prevot V, Delagrange P, Jockers R. Convergence of melatonin and serotonin (5-HT) signaling at MT2/5-HT2C receptor heteromers. The Journal of Biological Chemistry. 2015;**290**:11537-11546. DOI: 10.1074/jbc.M114.559542

[67] Ayoub MA, Couturier C, Lucas-Meunier E, Angers S, Fossier P, Bouvier M, Jockers R. Monitoring of ligand-independent dimerization and ligand-induced conformational changes of melatonin receptors in living cells by bioluminescence resonance energy transfer. The Journal of Biological Chemistry. 2002;**277**:21522-21528. DOI: 10.1074/jbc.M200729200

[68] Levoye A, Dam J, Ayoub MA, Guillaume J-L, Couturier C, Delagrange P, Jockers R. The orphan GPR50 receptor specifically inhibits MT1 melatonin receptor function through heterodimerization. The EMBO Journal. 2006;**25**:3012-3023. DOI: 10.1038/sj.emboj.7601193

[69] Reppert SM, Weaver DR, Ebisawa T, Mahle CD, Kolakowski LF. Cloning of a melatonin-related receptor from human pituitary. FEBS Letters. 1996;**386**:219-224

[70] Wojciech S, Ahmad R, Belaid-Choucair Z, Journé A-S, Gallet S, Dam J, Daulat A, Ndiaye-Lobry D, Lahuna O, Karamitri A, Guillaume J-L, Do Cruzeiro M, Guillonneau F, Saade A, Clément N, Courivaud T, Kaabi N, Tadagaki K, Delagrange P, Prévot V, Hermine O, Prunier C, Jockers R. The orphan GPR50 receptor promotes constitutive TGFβ receptor signaling and protects against cancer development. Nature Communications. 2018;**9**:685. DOI: 10.1038/s41467-018-03609-x

[71] Damian M, Pons V, Renault P, M'Kadmi C, Delort B, Hartmann L, Kaya AI, Louet M, Gagne D, Ben Haj Salah K, Denoyelle S, Ferry G, Boutin JA, Wagner R, Fehrentz J-A, Martinez J, Marie J, Floquet N, Galès C, Mary S, Hamm HE, Banères J-L. GHSR-D2R heteromerization modulates dopamine signaling through an effect on G protein conformation. Proceedings of the National Academy of Sciences of the United States of America. 2018;**115**:4501-4506. DOI: 10.1073/pnas.1712725115

[72] Pala D, Beuming T, Sherman W, Lodola A, Rivara S, Mor M. Structure-based virtual screening of MT2 melatonin receptor: Influence of template choice and structural refinement. Journal of Chemical Information and Modeling. 2013;**53**:821-835. DOI: 10.1021/ci4000147

[73] Rivara S, Lorenzi S, Mor M, Plazzi PV, Spadoni G, Bedini A, Tarzia G. Analysis of structure-activity relationships for MT2 selective antagonists by melatonin MT1 and MT2 receptor models. Journal of Medicinal Chemistry. 2005;**48**:4049-4060. DOI: 10.1021/jm048956y

[74] Pala D, Lodola A, Bedini A, Spadoni G, Rivara S. Homology models of melatonin receptors: Challenges and recent advances. International Journal of Molecular Sciences. 2013;**14**:8093-8121. DOI: 10.3390/ijms14048093

[75] Logez C, Berger S, Legros C, Banères J-L, Cohen W, Delagrange P, Nosjean O, Boutin JA, Ferry G, Simonin F, Wagner R. Recombinant human melatonin receptor MT1 isolated in mixed detergents shows pharmacology similar to that in mammalian cell membranes. PLoS One. 2014;**9**:e100616. DOI: 10.1371/journal.pone.0100616

[76] Logez C, Damian M, Legros C, Dupré C, Guéry M, Mary S, Wagner R, M'Kadmi C, Nosjean O, Fould B, Marie J, Fehrentz J-A, Martinez J, Ferry G, Boutin JA, Banères J-L. Detergent-free isolation of functional G protein-coupled receptors into nanometric lipid particles. Biochemistry. 2016;**55**:38-48. DOI: 10.1021/acs.biochem.5b01040

[77] Hardeland R. Taxon- and site-specific melatonin catabolism. Molecules (Basel, Switzerland). 2017;**22**:e2015. DOI: 10.3390/molecules22112015

[78] Semak I, Naumova M, Korik E, Terekhovich V, Wortsman J, Slominski A. A novel metabolic pathway of melatonin: Oxidation by cytochrome c. Biochemistry. 2005;**44**:9300-9307. DOI: 10.1021/bi050202d

[79] Ferry G, Ubeaud C, Lambert P-H, Bertin S, Cogé F, Chomarat P, Delagrange P, Serkiz B, Bouchet J-P, Truscott RJW, Boutin JA. Molecular evidence that melatonin is enzymatically oxidized in a different manner than tryptophan: Investigations with both indoleamine 2,3-dioxygenase and myeloperoxidase. The Biochemical Journal. 2005;**388**:205-215. DOI: 10.1042/BJ20042075

[80] Niu S, Li F, Tan D-X, Zhang L, Idle JR, Gonzalez FJ, Ma X. Analysis of N1-acetyl-N2-formyl-5-methoxykynuramine/N1-acetyl-5-methoxy-kynuramine formation from melatonin in mice. Journal of Pineal Research. 2010;**49**:106-114. DOI: 10.1111/j.1600-079x.2010.00771.x

[81] Andersen LPH, Gögenur I, Rosenberg J, Reiter RJ. The safety of melatonin in humans. Clinical Drug Investigation. 2016;**36**:169-175. DOI: 10.1007/s40261-015-0368-5

[82] Sánchez-Barceló EJ, Mediavilla MD, Tan DX, Reiter RJ. Clinical uses of melatonin: Evaluation of human trials. Current Medicinal Chemistry. 2010;**17**:2070-2095

[83] Ji Z-Z, Xu Y-C. Melatonin protects podocytes from angiotensin II-induced injury in an in vitro diabetic nephropathy model. Molecular Medicine Reports. 2016;**14**:920-926. DOI: 10.3892/mmr.2016.5313

[84] Miao Y, Zhou C, Bai Q, Cui Z, ShiYang X, Lu Y, Zhang M, Dai X, Xiong B. The protective role of melatonin in porcine oocyte meiotic failure caused by the exposure to benzo(a) pyrene. Human Reproduction (Oxford, England). 2018;**33**:116-127. DOI: 10.1093/humrep/dex331

[85] Mehrzadi S, Safa M, Kamrava SK, Darabi R, Hayat P, Motevalian M. Protective mechanisms of melatonin against hydrogen-peroxide-induced toxicity in human bone-marrow-derived mesenchymal stem cells. Canadian Journal of Physiology and Pharmacology. 2017;**95**:773-786. DOI: 10.1139/cjpp-2016-0409

[86] Sagrillo-Fagundes L, Clabault H, Laurent L, Hudon-Thibeault A-A, Salustiano EMA, Fortier M, Bienvenue-Pariseault J, Wong Yen P, Sanderson JT, Vaillancourt C. Human primary trophoblast cell culture model to study the protective effects of melatonin against hypoxia/reoxygenation-induced disruption. Journal of Visualized Experiments: JoVE. DOI: 10.3791/54228

[87] Xie S, Deng Y, Pan Y-Y, Wang Z-H, Ren J, Guo X-L, Yuan X, Shang J, Liu H-G. Melatonin protects against chronic intermittent hypoxia-induced cardiac hypertrophy by modulating autophagy through the 5′ adenosine monophosphate-activated protein kinase pathway. Biochemical and Biophysical Research Communications. 2015;**464**:975-981. DOI: 10.1016/j.bbrc.2015.06.149

[88] Boutin JA. Quinone reductase 2 as a promising target of melatonin therapeutic actions. Expert Opinion on Therapeutic Targets. 2015;**20**:303-317. DOI: 10.1517/14728222.2016.1091882

[89] Goldberg DM, Yan J, Soleas GJ. Absorption of three wine-related polyphenols in three different matrices by healthy subjects. Clinical Biochemistry. 2003;**36**:79-87

[90] Legros C, Brasseur C, Delagrange P, Ducrot P, Nosjean O, Boutin JA. Alternative radioligands for investigating the molecular pharmacology of melatonin receptors. The Journal of Pharmacology and Experimental Therapeutics. 2016;**356**:681-692. DOI: 10.1124/jpet.115.229989

[91] Sáenz de Miera C, Sage-Ciocca D, Simonneaux V, Pévet P, Monecke S. Melatonin-independent photoperiodic entrainment of the Circannual TSH rhythm in the pars Tuberalis of the European hamster. Journal of Biological Rhythms. 2018;**33**(3):302-317. DOI: 10.1177/0748730418766601

[92] Zampol MA, Barros MH. Melatonin improves survival and respiratory activity of yeast cells challenged by alpha-synuclein and menadione. Yeast (Chichester, England). 2018;**35**:281-290. DOI: 10.1002/yea.3296

[93] Jiao J, Ma Y, Chen S, Liu C, Song Y, Qin Y, Yuan C, Liu Y. Melatonin-producing endophytic bacteria from grapevine roots promote the abiotic stress-induced production of endogenous melatonin in their hosts. Frontiers in Plant Science. 2016;**7**:1387. DOI: 10.3389/fpls.2016.01387

[94] Díaz-Casado ME, Rusanova I, Aranda P, Fernández-Ortiz M, Sayed RKA, Fernández-Gil BI, Hidalgo-Gutiérrez A, Escames G, López LC, Acuña-Castroviejo D. In vivo determination of mitochondrial respiration in 1-methyl-4-phenyl-1,2,3,6-tetrahydropyridine-treated zebrafish reveals the efficacy of melatonin in restoring mitochondrial normalcy. Zebrafish. 2018;**15**:15-26. DOI: 10.1089/zeb.2017.1479

[95] Hardeland R. Melatonin in plants - diversity of levels and multiplicity of functions. Frontiers in Plant Science. 2016;**7**:198. DOI: 10.3389/fpls.2016.00198

[96] Tan D-X, Zheng X, Kong J, Manchester LC, Hardeland R, Kim SJ, Xu X, Reiter RJ. Fundamental issues related to the origin of melatonin and melatonin isomers during evolution: Relation to their biological functions. International Journal of Molecular Sciences. 2014;**15**:15858-15890. DOI: 10.3390/ijms150915858

[97] Tekbas OF, Ogur R, Korkmaz A, Kilic A, Reiter RJ. Melatonin as an antibiotic: New insights into the actions of this ubiquitous molecule. Journal of Pineal Research. 2008;**44**:222-226. DOI: 10.1111/j.1600-079X.2007.00516.x

[98] Anderson G, Maes M, Markus RP, Rodriguez M. Ebola virus: Melatonin as a readily available treatment option. Journal of Medical Virology. 2015;**87**:537-543. DOI: 10.1002/jmv.24130

[99] Roy J, Galano J-M, Durand T, Le Guennec J-Y, Lee JC-Y. Physiological role of reactive oxygen species as promoters of natural defenses. FASEB Journal : Official Publication of the Federation of American Societies for Experimental Biology. 2017;**31**:3729-3745. DOI: 10.1096/fj.201700170R

[100] Abdel Moneim AE, Ortiz F, Leonardo-Mendonca RC, Vergano-Villodres R, Guerrero-Martinez JA, Lopez LC, Acuna-Castroviejo D, Escames G. Protective effects of melatonin against oxidative damage induced by Egyptian cobra (Naja haje) crude venom in rats. Acta Tropica. 2015;**143**:58-65. DOI: 10.1016/j.actatropica.2014.12.007

[101] Allagui MS, Hachani R, Saidi S, Feriani A, Murat JC, Kacem K, El Feki A. Pleiotropic protective roles of melatonin against aluminium-induced toxicity in rats. General Physiology and Biophysics. 2015;**34**:415-424. DOI: 10.4149/gpb_2015028

[102] Al-Olayan EM, El-Khadragy MF, Abdel Moneim AE. The protective properties of melatonin against aluminium-induced neuronal injury. International Journal of Experimental Pathology. 2015;**96**:196-202. DOI: 10.1111/iep.12122

[103] Al-Rasheed N, Faddah L, Al-Rasheed N, Bassiouni YA, Hasan IH, Mahmoud AM, Mohamad RA, Yacoub HI. Protective effects of silymarin, alone or in combination with chlorogenic acid and/or melatonin, against carbon tetrachloride-induced hepatotoxicity. Pharmacognosy Magazine. 2016;**12**:S337-S345. DOI: 10.4103/0973-1296.185765

[104] Amin AH, El-Missiry MA, Othman AI. Melatonin ameliorates metabolic risk factors, modulates apoptotic proteins, and protects the rat heart against diabetes-induced apoptosis. European Journal of Pharmacology. 2015;**747**:166-173. DOI: 10.1016/j.ejphar.2014.12.002

[105] Asghari MH, Moloudizargari M, Abdollahi M. In response to the comments on our recently published paper entitled "on the mechanisms of melatonin in protection of aluminum phosphide cardiotoxicity". Archives of Toxicology. 2017;**91**:3457-3458. DOI: 10.1007/s00204-017-2029-3

[106] Banaei S, Ahmadiasl N, Alihemmati A. Comparison of the protective effects of erythropoietin and melatonin on renal ischemia-reperfusion injury. Trauma Monthly. 2016; **21**:e23005. DOI: 10.5812/traumamon.23005

[107] Barberino RS, Menezes VG, Ribeiro AEAS, Palheta RC, Jiang X, Smitz JEJ, Matos MHT. Melatonin protects against cisplatin-induced ovarian damage in mice via the MT1 receptor and antioxidant activity. Biology of Reproduction. 2017;**96**:1244-1255. DOI: 10.1093/biolre/iox053

[108] Berkiks I, Benmhammed H, Mesfioui A, Ouichou A, El Hasnaoui A, Mouden S, Touil T, Bahbiti Y, Nakache R, El Hessni A. Postnatal melatonin treatment protects against affective disorders induced by early-life immune stimulation by reducing the microglia cell activation and oxidative stress. The International Journal of Neuroscience. 2017: 1-10. DOI: 10.1080/00207454.2017.1398156

[109] Cao S, Shrestha S, Li J, Yu X, Chen J, Yan F, Ying G, Gu C, Wang L, Chen G. Melatonin-mediated mitophagy protects against early brain injury after subarachnoid hemorrhage through inhibition of NLRP3 inflammasome activation. Scientific Reports. 2017;**7**:2417. DOI: 10.1038/s41598-017-02679-z

[110] Cebi Sen C, Yumusak N, Atilgan HI, Sadic M, Koca G, Korkmaz M. The protective effect of melatonin on sperm quality in rat after radioiodine treatment. Andrologia. DOI: 10.1111/and.12962

[111] Chang Y-C, Hsu S-Y, Yang C-C, Sung P-H, Chen Y-L, Huang T-H, Kao G-S, Chen S-Y, Chen K-H, Chiang H-J, Yip H-K, Lee F-Y. Enhanced protection against renal ischemia-reperfusion injury with combined melatonin and exendin-4 in a rodent model. Experimental Biology and Medicine (Maywood, N.J.). 2016;**241**:1588-1602. DOI: 10.1177/1535370216642528

[112] Chang C-L, Sung P-H, Sun C-K, Chen C-H, Chiang H-J, Huang T-H, Chen Y-L, Zhen Y-Y, Chai H-T, Chung S-Y, Tong M-S, Chang H-W, Chen H-H, Yip H-K. Protective effect of melatonin-supported adipose-derived mesenchymal stem cells against small bowel ischemia-reperfusion injury in rat. Journal of Pineal Research. 2015;**59**:206-220. DOI: 10.1111/jpi.12251

[113] Chen Y, Zhang J, Zhao Q, Chen Q, Sun Y, Jin Y, Wu J. Melatonin induces anti-inflammatory effects to play a protective role via endoplasmic reticulum stress in acute pancreatitis. Cellular Physiology and Biochemistry: International Journal of Experimental Cellular Physiology, Biochemistry, and Pharmacology. 2016;**40**:1094-1104. DOI: 10.1159/000453164

[114] Chen K-H, Yang C-H, Wallace CG, Lin C-R, Liu C-K, Yin T-C, Huang T-H, Chen Y-L, Sun C-K, Yip H-K. Combination therapy with extracorporeal shock wave and melatonin markedly attenuated neuropathic pain in rat. American Journal of Translational Research. 2017;**9**:4593-4606

[115] Czechowska G, Celinski K, Korolczuk A, Wojcicka G, Dudka J, Bojarska A, Reiter RJ. Protective effects of melatonin against thioacetamide-induced liver fibrosis in rats. Journal of Physiology and Pharmacology : An Official Journal of the Polish Physiological Society. 2015;**66**:567-579

[116] Das N, Mandala A, Naaz S, Giri S, Jain M, Bandyopadhyay D, Reiter RJ, Roy SS. Melatonin protects against lipid-induced mitochondrial dysfunction in hepatocytes and inhibits stellate cell activation during hepatic fibrosis in mice. Journal of Pineal Research. 2017;**62**:e12404. DOI: 10.1111/jpi.12404

[117] Ding M, Ning J, Feng N, Li Z, Liu Z, Wang Y, Wang Y, Li X, Huo C, Jia X, Xu R, Fu F, Wang X, Pei J. Dynamin-related protein 1-mediated mitochondrial fission contributes to post-traumatic cardiac dysfunction in rats and the protective effect of melatonin. Journal of Pineal Research. 2018;**64**:e12447. DOI: 10.1111/jpi.12447

[118] Ding K, Xu J, Wang H, Zhang L, Wu Y, Li T. Melatonin protects the brain from apoptosis by enhancement of autophagy after traumatic brain injury in mice. Neurochemistry International. 2015;**91**:46-54. DOI: 10.1016/j.neuint.2015.10.008

[119] Dos Santos M, Favero G, Bonomini F, Stacchiotti A, Rodella LF, Veronese FV, Rezzani R. Oral supplementation of melatonin protects against lupus nephritis renal injury in a pristane-induced lupus mouse model. Life Sciences. 2018;**193**:242-251. DOI: 10.1016/j.lfs.2017.10.038

[120] Drąg-Kozak E, Socha M, Gosiewski G, Łuszczek-Trojnar E, Chyb J, Popek W. Protective effect of melatonin on cadmium-induced changes in some maturation and reproductive parameters of female Prussian carp (*Carassius gibelio* B.). Environmental Science and Pollution Research International. DOI: 10.1007/s11356-018-1308-8

[121] Ewida SF, Al-Sharaky DR. Implication of renal aquaporin-3 in fructose-induced metabolic syndrome and melatonin protection. Journal of Clinical and Diagnostic Research: JCDR. 2016;**10**:CF06-CF11. DOI: 10.7860/JCDR/2016/18362.7656

[122] Favero G, Trapletti V, Bonomini F, Stacchiotti A, Lavazza A, Rodella LF, Rezzani R. Oral supplementation of melatonin protects against fibromyalgia-related skeletal muscle alterations in reserpine-induced myalgia rats. International Journal of Molecular Sciences. 2017;**18**:e1389. DOI: 10.3390/ijms18071389

[123] Fernández-Gil B, Moneim AEA, Ortiz F, Shen Y-Q, Soto-Mercado V, Mendivil-Perez M, Guerra-Librero A, Acuña-Castroviejo D, Molina-Navarro MM, García-Verdugo JM, Sayed RKA, Florido J, Luna JD, López LC, Escames G. Melatonin protects rats from radiotherapy-induced small intestine toxicity. PLoS One. 2017;**12**:e0174474. DOI: 10.1371/journal.pone.0174474

[124] Galley HF, McCormick B, Wilson KL, Lowes DA, Colvin L, Torsney C. Melatonin limits paclitaxel-induced mitochondrial dysfunction in vitro and protects against paclitaxel-induced neuropathic pain in the rat. Journal of Pineal Research. 2017;**63**:e12444. DOI: 10.1111/jpi.12444

[125] Ghaznavi H, Mehrzadi S, Dormanesh B, Tabatabaei SMTH, Vahedi H, Hosseinzadeh A, Pazoki-Toroudi H, Rashidian A. Comparison of the protective effects of melatonin and silymarin against gentamicin-induced nephrotoxicity in rats. Journal of Evidence-based Complementary & Alternative Medicine. 2016;**21**:NP49-NP55. DOI: 10.1177/2156587215621672

[126] Ghosh AK, Naaz S, Bhattacharjee B, Ghosal N, Chattopadhyay A, Roy S, Reiter RJ, Bandyopadhyay D. Mechanism of melatonin protection against copper-ascorbate-induced oxidative damage in vitro through isothermal titration calorimetry. Life Sciences. 2017;**180**:123-136. DOI: 10.1016/j.lfs.2017.05.022

[127] Goc Z, Szaroma W, Kapusta E, Dziubek K. Protective effects of melatonin on the activity of SOD, CAT, GSH-Px and GSH content in organs of mice after administration of SNP. The Chinese Journal of Physiology. 2017;**60**:1-10. DOI: 10.4077/CJP.2017.BAF435

[128] Goudarzi M, Khodayar MJ, Hosseini Tabatabaei SMT, Ghaznavi H, Fatemi I, Mehrzadi S. Pretreatment with melatonin protects against cyclophosphamide-induced oxidative stress and renal damage in mice. Fundamental & Clinical Pharmacology. 2017;**31**: 625-635. DOI: 10.1111/fcp.12303

[129] Hermoso DAM, Shimada LBC, Gilglioni EH, Constantin J, Mito MS, Hermoso APM, Salgueiro-Pagadigorria CL, Iwamoto ELI. Melatonin protects female rats against steatosis and liver oxidative stress induced by oestrogen deficiency. Life Sciences. 2016;**157**:178-186. DOI: 10.1016/j.lfs.2016.05.044

[130] Hsu J-T, Le P-H, Lin C-J, Chen T-H, Kuo C-J, Chiang K-C, Yeh T-S. Mechanism of salutary effects of melatonin-mediated liver protection after trauma-hemorrhage: P38 MAPK-dependent iNOS/HIF-1α pathway. American Journal of Physiology. Gastrointestinal and Liver Physiology. 2017;**312**:G427-G433. DOI: 10.1152/ajpgi.00440.2016

[131] Hu Y, Wang Z, Pan S, Zhang H, Fang M, Jiang H, Zhang H, Gao Z, Xu K, Li Z, Xiao J, Lin Z. Melatonin protects against blood-brain barrier damage by inhibiting the TLR4/ NF-κB signaling pathway after LPS treatment in neonatal rats. Oncotarget. 2017;**8**:31638-31654. DOI: 10.18632/oncotarget.15780

[132] Ji M-H, Xia D-G, Zhu L-Y, Zhu X, Zhou X-Y, Xia J-Y, Yang J-J. Short- and long-term protective effects of melatonin in a mouse model of sepsis-associated encephalopathy. Inflammation. 2018;**41**:515-529. DOI: 10.1007/s10753-017-0708-0

[133] Jiang T, Chang Q, Cai J, Fan J, Zhang X, Xu G. Protective effects of melatonin on retinal inflammation and oxidative stress in experimental diabetic retinopathy. Oxidative Medicine and Cellular Longevity. 2016;**2016**:3528274. DOI: 10.1155/2016/3528274

[134] Jin CJ, Engstler AJ, Sellmann C, Ziegenhardt D, Landmann M, Kanuri G, Lounis H, Schroder M, Vetter W, Bergheim I. Sodium butyrate protects mice from the development of the early signs of non-alcoholic fatty liver disease: Role of melatonin and lipid peroxidation. The British Journal of Nutrition. 2016;**116**:1682-1693. DOI: 10.1017/S0007114516004025

[135] Karaer I, Simsek G, Gul M, Bahar L, Gurocak S, Parlakpinar H, Nuransoy A. Melatonin protects inner ear against radiation damage in rats. The Laryngoscope. 2015;**125**:E345-E349. DOI: 10.1002/lary.25376

[136] Karimfar MH, Niazvand F, Haghani K, Ghafourian S, Shirazi R, Bakhtiyari S. The protective effects of melatonin against cryopreservation-induced oxidative stress in human sperm. International Journal of Immunopathology and Pharmacology. 2015;**28**:69-76. DOI: 10.1177/0394632015572080

[137] Khaksar M, Oryan A, Sayyari M, Rezabakhsh A, Rahbarghazi R. Protective effects of melatonin on long-term administration of fluoxetine in rats. Experimental and Toxicologic Pathology : Official Journal of the Gesellschaft fur Toxikologische Pathologie. 2017;**69**:564-574. DOI: 10.1016/j.etp.2017.05.002

[138] Khalil WKB, Abdu F. Protective effect of melatonin against zonisamide-induced reproductive disorders in male rats. Archives of Medical Science. AMS. 2015;**11**:660-669. DOI: 10.5114/aoms.2013.39384

[139] Koc S, Cayli S, Aksakal C, Ocakli S, Soyalic H, Somuk BT, Yuce S. Protective effects of melatonin and selenium against apoptosis of olfactory sensory neurons: A rat model study. American Journal of Rhinology & Allergy. 2016;**30**:62-66. DOI: 10.2500/ajra.2016.30.4313

[140] Lebda MA, Sadek KM, Abouzed TK, Tohamy HG, El-Sayed YS. Melatonin mitigates thioacetamide-induced hepatic fibrosis via antioxidant activity and modulation of proinflammatory cytokines and fibrogenic genes. Life Sciences. 2018;**192**:136-143. DOI: 10.1016/j.lfs.2017.11.036

[141] Lee J-H, Moon J-H, Nazim UM, Lee Y-J, Seol J-W, Eo S-K, Lee J-H, Park S-Y. Melatonin protects skin keratinocyte from hydrogen peroxide-mediated cell death via the SIRT1 pathway. Oncotarget. 2016;**7**:12075-12088. DOI: 10.18632/oncotarget.7679

[142] Li R, Luo X, Li L, Peng Q, Yang Y, Zhao L, Ma M, Hou Z. The protective effects of melatonin against oxidative stress and inflammation induced by acute cadmium exposure in mice testis. Biological Trace Element Research. 2016;**170**:152-164. DOI: 10.1007/s12011-015-0449-6

[143] Li Y, Zhang Z, He C, Zhu K, Xu Z, Ma T, Tao J, Liu G. Melatonin protects porcine oocyte in vitro maturation from heat stress. Journal of Pineal Research. 2015;**59**:365-375. DOI: 10.1111/jpi.12268

[144] Lopez A, Ortiz F, Doerrier C, Venegas C, Fernandez-Ortiz M, Aranda P, Diaz-Casado ME, Fernandez-Gil B, Barriocanal-Casado E, Escames G, Lopez LC, Acuna-Castroviejo D. Mitochondrial impairment and melatonin protection in parkinsonian mice do not depend of inducible or neuronal nitric oxide synthases. PLoS One. 2017;**12**:e0183090. DOI: 10.1371/journal.pone.0183090

[145] Lv Y, Zhang P, Guo J, Zhu Z, Li X, Xu D, Zeng W. Melatonin protects mouse spermatogonial stem cells against hexavalent chromium-induced apoptosis and epigenetic histone modification. Toxicology and Applied Pharmacology. 2018;**340**:30-38. DOI: 10.1016/j.taap.2017.12.017

[146] Ma Q, Yang J, Huang X, Guo W, Li S, Zhou H, Li J, Cao F, Chen Y. Poly(Lactide-co-Glycolide)-Monomethoxy-poly-(polyethylene glycol) nanoparticles loaded with melatonin protect adipose-derived stem cells transplanted in infarcted heart tissue. Stem cells (Dayton, Ohio). DOI: 10.1002/stem.2777

[147] Ma M, Chen X-Y, Li B, Li X-T. Melatonin protects premature ovarian insufficiency induced by tripterygium glycosides: Role of SIRT1. American Journal of Translational Research. 2017;**9**:1580-1602

[148] Ma C, Li LX, Zhang Y, Xiang C, Ma T, Ma ZQ, Zhang ZP. Protective and sensitive effects of melatonin combined with adriamycin on ER+ (estrogen receptor) breast cancer. European Journal of Gynaecological Oncology. 2015;**36**:197-202

[149] Mehrzadi S, Kamrava SK, Dormanesh B, Motevalian M, Hosseinzadeh A, Hosseini Tabatabaei SMT, Ghaznavi H. Melatonin synergistically enhances protective effect of atorvastatin against gentamicin-induced nephrotoxicity in rat kidney. Canadian Journal of Physiology and Pharmacology. 2016;**94**:265-271. DOI: 10.1139/cjpp-2015-0277

[150] Mirhoseini M, Talebpour Amiri F, Karimpour Malekshah AA, Rezanejad Gatabi Z, Ghaffari E. Protective effects of melatonin on testis histology following acute torsion-detorsion in rats. International Journal of Reproductive Biomedicine (Yazd, Iran). 2017;**15**:141-146

[151] Montasser AOS, Saleh H, Ahmed-Farid OA, Saad A, Marie M-AS. Protective effects of Balanites aegyptiaca extract, melatonin and Ursodeoxycholic acid against hepatotoxicity induced by methotrexate in male rats. Asian Pacific Journal of Tropical Medicine. 2017;**10**:557-565. DOI: 10.1016/j.apjtm.2017.06.003

[152] Mukherjee D, Ghosh AK, Dutta M, Mitra E, Mallick S, Saha B, Reiter RJ, Bandyopadhyay D. Mechanisms of isoproterenol-induced cardiac mitochondrial damage: Protective actions of melatonin. Journal of Pineal Research. 2015;**58**:275-290. DOI: 10.1111/jpi.12213

[153] Munoz MF, Arguelles S, Cano M, Marotta F, Ayala A. Aging and oxidative stress decrease pineal elongation factor 2: In vivo protective effect of melatonin in young rats treated with cumene hydroperoxide. Journal of Cellular Biochemistry. 2017;**118**: 182-190. DOI: 10.1002/jcb.25624

[154] Naseri S, Moghahi SMHN, Mokhtari T, Roghani M, Shirazi AR, Malek F, Rastegar T. Radio-protective effects of melatonin on subventricular zone in irradiated rat: Decrease in apoptosis and upregulation of nestin. Journal of Molecular Neuroscience : MN. 2017;**63**:198-205. DOI: 10.1007/s12031-017-0970-5

[155] Naskar A, Prabhakar V, Singh R, Dutta D, Mohanakumar KP. Melatonin enhances L-DOPA therapeutic effects, helps to reduce its dose, and protects dopaminergic neurons in 1-methyl-4-phenyl-1,2,3,6-tetrahydropyridine-induced parkinsonism in mice. Journal of Pineal Research. 2015;**58**:262-274. DOI: 10.1111/jpi.12212

[156] O'Neal-Moffitt G, Delic V, Bradshaw PC, Olcese J. Prophylactic melatonin significantly reduces Alzheimer's neuropathology and associated cognitive deficits independent of antioxidant pathways in AβPPswe/PS1 mice. Molecular Neurodegeneration. 2015;**10**:813. DOI: 10.1186/s13024-015-0027-6

[157] Ortiz F, Acuna-Castroviejo D, Doerrier C, Dayoub JC, Lopez LC, Venegas C, Garcia JA, Lopez A, Volt H, Luna-Sanchez M, Escames G. Melatonin blunts the mitochondrial/NLRP3 connection and protects against radiation-induced oral mucositis. Journal of Pineal Research. 2015;**58**:34-49. DOI: 10.1111/jpi.12191

[158] Othman AI, Edrees GM, El-Missiry MA, Ali DA, Aboel-Nour M, Dabdoub BR. Melatonin controlled apoptosis and protected the testes and sperm quality against bisphenol A-induced oxidative toxicity. Toxicology and Industrial Health. 2016;**32**:1537-1549. DOI: 10.1177/0748233714561286

[159] Ozsoy M, Gonul Y, Ozkececi ZT, Bali A, Celep RB, Kocak A, Adali F, Tosun M, Celik S. The protective effect of melatonin on remote organ liver ischemia and reperfusion injury following aortic clamping. Annali Italiani di Chirurgia. 2016;**87**:271-279

[160] Ozsoy O, Yildirim FB, Ogut E, Kaya Y, Tanriover G, Parlak H, Agar A, Aslan M. Melatonin is protective against 6-hydroxydopamine-induced oxidative stress in a hemiparkinsonian rat model. Free Radical Research. 2015;**49**:1004-1014. DOI: 10.3109/10715762.2015.1027198

[161] Pal R, Gulati K, Banerjee BD, Ray A. Pharmacological and biochemical studies on the protective effects of melatonin during stress-induced behavioral and immunological changes in relation to oxidative stress in rats. Canadian Journal of Physiology and Pharmacology. 2016;**94**:296-301. DOI: 10.1139/cjpp-2015-0240

[162] Pang Y-W, Sun Y-Q, Jiang X-L, Huang Z-Q, Zhao S-J, Du W-H, Hao H-S, Zhao X-M, Zhu H-B. Protective effects of melatonin on bovine sperm characteristics and subsequent in vitro embryo development. Molecular Reproduction and Development. 2016; **83**:993-1002. DOI: 10.1002/mrd.22742

[163] Patino P, Parada E, Farre-Alins V, Molz S, Cacabelos R, Marco-Contelles J, Lopez MG, Tasca CI, Ramos E, Romero A, Egea J. Melatonin protects against oxygen and glucose deprivation by decreasing extracellular glutamate and Nox-derived ROS in rat hippocampal slices. Neurotoxicology. 2016;**57**:61-68. DOI: 10.1016/j.neuro.2016.09.002

[164] Paul R, Phukan BC, Justin Thenmozhi A, Manivasagam T, Bhattacharya P, Borah A. Melatonin protects against behavioral deficits, dopamine loss and oxidative stress in homocysteine model of Parkinson's disease. Life Sciences. 2018;**192**:238-245. DOI: 10.1016/j.lfs.2017.11.016

[165] Rajput P, Jangra A, Kwatra M, Mishra A, Lahkar M. Alcohol aggravates stress-induced cognitive deficits and hippocampal neurotoxicity: Protective effect of melatonin. Biomedicine & pharmacotherapy = Biomedecine & pharmacotherapie. 2017;**91**:457-466. DOI: 10.1016/j.biopha.2017.04.077

[166] Sadek AS, Khattab RT. The protective role of melatonin on L-arginine-induced acute pancreatitis in adult male albino rats. Folia Morphologica. 2017;**76**:66-73. DOI: 10.5603/FM.a2016.0029

[167] Sarihan ME, Parlakpinar H, Ciftci O, Yilmaz F, Sagir M, Yilmaz O, Ceker G. Protective effects of melatonin against 2,3,7,8-tetrachlorodibenzo-p-dioxin-induced cardiac injury in rats. European Journal of Pharmacology. 2015;**762**:214-220. DOI: 10.1016/j.ejphar.2015.04.054

[168] Scheuer C, Pommergaard H-C, Rosenberg J, Gogenur I. Dose dependent sun protective effect of topical melatonin: A randomized, placebo-controlled, double-blind study. Journal of Dermatological Science. 2016;**84**:178-185. DOI: 10.1016/j.jdermsci.2016.08.007

[169] Shahrokhi N, Khaksari M, Nourizad S, Shahrokhi N, Soltani Z, Gholamhosseinian A. Protective effects of an interaction between vagus nerve and melatonin on gastric ischemia/reperfusion: The role of oxidative stress. Iranian Journal of Basic Medical Sciences. 2016;**19**:72-79

[170] Shang B, Shi H, Wang X, Guo X, Wang N, Wang Y, Dong L. Protective effect of melatonin on myenteric neuron damage in experimental colitis in rats. Fundamental & Clinical Pharmacology. 2016;**30**:117-127. DOI: 10.1111/fcp.12181

[171] Shao G, Tian Y, Wang H, Liu F, Xie G. Protective effects of melatonin on lipopolysaccharide-induced mastitis in mice. International Immunopharmacology. 2015;**29**:263-268. DOI: 10.1016/j.intimp.2015.11.011

[172] Shokri S, Kazemi M, Firouzjaei MA, Hemadi M, Moayeri A, Ganjkhani M, Nejatbakhsh R. Melatonin protects testes against lithium-pilocarpine-induced temporal lobe epilepsy in rats: A time course study. Andrologia. 2015;**47**:343-353. DOI: 10.1111/and.12269

[173] Shokrzadeh M, Chabra A, Naghshvar F, Ahmadi A, Jafarinejhad M, Hasani-Nourian Y. Protective effects of melatonin against cyclophosphamide-induced oxidative lung toxicity in mice. Drug Research. 2015;**65**:281-286. DOI: 10.1055/s-0034-1371801

[174] Sinha B, Wu Q, Li W, Tu Y, Sirianni AC, Chen Y, Jiang J, Zhang X, Chen W, Zhou S, Reiter RJ, Manning SM, Patel NJ, Aziz-Sultan AM, Inder TE, Friedlander RM, Fu J, Wang X. Protection of melatonin in experimental models of newborn hypoxic-ischemic brain injury through MT1 receptor. Journal of Pineal Research. 2018;**64**:e12443. DOI: 10.1111/jpi.12443

[175] Tanabe M, Tamura H, Taketani T, Okada M, Lee L, Tamura I, Maekawa R, Asada H, Yamagata Y, Sugino N. Melatonin protects the integrity of granulosa cells by reducing oxidative stress in nuclei, mitochondria, and plasma membranes in mice. The Journal of Reproduction and Development. 2015;**61**:35-41. DOI: 10.1262/jrd.2014-105

[176] Tang L, Cong Z, Hao S, Li P, Huang H, Shen Y, Li K, Jing H. Protective effect of melatonin on the development of abdominal aortic aneurysm in a rat model. The Journal of Surgical Research. 2017;**209**:266-278.e1. DOI: 10.1016/j.jss.2016.06.018

[177] Tas U, Ayan M, Sogut E, Kuloglu T, Uysal M, Tanriverdi HI, Senel U, Ozyurt B, Sarsilmaz M. Protective effects of thymoquinone and melatonin on intestinal ischemia-reperfusion injury. Saudi Journal of Gastroenterology : Official Journal of the Saudi Gastroenterology Association. 2015;**21**:284-289. DOI: 10.4103/1319-3767.166203

[178] Torabi F, Malekzadeh Shafaroudi M, Rezaei N. Combined protective effect of zinc oxide nanoparticles and melatonin on cyclophosphamide-induced toxicity in testicular histology and sperm parameters in adult Wistar rats. International Journal of Reproductive Biomedicine (Yazd, Iran). 2017;**15**:403-412

[179] Uygur R, Aktas C, Caglar V, Uygur E, Erdogan H, Ozen OA. Protective effects of melatonin against arsenic-induced apoptosis and oxidative stress in rat testes. Toxicology and Industrial Health. 2016;**32**:848-859. DOI: 10.1177/0748233713512891

[180] Vazan R, Ravingerova T. Protective effect of melatonin against myocardial injury induced by epinephrine. Journal of Physiology and Biochemistry. 2015;**71**:43-49. DOI: 10.1007/s13105-014-0377-5

[181] Vinod C, Jagota A. Daily NO rhythms in peripheral clocks in aging male Wistar rats: Protective effects of exogenous melatonin. Biogerontology. 2016;**17**:859-871. DOI: 10.1007/s10522-016-9656-6

[182] Wang Z, Zhou F, Dou Y, Tian X, Liu C, Li H, Shen H, Chen G. Melatonin alleviates intracerebral hemorrhage-induced secondary brain injury in rats via suppressing apoptosis, inflammation, oxidative stress, dna damage, and mitochondria injury. Translational Stroke Research. 2018;**9**:74-91. DOI: 10.1007/s12975-017-0559-x

[183] Wang Z, Ni L, Wang J, Lu C, Ren M, Han W, Liu C. The protective effect of melatonin on smoke-induced vascular injury in rats and humans: A randomized controlled trial. Journal of Pineal Research. 2016;**60**:217-227. DOI: 10.1111/jpi.12305

[184] Xue F, Shi C, Chen Q, Hang W, Xia L, Wu Y, Tao SZ, Zhou J, Shi A, Chen J. Melatonin mediates protective effects against kainic acid-induced neuronal death through safeguarding ER stress and mitochondrial disturbance. Frontiers in Molecular Neuroscience. 2017;**10**:49. DOI: 10.3389/fnmol.2017.00049

[185] Yang S, Tang W, He Y, Wen L, Sun B, Li S. Long non-coding RNA and microRNA-675/let-7a mediates the protective effect of melatonin against early brain injury after subarachnoid hemorrhage via targeting TP53 and neural growth factor. Cell Death & Disease. 2018;**9**:99. DOI: 10.1038/s41419-017-0155-8

[186] Yi W-J, Kim TS. Melatonin protects mice against stress-induced inflammation through enhancement of M2 macrophage polarization. International Immunopharmacology. 2017;**48**:146-158. DOI: 10.1016/j.intimp.2017.05.006

[187] Yildirim ME, Badem H, Cakmak M, Yilmaz H, Kosem B, Karatas OF, Bayrak R, Cimentepe E. Melatonin protects kidney against apoptosis induced by acute unilateral ureteral obstruction in rats. Central European Journal of Urology. 2016;**69**:225-230. DOI: 10.5173/ceju.2016.770

[188] Yu L-M, Di W-C, Dong X, Li Z, Zhang Y, Xue X-D, Xu Y-L, Zhang J, Xiao X, Han J-S, Liu Y, Yang Y, Wang H-S. Melatonin protects diabetic heart against ischemia-reperfusion injury, role of membrane receptor-dependent cGMP-PKG activation. Biochimica et Biophysica Acta. 2018;**1864**:563-578. DOI: 10.1016/j.bbadis.2017.11.023

[189] Yu Z, Wang T, Lan M, Zang X-W, Li Y-L, Cui X-S, Kim N-H, Sun S-C. Melatonin protects oocytes from MEHP exposure-induced meiosis defects in porcine. Biology of Reproduction. DOI: 10.1093/biolre/iox185

[190] Yu L, Liang H, Dong X, Zhao G, Jin Z, Zhai M, Yang Y, Chen W, Liu J, Yi W, Yang J, Yi D, Duan W, Yu S. Reduced silent information regulator 1 signaling exacerbates myocardial ischemia-reperfusion injury in type 2 diabetic rats and the protective effect of melatonin. Journal of Pineal Research. 2015;**59**:376-390. DOI: 10.1111/jpi.12269

[191] Yu L, Liang H, Lu Z, Zhao G, Zhai M, Yang Y, Yang J, Yi D, Chen W, Wang X, Duan W, Jin Z, Yu S. Membrane receptor-dependent Notch1/Hes1 activation by melatonin protects against myocardial ischemia-reperfusion injury: In vivo and in vitro studies. Journal of Pineal Research. 2015;**59**:420-433. DOI: 10.1111/jpi.12272

[192] Zasada K, Karbownik-Lewinska M. Comparison of potential protective effects of melatonin and propylthiouracil against lipid peroxidation caused by nitrobenzene in

the thyroid gland. Toxicology and Industrial Health. 2015;**31**:1195-1201. DOI: 10.1177/0748233713491799

[193] Zhai M, Liu Z, Zhang B, Jing L, Li B, Li K, Chen X, Zhang M, Yu B, Ren K, Yang Y, Yi W, Yang J, Liu J, Yi D, Liang H, Jin Z, Reiter RJ, Duan W, Yu S. Melatonin protects against the pathological cardiac hypertrophy induced by transverse aortic constriction through activating PGC-1beta: In vivo and in vitro studies. Journal of Pineal Research. 2017;**63**:e12433. DOI: 10.1111/jpi.12433

[194] Zhang M, Dai X, Lu Y, Miao Y, Zhou C, Cui Z, Liu H, Xiong B. Melatonin protects oocyte quality from Bisphenol A-induced deterioration in the mouse. Journal of Pineal Research. 2017;**62**:e12396. DOI: 10.1111/jpi.12396

[195] Zhang M, Lin J, Wang S, Cheng Z, Hu J, Wang T, Man W, Yin T, Guo W, Gao E, Reiter RJ, Wang H, Sun D. Melatonin protects against diabetic cardiomyopathy through Mst1/Sirt3 signaling. Journal of Pineal Research. 2017;**63**:e12418. DOI: 10.1111/jpi.12418

[196] Zhang Y, Wei Z, Liu W, Wang J, He X, Huang H, Zhang J, Yang Z. Melatonin protects against arsenic trioxide-induced liver injury by the upregulation of Nrf2 expression through the activation of PI3K/AKT pathway. Oncotarget. 2017;**8**:3773-3780. DOI: 10.18632/oncotarget.13931

[197] Zhang S, Wang P, Ren L, Hu C, Bi J. Protective effect of melatonin on soluble Abeta1-42-induced memory impairment, astrogliosis, and synaptic dysfunction via the Musashi1/Notch1/Hes1 signaling pathway in the rat hippocampus. Alzheimer's Research & Therapy. 2016;**8**:40. DOI: 10.1186/s13195-016-0206-x

[198] Zhao J, Fu B, Peng W, Mao T, Wu H, Zhang Y. Melatonin protect the development of preimplantation mouse embryos from sodium fluoride-induced oxidative injury. Environmental Toxicology and Pharmacology. 2017;**54**:133-141. DOI: 10.1016/j.etap.2017.06.014

[199] Zhou H, Zhang Y, Hu S, Shi C, Zhu P, Ma Q, Jin Q, Cao F, Tian F, Chen Y. Melatonin protects cardiac microvasculature against ischemia/reperfusion injury via suppression of mitochondrial fission-VDAC1-HK2-mPTP-mitophagy axis. Journal of Pineal Research. 2017;**63**:e12413. DOI: 10.1111/jpi.12413

[200] Zhu H, Jin Q, Li Y, Ma Q, Wang J, Li D, Zhou H, Chen Y. Melatonin protected cardiac microvascular endothelial cells against oxidative stress injury via suppression of IP3R-Ca2+c/VDAC-Ca2+m axis by activation of MAPK/ERK signaling pathway. Cell Stress & Chaperones. 2018;**23**:101-113. DOI: 10.1007/s12192-017-0827-4

[201] Kobylinska A, Reiter RJ, Posmyk MM. Melatonin protects cultured tobacco cells against lead-induced cell death via inhibition of cytochrome c translocation. Frontiers in Plant Science. 2017;**8**:1560. DOI: 10.3389/fpls.2017.01560

[202] Wang L, Feng C, Zheng X, Guo Y, Zhou F, Shan D, Liu X, Kong J. Plant mitochondria synthesize melatonin and enhance the tolerance of plants to drought stress. Journal of Pineal Research. 2017;**63**:e12429. DOI: 10.1111/jpi.12429

[203] Xu W, Cai S-Y, Zhang Y, Wang Y, Ahammed GJ, Xia X-J, Shi K, Zhou Y-H, Yu J-Q, Reiter RJ, Zhou J. Melatonin enhances thermotolerance by promoting cellular protein protection in tomato plants. Journal of Pineal Research. 2016;**61**:457-469. DOI: 10.1111/jpi.12359

[204] Zheng X, Tan DX, Allan AC, Zuo B, Zhao Y, Reiter RJ, Wang L, Wang Z, Guo Y, Zhou J, Shan D, Li Q, Han Z, Kong J. Chloroplastic biosynthesis of melatonin and its involvement in protection of plants from salt stress. Scientific Reports. 2017;**7**:41236. DOI: 10.1038/srep41236

[205] Baburina Y, Odinokova I, Azarashvili T, Akatov V, Lemasters JJ, Krestinina O. 2′,3′-cyclic nucleotide 3′-phosphodiesterase as a messenger of protection of the mitochondrial function during melatonin treatment in aging. Biochimica et Biophysica Acta. 2017;**1859**:94-103. DOI: 10.1016/j.bbamem.2016.11.003

[206] Bardak H, Uğuz AC, Bardak Y. Protective effects of melatonin and memantine in human retinal pigment epithelium (ARPE-19) cells against 2-ethylpyridine-induced oxidative stress: Implications for age-related macular degeneration. Cutaneous and Ocular Toxicology. 2018;**37**:112-120. DOI: 10.1080/15569527.2017.1354218

[207] Charao MF, Baierle M, Gauer B, Goethel G, Fracasso R, Paese K, Brucker N, Moro AM, Bubols GB, Dias BB, Matte US, Guterres SS, Pohlmann AR, Garcia SC. Protective effects of melatonin-loaded lipid-core nanocapsules on paraquat-induced cytotoxicity and genotoxicity in a pulmonary cell line. Mutation Research, Genetic Toxicology and Environmental Mutagenesis. 2015;**784-785**:1-9. DOI: 10.1016/j.mrgentox.2015.04.006

[208] Chen Y, Qing W, Sun M, Lv L, Guo D, Jiang Y. Melatonin protects hepatocytes against bile acid-induced mitochondrial oxidative stress via the AMPK-SIRT3-SOD2 pathway. Free Radical Research. 2015;**49**:1275-1284. DOI: 10.3109/10715762.2015.1067806

[209] Fu J, Xia X, Liu Z, Wang Y, Wang Y, Shi Q, Song X, Song E, Song Y. The acute exposure of tetrachloro-p-benzoquinone (a.K.A. chloranil) triggers inflammation and neurological dysfunction via toll-like receptor 4 signaling: The protective role of melatonin preconditioning. Toxicology. 2017;**381**:39-50. DOI: 10.1016/j.tox.2017.02.015

[210] Gurer-Orhan H, Karaaslan C, Ozcan S, Firuzi O, Tavakkoli M, Saso L, Suzen S. Novel indole-based melatonin analogues: Evaluation of antioxidant activity and protective effect against amyloid beta-induced damage. Bioorganic & Medicinal Chemistry. 2016;**24**:1658-1664. DOI: 10.1016/j.bmc.2016.02.039

[211] Han L, Wang H, Li L, Li X, Ge J, Reiter RJ, Wang Q. Melatonin protects against maternal obesity-associated oxidative stress and meiotic defects in oocytes via the SIRT3-SOD2-dependent pathway. Journal of Pineal Research. 2017;**63**:e12431. DOI: 10.1111/jpi.12431

[212] Janjetovic Z, Jarrett SG, Lee EF, Duprey C, Reiter RJ, Slominski AT. Melatonin and its metabolites protect human melanocytes against UVB-induced damage: Involvement of NRF2-mediated pathways. Scientific Reports. 2017;**7**:1274. DOI: 10.1038/s41598-017-01305-2

[213] Jumnongprakhon P, Govitrapong P, Tocharus C, Pinkaew D, Tocharus J. Melatonin protects methamphetamine-induced Neuroinflammation through NF-kappaB and Nrf2 pathways in Glioma cell line. Neurochemical Research. 2015;**40**:1448-1456. DOI: 10.1007/s11064-015-1613-2

[214] Liu X-W, Zi Y, Liu Y-E, Zhang Y-B, Xiang L-B, Hou M-x. Melatonin exerts protective effect on N2a cells under hypoxia conditions through Zip1/ERK pathway. Neuroscience Letters. 2015;**595**:74-80. DOI: 10.1016/j.neulet.2015.04.013

[215] Lu Q, Yi X, Cheng X, Sun X, Yang X. Melatonin protects against myocardial hypertrophy induced by lipopolysaccharide. In Vitro Cellular & Developmental Biology. Animal. 2015;**51**:353-360. DOI: 10.1007/s11626-014-9844-0

[216] Maarman GJ, Andrew BM, Blackhurst DM, Ojuka EO. Melatonin protects against uric acid-induced mitochondrial dysfunction, oxidative stress, and triglyceride accumulation in C2C12 myotubes. Journal of Applied Physiology (Bethesda, Md. : 1985). 2017;**122**:1003-1010. DOI: 10.1152/japplphysiol.00873.2016

[217] Ozerkan D, Ozsoy N, Yilmaz E. Vitamin D and melatonin protect the cell's viability and ameliorate the CCl4 induced cytotoxicity in HepG2 and Hep3B hepatoma cell lines. Cytotechnology. 2015;**67**:995-1002. DOI: 10.1007/s10616-014-9738-8

[218] Pang Y, Zhao S, Sun Y, Jiang X, Hao H, Du W, Zhu H. Protective effects of melatonin on the in vitro developmental competence of bovine oocytes. Animal science journal = Nihon chikusan Gakkaiho. DOI: 10.1111/asj.12970

[219] Sanchez-Bretano A, Baba K, Janjua U, Piano I, Gargini C, Tosini G. Melatonin partially protects 661W cells from H_2O_2-induced death by inhibiting Fas/FasL-caspase-3. Molecular Vision. 2017;**23**:844-852

[220] Song J, Kang SM, Lee KM, Lee JE. The protective effect of melatonin on neural stem cell against LPS-induced inflammation. BioMed Research International. 2015;**2015**:854359. DOI: 10.1155/2015/854359

[221] Tan SS, Han X, Sivakumaran P, Lim SY, Morrison WA. Melatonin protects human adipose-derived stem cells from oxidative stress and cell death. Archives of Plastic Surgery. 2016;**43**:237-241. DOI: 10.5999/aps.2016.43.3.237

[222] Waseem M, Sahu U, Salman M, Choudhury A, Kar S, Tabassum H, Parvez S, Ghavami S. Melatonin pre-treatment mitigates SHSY-5Y cells against oxaliplatin induced mitochondrial stress and apoptotic cell death. PLoS One. 2017;**12**:e0180953. DOI: 10.1371/journal.pone.0180953

[223] Wongprayoon P, Govitrapong P. Melatonin protects SH-SY5Y neuronal cells against methamphetamine-induced endoplasmic reticulum stress and apoptotic cell death. Neurotoxicity Research. 2017;**31**:1-10. DOI: 10.1007/s12640-016-9647-z

[224] Yang F, Yang L, Li Y, Yan G, Feng C, Liu T, Gong R, Yuan Y, Wang N, Idiiatullina E, Bikkuzin T, Pavlov V, Li Y, Dong C, Wang D, Cao Y, Han Z, Zhang L, Huang Q, Ding F,

Bi Z, Cai B. Melatonin protects bone marrow mesenchymal stem cells against iron overload-induced aberrant differentiation and senescence. Journal of Pineal Research. 2017;**63**:e124. DOI: 10.1111/jpi.12422

[225] Yang W, Kang X, Qin N, Li F, Jin X, Ma Z, Qian Z, Wu S. Melatonin protects chondrocytes from impairment induced by glucocorticoids via NAD(+)-dependent SIRT1. Steroids. 2017;**126**:24-29. DOI: 10.1016/j.steroids.2017.08.005

[226] Yu X, Li Z, Zheng H, Ho J, Chan MTV, Wu WKK. Protective roles of melatonin in central nervous system diseases by regulation of neural stem cells. Cell Proliferation. 2017;**50**:e12323. DOI: 10.1111/cpr.12323

[227] Zhao Y, Zhao R, Wu J, Wang Q, Pang K, Shi Q, Gao Q, Hu Y, Dong X, Zhang J, Sun J. Melatonin protects against Aβ-induced neurotoxicity in primary neurons via miR-132/PTEN/AKT/FOXO3a pathway. BioFactors (Oxford, England). DOI: 10.1002/biof.1411

[228] Zhou H, Ma Q, Zhu P, Ren J, Reiter RJ, Chen Y. Protective role of melatonin in cardiac ischemia-reperfusion injury: From pathogenesis to targeted therapy. Journal of Pineal Research. 2018;**64**:e12471. DOI: 10.1111/jpi.12471

[229] Zhu P, Liu J, Shi J, Zhou Q, Liu J, Zhang X, Du Z, Liu Q, Guo Y. Melatonin protects ADSCs from ROS and enhances their therapeutic potency in a rat model of myocardial infarction. Journal of Cellular and Molecular Medicine. 2015;**19**:2232-2243. DOI: 10.1111/jcmm.12610

[230] Forman HJ, Davies KJA, Ursini F. How do nutritional antioxidants really work: Nucleophilic tone and Para-hormesis versus free radical scavenging in vivo. Free Radical Biology & Medicine. 2014;**66**:24-35. DOI: 10.1016/j.freeradbiomed.2013.05.045

[231] Forman HJ, Augusto O, Brigelius-Flohe R, Dennery PA, Kalyanaraman B, Ischiropoulos H, Mann GE, Radi R, Roberts LJ, Vina J, Davies KJA. Even free radicals should follow some rules: A guide to free radical research terminology and methodology. Free Radical Biology & Medicine. 2015;**78**:233-235. DOI: 10.1016/j.freeradbiomed.2014.10.504

[232] Galano A, Castaneda-Arriaga R, Perez-Gonzalez A, Tan D-X, Reiter RJ. Phenolic melatonin-related compounds: Their role as chemical protectors against oxidative stress. Molecules (Basel, Switzerland). DOI: 10.3390/molecules21111442

[233] Cano A, Alcaraz O, Arnao MB. Free radical-scavenging activity of indolic compounds in aqueous and ethanolic media. Analytical and Bioanalytical Chemistry. 2003;**376**:33-37. DOI: 10.1007/s00216-003-1848-7

[234] Rodriguez C, Mayo JC, Sainz RM, Antolín I, Herrera F, Martín V, Reiter RJ. Regulation of antioxidant enzymes: A significant role for melatonin. Journal of Pineal Research. 2004;**36**:1-9

[235] Chetsawang B, Putthaprasart C, Phansuwan-Pujito P, Govitrapong P. Melatonin protects against hydrogen peroxide-induced cell death signaling in SH-SY5Y cultured cells: Involvement of nuclear factor kappa B, Bax and Bcl-2. Journal of Pineal Research. 2006;**41**:116-123. DOI: 10.1111/j.1600-079X.2006.00335.x

[236] Jung KH, Hong S-W, Zheng H-M, Lee D-H, Hong S-S. Melatonin downregulates nuclear erythroid 2-related factor 2 and nuclear factor-kappaB during prevention of oxidative liver injury in a dimethylnitrosamine model. Journal of Pineal Research. 2009;**47**: 173-183. DOI: 10.1111/j.1600-079X.2009.00698.x

[237] Prochaska HJ, Talalay P. Regulatory mechanisms of monofunctional and bifunctional anticarcinogenic enzyme inducers in murine liver. Cancer Research. 1988;**48**:4776-4782

[238] Liu C, Weaver DR, Jin X, Shearman LP, Pieschl RL, Gribkoff VK, Reppert SM. Molecular dissection of two distinct actions of melatonin on the suprachiasmatic circadian clock. Neuron. 1997;**19**:91-102

[239] Jin X, von Gall C, Pieschl RL, Gribkoff VK, Stehle JH, Reppert SM, Weaver DR. Targeted disruption of the mouse Mel(1b) melatonin receptor. Molecular and Cellular Biology. 2003;**23**:1054-1060

[240] O'Neal-Moffitt G, Pilli J, Kumar SS, Olcese J. Genetic deletion of MT_1/MT_2 melatonin receptors enhances murine cognitive and motor performance. Neuroscience. 2014;**277**:506-521. DOI: 10.1016/j.neuroscience.2014.07.018

[241] Dubocovich ML, Hudson RL, Sumaya IC, Masana MI, Manna E. Effect of MT1 melatonin receptor deletion on melatonin-mediated phase shift of circadian rhythms in the C57BL/6 mouse. Journal of Pineal Research. 2005;**39**:113-120. DOI: 10.1111/j.1600-079X.2005.00230.x

[242] Hutchinson AJ, Hudson RL, Dubocovich ML. Genetic deletion of MT(1) and MT(2) melatonin receptors differentially abrogates the development and expression of methamphetamine-induced locomotor sensitization during the day and the night in C3H/HeN mice. Journal of Pineal Research. 2012;**53**:399-409. DOI: 10.1111/j.1600-079X.2012.01010.x

[243] Kleber A, Altmeyer S, Wolf B, Wolf A, Volk T, Fink T, Kubulus D. Impact of melatonin receptor deletion on intracellular signaling in spleen cells of mice after polymicrobial sepsis. Inflammation Research: Official Journal of the European Histamine Research Society. 2014;**63**:1023-1033. DOI: 10.1007/s00011-014-0779-4

[244] Mühlbauer E, Gross E, Labucay K, Wolgast S, Peschke E. Loss of melatonin signalling and its impact on circadian rhythms in mouse organs regulating blood glucose. European Journal of Pharmacology. 2009;**606**:61-71. DOI: 10.1016/j.ejphar.2009.01.029

[245] Lardone PJ, Rubio A, Cerrillo I, Gómez-Corvera A, Carrillo-Vico A, Sanchez-Hidalgo M, Guerrero JM, Fernandez-Riejos P, Sanchez-Margalet V, Molinero P. Blocking of melatonin synthesis and MT(1) receptor impairs the activation of Jurkat T cells. Cellular and Molecular Life Sciences: CMLS. 2010;**67**:3163-3172. DOI: 10.1007/s00018-010-0374-y

[246] Posa L, de Gregorio D, Gobbi G, Comai S. Targeting melatonin MT2 receptors: A novel pharmacological avenue for inflammatory and neuropathic pain. Current Medicinal Chemistry. 2017;**24**. in press. DOI: 10.2174/0929867324666170209104926

[247] Liu D, Wei N, Man H-Y, Lu Y, Zhu L-Q, Wang J-Z. The MT2 receptor stimulates axonogenesis and enhances synaptic transmission by activating Akt signaling. Cell Death and Differentiation. 2015;**22**:583-596. DOI: 10.1038/cdd.2014.195

[248] Dubocovich ML. Pharmacology and function of melatonin receptors. FASEB Journal : Official Publication of the Federation of American Societies for Experimental Biology. 1988;**2**:2765-2773

[249] Molinari EJ, North PC, Dubocovich ML. 2-125Iiodo-5-methoxycarbonylamino-N-acetyltryptamine: A selective radioligand for the characterization of melatonin ML2 binding sites. European Journal of Pharmacology. 1996;**301**:159-168

[250] Paul P, Lahaye C, Delagrange P, Nicolas JP, Canet E, Boutin JA. Characterization of 2-125Iiodomelatonin binding sites in Syrian hamster peripheral organs. The Journal of Pharmacology and Experimental Therapeutics. 1999;**290**:334-340

[251] Liao S, Dulaney JT, Williams-Ashman HG. Purification and properties of a flavoprotein catalyzing the oxidation of reduced ribosyl nicotinamide. The Journal of Biological Chemistry. 1962;**237**:2981-2987

[252] Chomarat P, Cogé F, Guénin SP, Mailliet F, Vella F, Mallet C, Giraudet S, Nagel N, Leonce S, Ferry G, Delagrange P, Boutin JA. Cellular knock-down of quinone reductase 2: A laborious road to successful inhibition by RNA interference. Biochimie. 2007;**89**:1264-1275. DOI: 10.1016/j.biochi.2007.07.004

[253] Mailliet F, Ferry G, Vella F, Thiam K, Delagrange P, Boutin JA. Organs from mice deleted for NRH:Quinone oxidoreductase 2 are deprived of the melatonin binding site MT3. FEBS Letters. 2004;**578**:116-120. DOI: 10.1016/j.febslet.2004.10.083

[254] Vella F, Ferry G, Delagrange P, Boutin JA. NRH: Quinone reductase 2: An enzyme of surprises and mysteries. Biochemical Pharmacology. 2005;**71**:1-12. DOI: 10.1016/j.bcp.2005.09.019

[255] Manchester LC, Coto-Montes A, Boga JA, Andersen LPH, Zhou Z, Galano A, Vriend J, Tan D-X, Reiter RJ. Melatonin: An ancient molecule that makes oxygen metabolically tolerable. Journal of Pineal Research. 2015;**59**:403-419. DOI: 10.1111/jpi.12267

[256] Reiter RJ, Rosales-Corral S, Tan DX, Jou MJ, Galano A, Xu B. Melatonin as a mitochondria-targeted antioxidant: One of evolution's best ideas. Cellular and Molecular Life Sciences: CMLS. 2017;**74**:3863-3881. DOI: 10.1007/s00018-017-2609-7

[257] Reiter RJ, Tan DX, Rosales-Corral S, Galano A, Zhou XJ, Xu B. Mitochondria: Central organelles for melatonin's antioxidant and anti-aging actions. Molecules (Basel, Switzerland). DOI: 10.3390/molecules23020509

[258] Xu M, Ashraf M. Melatonin protection against lethal myocyte injury induced by doxorubicin as reflected by effects on mitochondrial membrane potential. Journal of Molecular and Cellular Cardiology. 2002;**34**:75-79. DOI: 10.1006/jmcc.2001.1485

[259] Jou M-J, Peng T-I, Reiter RJ, Jou S-B, Wu H-Y, Wen S-T. Visualization of the antioxidative effects of melatonin at the mitochondrial level during oxidative stress-induced apoptosis of rat brain astrocytes. Journal of Pineal Research. 2004;**37**:55-70. DOI: 10.1111/j.1600-079X.2004.00140.x

[260] Escames G, López LC, Tapias V, Utrilla P, Reiter RJ, Hitos AB, León J, Rodríguez MI, Acuña-Castroviejo D. Melatonin counteracts inducible mitochondrial nitric oxide synthase-dependent mitochondrial dysfunction in skeletal muscle of septic mice. Journal of Pineal Research. 2006;**40**:71-78. DOI: 10.1111/j.1600-079X.2005.00281.x

[261] Han Y-x, Zhang S-h, Wang X-m, Wu J-b. Inhibition of mitochondria responsible for the anti-apoptotic effects of melatonin during ischemia-reperfusion. Journal of Zhejiang University. Science. B. 2006;**7**:142-147. DOI: 10.1631/jzus.2006.B0142

[262] Petrosillo G, Di Venosa N, Pistolese M, Casanova G, Tiravanti E, Colantuono G, Federici A, Paradies G, Ruggiero FM. Protective effect of melatonin against mitochondrial dysfunction associated with cardiac ischemia- reperfusion: Role of cardiolipin. FASEB Journal : Official Publication of the Federation of American Societies for Experimental Biology. 2006;**20**:269-276. DOI: 10.1096/fj.05-4692com

[263] Luchetti F, Canonico B, Mannello F, Masoni C, D'Emilio A, Battistelli M, Papa S, Falcieri E. Melatonin reduces early changes in intramitochondrial cardiolipin during apoptosis in U937 cell line. Toxicology in vitro: An International Journal Published in Association with BIBRA. 2007;**21**:293-301. DOI: 10.1016/j.tiv.2006.08.003

[264] Jou M-J, Peng T-I, Yu P-Z, Jou S-B, Reiter RJ, Chen J-Y, Wu H-Y, Chen C-C, Hsu L-F. Melatonin protects against common deletion of mitochondrial DNA-augmented mitochondrial oxidative stress and apoptosis. Journal of Pineal Research. 2007;**43**: 389-403. DOI: 10.1111/j.1600-079X.2007.00490.x

[265] Fischer TW, Zmijewski MA, Wortsman J, Slominski A. Melatonin maintains mitochondrial membrane potential and attenuates activation of initiator (casp-9) and effector caspases (casp-3/casp-7) and PARP in UVR-exposed HaCaT keratinocytes. Journal of Pineal Research. 2008;**44**:397-407. DOI: 10.1111/j.1600-079X.2007.00542.x

[266] Petrosillo G, Fattoretti P, Matera M, Ruggiero FM, Bertoni-Freddari C, Paradies G. Melatonin prevents age-related mitochondrial dysfunction in rat brain via cardiolipin protection. Rejuvenation Research. 2008;**11**:935-943. DOI: 10.1089/rej.2008.0772

[267] Hibaoui Y, Roulet E, Ruegg UT. Melatonin prevents oxidative stress-mediated mitochondrial permeability transition and death in skeletal muscle cells. Journal of Pineal Research. 2009;**47**:238-252. DOI: 10.1111/j.1600-079X.2009.00707.x

[268] Jou M-J, Peng T-I, Hsu L-F, Jou S-B, Reiter RJ, Yang C-M, Chiao C-C, Lin Y-F, Chen C-C. Visualization of melatonin's multiple mitochondrial levels of protection against mitochondrial Ca(2+)-mediated permeability transition and beyond in rat brain astrocytes. Journal of Pineal Research. 2010;**48**:20-38. DOI: 10.1111/j.1600-079X.2009.00721.x

[269] Jou M-J. Melatonin preserves the transient mitochondrial permeability transition for protection during mitochondrial Ca(2+) stress in astrocyte. Journal of Pineal Research. 2011;**50**:427-435. DOI: 10.1111/j.1600-079X.2011.00861.x

[270] Anjum S, Rahman S, Kaur M, Ahmad F, Rashid H, Ansari RA, Raisuddin S. Melatonin ameliorates bisphenol A-induced biochemical toxicity in testicular mitochondria of

mouse. Food and chemical toxicology: An international journal published for the British industrial. Biological Research Association. 2011;**49**:2849-2854. DOI: 10.1016/j.fct.2011.07.062

[271] Cheshchevik VT, Lapshina EA, Dremza IK, Zabrodskaya SV, Reiter RJ, Prokopchik NI, Zavodnik IB. Rat liver mitochondrial damage under acute or chronic carbon tetrachloride-induced intoxication: Protection by melatonin and cranberry flavonoids. Toxicology and Applied Pharmacology. 2012;**261**:271-279. DOI: 10.1016/j.taap.2012.04.007

[272] Mukherjee D, Ghosh AK, Bandyopadhyay A, Basu A, Datta S, Pattari SK, Reiter RJ, Bandyopadhyay D. Melatonin protects against isoproterenol-induced alterations in cardiac mitochondrial energy-metabolizing enzymes, apoptotic proteins, and assists in complete recovery from myocardial injury in rats. Journal of Pineal Research. 2012;**53**:166-179

[273] Yang Y, Duan W, Jin Z, Yi W, Yan J, Zhang S, Wang N, Liang Z, Li Y, Chen W, Yi D, Yu S. JAK2/STAT3 activation by melatonin attenuates the mitochondrial oxidative damage induced by myocardial ischemia/reperfusion injury. Journal of Pineal Research. 2013;**55**:275-286. DOI: 10.1111/jpi.12070

[274] Canonico B, Luchetti F, Ambrogini P, Arcangeletti M, Betti M, Cesarini E, Lattanzi D, Ciuffoli S, Palma F, Cuppini R, Papa S. Pharmacological doses of melatonin induce alterations in mitochondrial mass and potential, bcl-2 levels and K+ currents in UVB-exposed U937 cells. Cell Biology International. 2013;**37**:213-226. DOI: 10.1002/cbin.10030

[275] Kashani IR, Rajabi Z, Akbari M, Hassanzadeh G, Mohseni A, Eramsadati MK, Rafiee K, Beyer C, Kipp M, Zendedel A. Protective effects of melatonin against mitochondrial injury in a mouse model of multiple sclerosis. Experimental Brain Research. 2014;**232**:2835-2846. DOI: 10.1007/s00221-014-3946-5

[276] Guo P, Pi H, Xu S, Zhang L, Li Y, Li M, Cao Z, Tian L, Xie J, Li R, He M, Lu Y, Liu C, Duan W, Yu Z, Zhou Z. Melatonin improves mitochondrial function by promoting MT1/SIRT1/PGC-1 alpha-dependent mitochondrial biogenesis in cadmium-induced hepatotoxicity in vitro. Toxicological Sciences: An Official Journal of the Society of Toxicology. 2014;**142**:182-195. DOI: 10.1093/toxsci/kfu164

[277] Yang Y, Jiang S, Dong Y, Fan C, Zhao L, Yang X, Li J, Di S, Yue L, Liang G, Reiter RJ, Qu Y. Melatonin prevents cell death and mitochondrial dysfunction via a SIRT1-dependent mechanism during ischemic-stroke in mice. Journal of Pineal Research. 2015;**58**:61-70. DOI: 10.1111/jpi.12193

[278] He C, Wang J, Zhang Z, Yang M, Li Y, Tian X, Ma T, Tao J, Zhu K, Song Y, Ji P, Liu G. Mitochondria synthesize melatonin to ameliorate its function and improve mice oocyte's quality under in vitro conditions. International Journal of Molecular Sciences. 2016;**17**:e939. DOI: 10.3390/ijms17060939

[279] Ahluwalia A, Brzozowska IM, Hoa N, Jones MK, Tarnawski AS. Melatonin signaling in mitochondria extends beyond neurons and neuroprotection: Implications for

angiogenesis and cardio/gastroprotection. Proceedings of the National Academy of Sciences of the United States of America. 2018;**115**:E1942-E1943. DOI: 10.1073/pnas.1722131115

[280] Mayo JC, Sainz RM, González-Menéndez P, Hevia D, Cernuda-Cernuda R. Melatonin transport into mitochondria. Cellular and Molecular Life Sciences: CMLS. 2017;**74**:3927-3940. DOI: 10.1007/s00018-017-2616-8

[281] Gautier C, Dufour E, Dupré C, Lizzo G, Caignard S, Riest-Fery I, Brasseur C, Legros C, Delagrange P, Nosjean O, Simonneaux V, Boutin JA, Guenin SP. Hamster melatonin receptors: Cloning and binding characterization of MT and attempt to clone MT_2. International Journal of Medical Sciences. 2018. [In press]

Permissions

All chapters in this book were first published in MMBCPA, by InTech Open; hereby published with permission under the Creative Commons Attribution License or equivalent. Every chapter published in this book has been scrutinized by our experts. Their significance has been extensively debated. The topics covered herein carry significant findings which will fuel the growth of the discipline. They may even be implemented as practical applications or may be referred to as a beginning point for another development.

The contributors of this book come from diverse backgrounds, making this book a truly international effort. This book will bring forth new frontiers with its revolutionizing research information and detailed analysis of the nascent developments around the world.

We would like to thank all the contributing authors for lending their expertise to make the book truly unique. They have played a crucial role in the development of this book. Without their invaluable contributions this book wouldn't have been possible. They have made vital efforts to compile up to date information on the varied aspects of this subject to make this book a valuable addition to the collection of many professionals and students.

This book was conceptualized with the vision of imparting up-to-date information and advanced data in this field. To ensure the same, a matchless editorial board was set up. Every individual on the board went through rigorous rounds of assessment to prove their worth. After which they invested a large part of their time researching and compiling the most relevant data for our readers.

The editorial board has been involved in producing this book since its inception. They have spent rigorous hours researching and exploring the diverse topics which have resulted in the successful publishing of this book. They have passed on their knowledge of decades through this book. To expedite this challenging task, the publisher supported the team at every step. A small team of assistant editors was also appointed to further simplify the editing procedure and attain best results for the readers.

Apart from the editorial board, the designing team has also invested a significant amount of their time in understanding the subject and creating the most relevant covers. They scrutinized every image to scout for the most suitable representation of the subject and create an appropriate cover for the book.

The publishing team has been an ardent support to the editorial, designing and production team. Their endless efforts to recruit the best for this project, has resulted in the accomplishment of this book. They are a veteran in the field of academics and their pool of knowledge is as vast as their experience in printing. Their expertise and guidance has proved useful at every step. Their uncompromising quality standards have made this book an exceptional effort. Their encouragement from time to time has been an inspiration for everyone.

The publisher and the editorial board hope that this book will prove to be a valuable piece of knowledge for researchers, students, practitioners and scholars across the globe.

List of Contributors

Marilena Vlachou and Angeliki Siamidi
School of Health Sciences, Department of Pharmacy, Division of Pharmaceutical Technology, National and Kapodistrian University of Athens, Athens, Greece

Cristina Manuela Drăgoi and Alina Crenguța Nicolae
Department of Biochemistry, Faculty of Pharmacy, University of Medicine and Pharmacy "Carol Davila," Bucharest, Romania

Andreea Letiția Arsene
Department of General and Pharmaceutical Microbiology, Faculty of Pharmacy, University of Medicine and Pharmacy "Carol Davila," Bucharest, Romania

Cristina Elena Dinu-Pîrvu
Department of Physical and Colloidal Chemistry, Faculty of Pharmacy, University of Medicine and Pharmacy "Carol Davila," Bucharest, Romania

Ion Bogdan Dumitrescu
Department of Pharmaceutical Physics and Informatics, Faculty of Pharmacy, University of Medicine and Pharmacy "Carol Davila," Bucharest, Romania

Daniela Elena Popa and George T.A. Burcea-Dragomiroiu
Department of Drug Control, Faculty of Pharmacy, University of Medicine and Pharmacy "Carol Davila," Bucharest, Romania

Denisa Ioana Udeanu
Department of Clinical Laboratory and Food Safety, Faculty of Pharmacy, University of Medicine and Pharmacy "Carol Davila," Bucharest, Romania

Olivia Carmen Timnea
Department of Medical Sciences, Faculty of Physical Education and Sports, Ecologic University of Bucharest, Romania

Bruno Stefan Velescu
Department of Pharmacology and Clinical Pharmacy, Faculty of Pharmacy, University of Medicine and Pharmacy "Carol Davila", Bucharest, Romania

Akikazu Takada
International Projects on Food and Health (NPO), Tokyo, Japan

Fumiko Shimizu
Faculty of Life and Environmental Sciences, Showa Women's University, Tokyo, Japan

Junichi Masuda
Global Application Development Center, Shimadzu Corporation, Kanagawa-ken, Japan

Tamer Awad Ramadan
Animal Production Research Institute, Agricultural Research Center, Giza, Egypt

Justyna Paprocka
Department of Child Neurology, School of Medicine in Katowice, Medical University of Silesia, Katowice, Poland

Marek Kijonka and Maria Sokół
Department of Medical Physics, Maria Skłodowska-Curie Memorial Cancer Center and Institute of Oncology, Gliwice Branch, Poland

Aysun Hacışevki and Burcu Baba
Department of Biochemistry, Faculty of Pharmacy, Gazi University, Etiler, Ankara, Turkey

Hanan Farouk Aly and Maha Zaki Rizk
Therapeutic Chemistry Department, National Research Centre, Giza-Dokki, Egypt

Hitomi Takeuchi and Tetsuo Harada
Laboratory of Environmental Physiology, Graduate School of Integrated Arts and Sciences, Kochi University, Akebono-cho, Kochi, Japan

Edyta Molik and Dorota Zięba-Przybylska
Department of Animal Biotechnology, Agricultural University in Krakow, Kraków, Poland
Mahsa Rastegar Moghaddam Mansouri and Sadegh Abbasian
2020 Olympic Sport School, Tehran, Iran
Center of Sport Talent Identification and Development, Department of Education, Malard, Tehran, Iran

Mohammad Khazaie
Center of Sport Talent Identification and Development, Department of Education, Malard,Tehran, Iran
Faculty of Physical Education and Sport Sciences, University of Tehran, Tehran, Iran

Jean A. Boutin
Institut de Recherches Internationales SERVIER, Suresnes, France

Index

P

Q

R

S

T

V

www.ingramcontent.com/pod-product-compliance
Lightning Source LLC
LaVergne TN
LVHW081038210926
848485LV00004B/1052